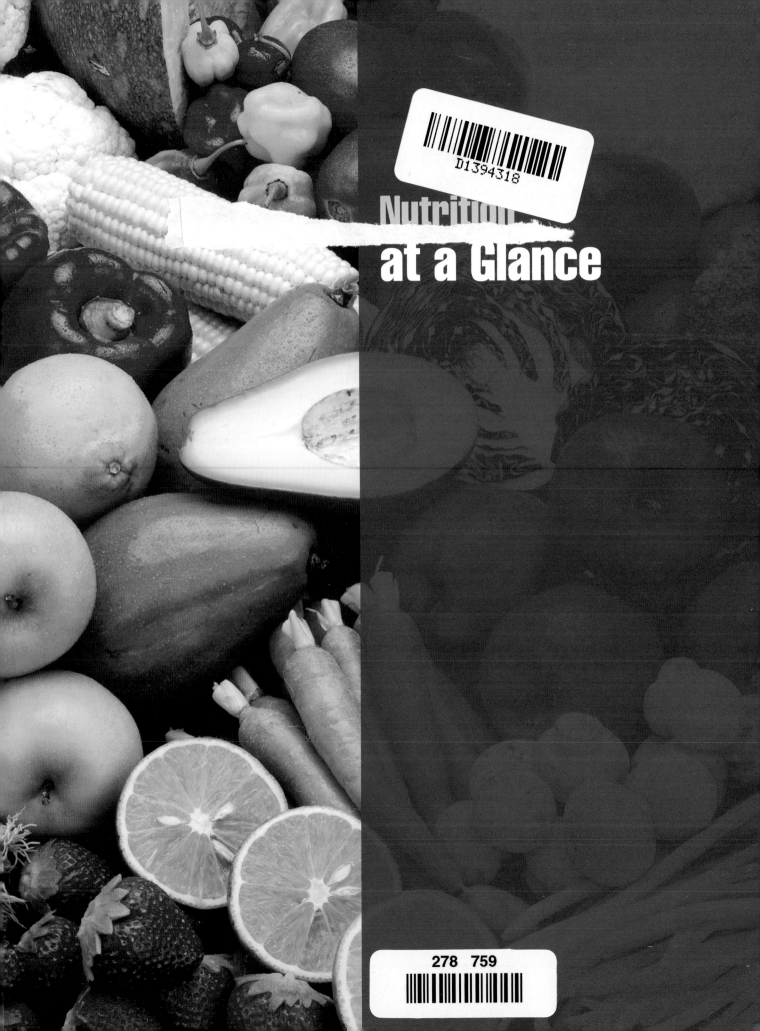

Nutrition
at a Glance

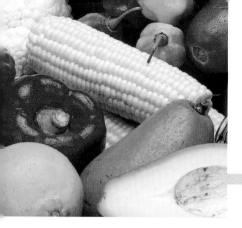

Dedication

This book is dedicated to Mary Barasi who was an amazing teacher, friend and supporter. Since my undergraduate days, Mary's belief in my ability to be a researcher and her dedication and encouragement to help me get there resulted in the happy position I am in today at the University of Alberta, in beautiful Canada. It just takes one person to tell you that you are capable and to help you navigate the system, and for me, that was Mary. I am eternally grateful to her and I am honoured to have had the opportunity to be the editor of this book.

I would like to thank from the bottom (to the top) of my heart my wonderful parents who have always supported and encouraged me in all my endeavours and especially in my love of nutrition and research.

This new edition is also available as an e-book.
For more details, please see
www.wiley.com/buy/
or scan this QR code:

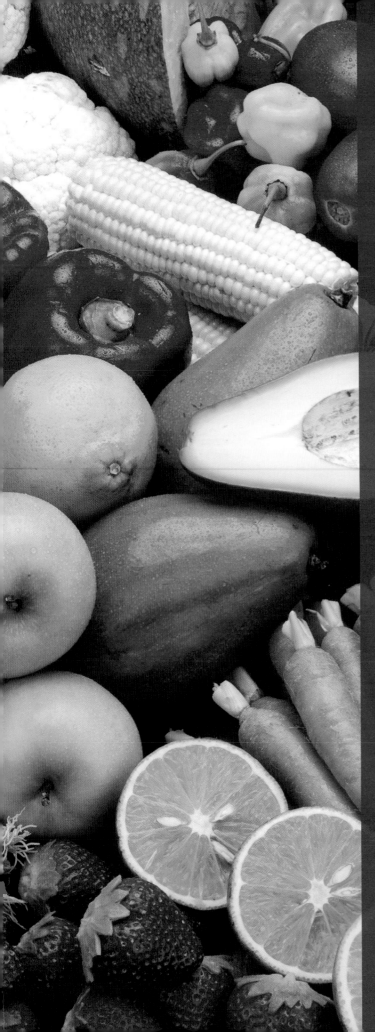

Nutrition at a Glance

Second Edition

Editor-in-Chief:

Sangita Sharma, PhD
Centennial Professor
Endowed Chair in Aboriginal Health
Professor of Aboriginal & Global Health Research
Aboriginal and Global Health Research Group
Department of Medicine
Faculty of Medicine & Dentistry
University of Alberta, Edmonton, Canada

Co-Editors:

Tony Sheehy, PhD
Lecturer
School of Food & Nutritional Sciences
University College Cork, Cork, Ireland

Fariba Kolahdooz, PhD
Nutritional Epidemiologist
Assistant Director – Research
Aboriginal and Global Health Research Group
Department of Medicine
Faculty of Medicine & Dentistry
University of Alberta, Edmonton, Canada

Founding editor:
Mary Barasi

WILEY Blackwell

This edition first published 2016 © 2016 John Wiley & Sons, Ltd.

Registered Office
John Wiley & Sons, Ltd, The Atrium, Southern Gate, Chichester, West Sussex, PO19 8SQ, UK

Editorial Offices
9600 Garsington Road, Oxford, OX4 2DQ, UK
1606 Golden Aspen Drive, Suites 103 and 104, Ames, Iowa 50010, USA

For details of our global editorial offices, for customer services and for information about how to apply for permission to reuse the copyright material in this book please see our website at www.wiley.com/wiley-blackwell

Library of Congress Cataloging-in-Publication Data

Nutrition at a glance / editor-in-chief, Sangita Sharma ; co-editors, Tony Sheehy, Fariba Kolahdooz ; founding editor, Mary Barasi. – Second edition.
    p. ; cm. – (At a glance series)
Preceded by: Nutrition at a glance / Mary E. Barasi. 2007.
Includes index.
ISBN 978-1-118-66101-7 (pbk.)
I. Sharma, Sangita (Professor in Aboriginal and global health research), editor. II. Sheehy, Tony, co-editor. III. Kolahdooz, Fariba., co-editor. IV. Barasi, Mary E., editor. V. Barasi, Mary E. Nutrition at a glance. Preceded by (work): VI. Series: At a glance series (Oxford, England)
[DNLM: 1. Nutritional Physiological Phenomena–Handbooks. 2. Nutrition Disorders–Handbooks. QU 39]
QP141.A1
612.3–dc23

                                        2015009590

A catalogue record for this book is available from the British Library.

Wiley also publishes its books in a variety of electronic formats. Some content that appears in print may not be available in electronic books.

Cover image: © fcafotodigital

Set in 9.5/11.5pt Minion by SPi Global, Pondicherry, India
Printed and bound in Singapore by Markono Print Media Pte Ltd

1 2016

Contents

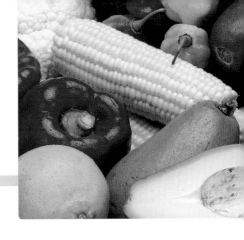

v

Part III   Nutrition throughout the life cycle   93

Part IV   The role of nutrition in key organs/systems   107

Part V   Nutrition-related diseases   119

Part VI   Public health and sports nutrition   143

Part VII   Foods, phytochemicals including functional and genetically modified foods   159

Appendices   168

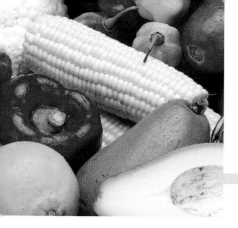

Acknowledgements

This book would never have been updated without the incredible help of two amazing co-editors and friends, Dr. Tony Sheehy and Dr. Fariba Kolahdooz. I am truly blessed to work with two such outstanding scientists.

I would like to acknowledge the Aboriginal and Global Health Research Group for their hard work and assistance. Thank you to Dr. Edwige Landais for her work on Chapter 35 on nutritional assessment methods and food frequency questionnaires and to Shaylene Bachelet for her assistance in writing Chapter 32 on research ethics. I am also grateful to Se Lim Jang for her contributions to Chapter 15 on dietary supplements, Chapter 66 on adverse reactions to food, Chapter 76 on genetically modified foods and Chapter 77 on food safety. Thank you as well to Michelle Wong, Yashar Rahimoghli Turk, and Kristine Tonks for their incredible assistance in the preparation of the final manuscript.

A special thanks goes to Dr. Gail Andrew, Dr. Shelley Birchard and Dr. Sharon Mitchell for their contributions to Chapter 28 on fetal alcohol spectrum disorder.

How to use your textbook

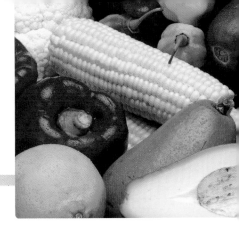

Features contained within your textbook

Each topic is presented in a double-page spread with clear, easy-to-follow diagrams supported by succinct explanatory text.

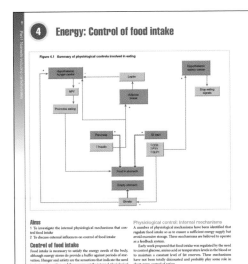

Your textbook is full of **photographs, illustrations and tables**.

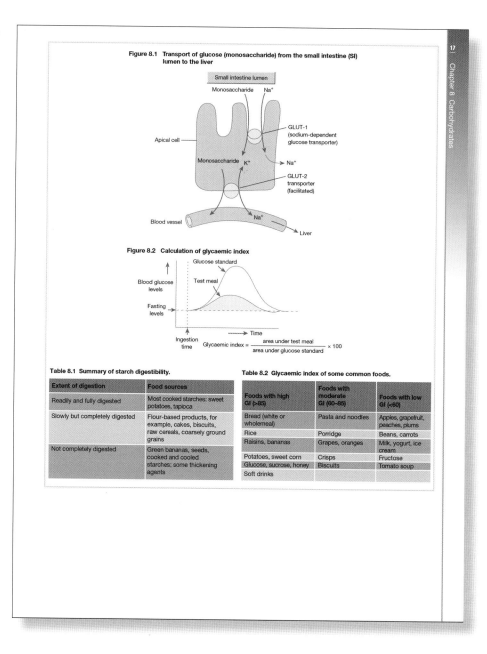

Figure 8.1 Transport of glucose (monosaccharide) from the small intestine (SI) lumen to the liver

Small intestine lumen

Monosaccharide   Na⁺

Apical cell

GLUT-1 (sodium-dependent glucose transporter)

Monosaccharide   K⁺

Na⁺

GLUT-2 transporter (facilitated)

Blood vessel

Na⁺

Liver

Figure 8.2 Calculation of glycaemic index

Glucose standard

Blood glucose levels

Test meal

Fasting levels

Time

Ingestion time

$$\text{Glycaemic index} = \frac{\text{area under test meal}}{\text{area under glucose standard}} \times 100$$

Table 8.1 Summary of starch digestibility.

Extent of digestion	Food sources
Readily and fully digested	Most cooked starches: sweet potatoes, tapioca
Slowly but completely digested	Flour-based products, for example, cakes, biscuits, raw cereals, coarsely ground grains
Not completely digested	Green bananas, seeds, cooked and cooled starches; some thickening agents

Table 8.2 Glycaemic index of some common foods.

Foods with high GI (>85)	Foods with moderate GI (60–85)	Foods with low GI (<60)
Bread (white or wholemeal)	Pasta and noodles	Apples, grapefruit, peaches, plums
Rice	Porridge	Beans, carrots
Raisins, bananas	Grapes, oranges	Milk, yogurt, ice cream
Potatoes, sweet corn	Crisps	Fructose
Glucose, sucrose, honey	Biscuits	Tomato soup
Soft drinks		

Self-assessment review questions, available on the book's companion website, help you test yourself after each chapter.

Part I: Nutrients including energy, carbohydrates, fat, proteins, vitamins, minerals and alcohol

Chapter 1 Introduction to the nutrients

1. Which one of the following statements is correct?

A. Carbohydrates are the body's major energy reserve.
B. When there is no further need for amino acids for growth or repair, they are broken down and used for energy. [True]
C. The carbohydrates glucose, sucrose and fructose are non-glycaemic carbohydrates.
D. In addition to carbon, hydrogen and oxygen, all fats contain nitrogen.

The correct answer is B.

2. Which one of the following statements is correct?

A. Vitamins are inorganic substances required by the body in small amounts for its normal functioning.
B. Vitamins are required in gram amounts each day, whereas trace elements are required in milligram amounts.
C. Carbohydrates, fats and proteins all have structural roles in the body. [True]
D. Excessive intake of one mineral has no effect on the uptake of another.

The correct answer is C.

3. Which one of the following components is not a type of carbohydrate?

A. Maltodextrins
B. Sterols [True]
C. Lactose
D. Dietary fibre

The correct answer is B.

4. How many essential amino acids are there for adults?

A. 4
B. 12
C. 20
D. None of the above [True]

The correct answer is D.

Chapter 2 The relationship between diet, health and disease

1. Which one of the following statements is incorrect?

A. Rickets is the major symptom of vitamin D deficiency.
B. Goitre is the major symptom of iodine deficiency.
C. Beriberi is the major symptom of vitamin B₁ deficiency. [True]
D. Scurvy is the major symptom of vitamin C deficiency.

The correct answer is C.

2. The scientific study of the relationship between exposure to a particular dietary factor and disease outcome is called:

A. Clinical nutrition
B. Public health nutrition
C. Nutritional epidemiology [True]
D. Food toxicology
E. None of the above

The correct answer is C.

3. Which of the following dietary factors are implicated in the development of cancer?

A. Red meat
B. Alcohol
C. Saturated fat
D. Excessive caloric intake
E. All of the above [True]

The correct answer is E.

Chapter 3 Energy intake: Food sources

1. Which one of the following statements is correct?

A. Proteins, fats and carbohydrates provide energy to the body, but alcohol does not
B. Minerals and vitamins do not provide energy themselves and are not required to release energy from foods.
C. The metabolisable energy content of a food is greater than its heat of combustion.
D. Dietary fibre combusts completely in a bomb calorimeter but is indigestible to humans. [True]

The correct answer is D.

2. A chocolate bar contains 57 g carbohydrate, 8 g protein and 31 g fat per 100 g. What is its energy content?

A. 525 kcal/100 g [True]
B. 667 kcal/100 g
C. 416 kcal/100 g
D. None of the above

The correct answer is A.

3. If the average energy content of one banana is 105 kcal, what is its energy content in kilojoules (kJ)?

A. 25
B. 439 [True]
C. 101
D. None of the above

The correct answer is B.

4. During a dietary intake study, one individual had an average daily intake of 95 g protein, 67 g fat and 275 g carbohydrate. What percentage of total calories was supplied by fat in this person's diet?

A. 20
B. 30 [True]
C. 40
D. 50

About the companion website

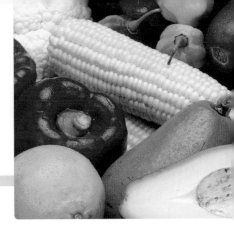

Don't forget to visit the companion website for this book:

www.ataglanceseries.com/nutrition

There, you will find valuable material designed to enhance your learning, including:

- Abbreviations and definitions
- Interactive multiple-choice questions
- References and suggested reading
- Global dietary guidelines and dietary reference intakes (DRIs)

Scan this QR code to visit the companion website:

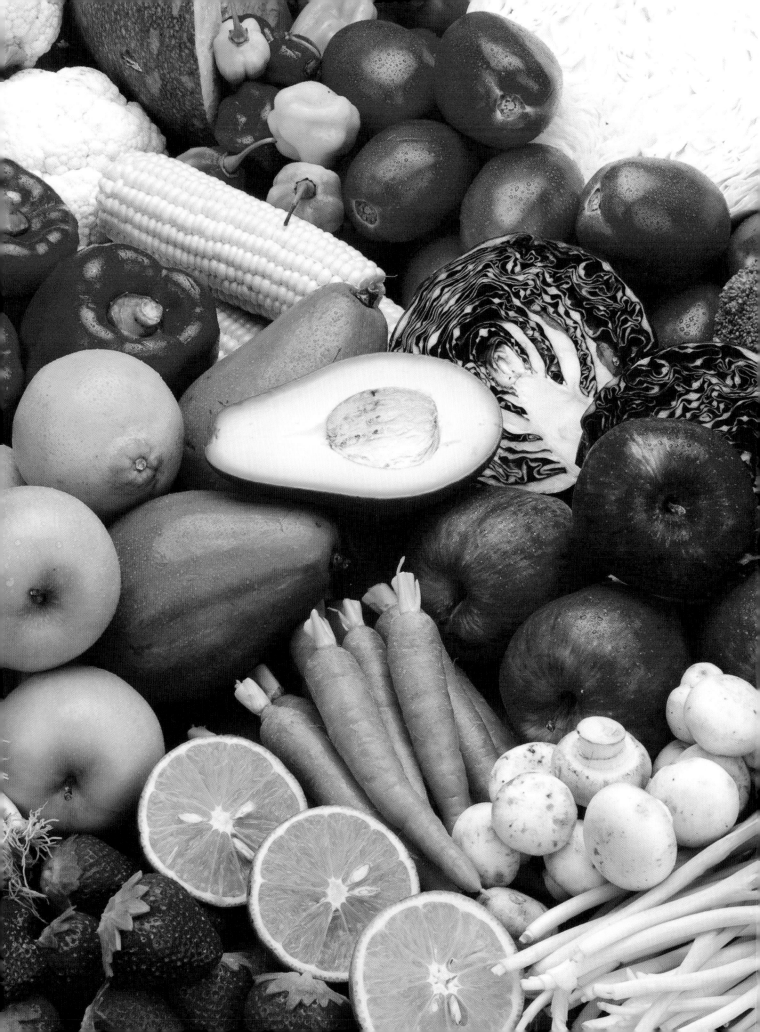

Nutrients including carbohydrates, fat, proteins, vitamins, minerals, and alcohol

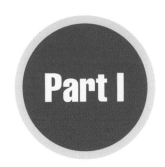

Part I

Chapters

1 Introduction to the nutrients

Aims

1 To show how nutrients are classified and discuss their main roles
2 To describe how nutrients may interact to fulfil similar roles

Food is composed of a large variety of chemical substances, some of which are recognised as nutrients. Over the past century or so, scientists have identified the roles of these nutrients in the body and the consequences of insufficient intakes. Many other substances are present in foods of plant origin that help promote the plant's growth, protect it against predators or contribute to its appearance or smell to attract animals that will spread its seeds. Although these substances (phytochemicals) are not recognised as nutrients, some may be biologically active in humans and could have either beneficial or harmful effects.

Classification of nutrients

Traditionally, the major nutrients have been classified according to the amounts in which they are required by the body, their chemical nature and their functions. The principal distinction is between **macronutrients** and **micronutrients**:

1 *Macronutrients* are required in relatively large amounts, usually expressed in terms of grams per day.
2 *Micronutrients* are required in small amounts, usually expressed in terms of milligrams or micrograms per day.

Some classifications also include *ultratrace nutrients*. These are found in the diet in very small amounts (typically <1 µg/g of dry food). For many of these substances, their roles are, as yet, uncertain.

Water is an essential component of the diet, as an adequate intake of fluid is vital to sustain life.

Macronutrients

This category comprises carbohydrates, fats and proteins:
• Carbohydrates and fats are the major *providers of energy*, although proteins can also be used to provide energy.
• They all have a *structural* role in the body, the most important in this respect being proteins.
• All contain *carbon*, *hydrogen* and *oxygen*. In addition, all proteins contain nitrogen, while some amino acids (cysteine and methionine) that are found in proteins contain sulphur.

Carbohydrates

Carbohydrates are the most important source of food energy in the world. Carbohydrates occur in the diet in various degrees of complexity, ranging from simple sugars (mono- and disaccharides) to larger units such as oligosaccharides and polysaccharides. Simple sugars include the monosaccharides glucose, fructose and galactose and the disaccharides sucrose and lactose. Oligosaccharides include maltodextrins and fructo-oligosaccharides. Important polysaccharides include starch and glycogen.

The main function of carbohydrates is to act as a source of energy, in the form of glucose. However, some carbohydrates resist digestion and are termed 'non-glycaemic' (see Chapter 8). They comprise the non-starch polysaccharides (NSP), which are part of the category known as 'dietary fibre'. These carbohydrates play an important role in bowel function.

Fats

Fats are a diverse group of lipid-soluble substances, the majority of which are triacylglycerols (TAGs). Other lipid-soluble substances including phospholipids and sterols (e.g. cholesterol) are also included in this group.

TAGs are broken down to yield energy and are the body's richest source of energy, having over twice the caloric content of carbohydrates and proteins. They are also the body's major energy reserve, stored in the adipose tissue. Specific fatty acids found in TAGs (called *essential fatty acids*) are important for cell membrane structure and function. Since the body lacks the ability to manufacture essential fatty acids, they must be supplied in the diet.

Proteins

Proteins consist of chains of *amino acids*. Food proteins typically contain 20 different amino acids, but because these can be arranged in countless ways, there is enormous diversity between different proteins in the diet in terms of their amino acid sequences. On digestion, individual amino acids are used for the synthesis of other amino acids and proteins required by the body. This process involves considerable recycling of the components.

There are eight *essential amino acids* (more in children), which must be supplied by the diet. Certain other amino acids may become *conditionally* essential in situations of physiological stress. Only when there is no further need for amino acids are they broken down and used as a source of energy. During that process, the nitrogen part of the amino acid is excreted via the urine as urea.

Micronutrients

The micronutrients consist of the vitamins and minerals (see Table 1.1).

Table 1.1 Classification of micronutrients by chemical properties.

Name	Main members of the group	Role(s)
Fat-soluble vitamins	Vitamins A, D, E, K	Structural role, cell integrity, homeostasis, antioxidant, nerve impulses
Water-soluble vitamins	B vitamins, vitamin C	Metabolism, cell division, antioxidant, cofactors for enzymes, synthesis of neurotransmitters
Minerals	Calcium, phosphorus, sodium, chloride, potassium, magnesium, iron, zinc, copper, manganese, iodine, selenium	Structural role, cofactors for enzymes, acid–base balance

Nutrition at a Glance, Second Edition. Edited by Sangita Sharma, Tony Sheehy and Fariba Kolahdooz.
© 2016 John Wiley & Sons, Ltd. Published 2016 by John Wiley & Sons, Ltd.

Vitamins

Vitamins are *organic* substances that are required by the body in very small amounts for its normal functioning. They are classified into the **fat-soluble vitamins** (A, D, E and K) and the **water-soluble vitamins** (B-group vitamins and vitamin C).

The body does have the capacity to synthesise some vitamins. For example, *vitamin D* is synthesised in the skin by the action of ultraviolet light on a precursor molecule, 7-dehydrocholesterol. Vitamin B_3 (niacin) can also be made in the body, from the amino acid tryptophan, which means that a separate supply of niacin may not be needed if protein intake is adequate. However, in the case of both of these vitamins, there are situations where synthesis is insufficient, and so a dietary need remains.

Minerals

Minerals are *inorganic* substances required by the body in small amounts, generally to function as part of the structure of other molecules (e.g. calcium in the bone or iron in haemoglobin) or to act as essential cofactors for the activity of enzymes (e.g. selenium in glutathione peroxidase).

For some minerals (e.g. iron), uptake from the diet must be carefully regulated as there is only a very limited capacity for excretion, and potential toxicity may result if large amounts accumulate in storage organs.

In addition, some minerals compete with each other for absorption, so excessive intakes of one may hinder the uptake of another (e.g. zinc and iron, or iron and calcium).

Water

Water provides the basic medium in which all the body's reactions occur. Inadequate fluid intakes will quickly compromise the metabolic functions of the body and disturb the homeostatic mechanisms that normally operate.

Alcohol

Alcohol is not considered a nutrient, but when ingested, it is broken down to provide energy. Some alcoholic beverages (e.g. beer) provide additional nutrients such as B vitamins, albeit in small amounts.

Grouping of nutrients by functional role

Many nutrients interact in carrying out their functional roles in the body, and this may also be used as a basis for classification:

• At the genetic level, nutrients are involved in regulating the transcription of genes, thus affecting the synthesis of proteins, including enzymes.

• At the cellular level, nutrients are involved as cofactors in controlling and regulating metabolic reactions and the release of energy. They are regulated by hormones and other chemical messengers, such as cytokines, which are also influenced by the nutrient environment.

• Immune and defence mechanisms function through the release of highly reactive molecules called *free radicals*, which must then be quenched by antioxidants, again supplied directly by the diet or indirectly as enzymes activated by dietary factors.

Interactions

When food is eaten, interactions may occur between nutrients and non-nutritional constituents at all stages of the processing and metabolism of the food. It is therefore unwise to study nutrients in isolation without considering some of the other factors that may influence their activity and how they may interact in whole body functioning.

Key characteristics of nutrients

In studying the nutrients, it is important to pay attention to:
• Their structure and chemical characteristics
• Which foods are major sources
• How they are digested, absorbed, transported and stored
• In what form they are used, what determines their use, how and in what circumstances they are mobilised and how surplus or metabolic end products are excreted
• What the physiological requirement for the nutrient is and how this can be translated into a recommended level of intake
• How the body responds to overconsumption and underconsumption
• How long it takes to develop a deficiency or a toxicity and what are the characteristic features
• Interaction between nutrients
• Which members of a population are vulnerable to deficiency
• Whether there are any therapeutic applications of the nutrient
• What are the gaps in knowledge requiring further study

2 The relationship between diet, health and disease

Aim

1 To gain an insight into the associations between diet, health and disease and to recognise the complexity of these relationships

Scientific approaches, such as nutritional epidemiology, can provide evidence on which dietary advice and public health policies can be based.

Historical perspective

Early studies in nutrition originated from observations of nutrient deficiencies, for which cures with a single nutrient were discovered. This led the way to the identification of many micronutrients (see Table 2.1). For example:

• **Scurvy** had been a significant cause of death among sailors on long sea voyages since the fifteenth century. In the eighteenth century, it was discovered that it could be treated by consuming citrus fruits. However, it was not identified as being due specifically to vitamin C deficiency until the early twentieth century, when the guinea pig was found to be susceptible to the disease and could thus be used as an experimental model.

• **Beriberi**, the disease caused by vitamin B_1 deficiency, was reported in Java, Indonesia, during the late nineteenth century among humans and birds fed refined rice. It could be cured by feeding rice bran, which was eventually shown to be rich in the vitamin.

• The association between low levels of iodine in food and drinking water and the swelling of the thyroid gland, known as **goitre**, was described in the early nineteenth century. The key role of iodine in the formation of thyroid hormones was not established until the early part of the twentieth century.

• Iron, folate and vitamin B_{12} deficiencies are associated with **anaemias** that have distinct cytological profiles. Although the common feature was anaemia, differential diagnosis and treatments were required to ensure the correct treatment.

• **Rickets** is due to vitamin D deficiency. Vitamin D can be obtained in the diet, but for most people, synthesis in the skin on exposure to sunlight is the most important source. Thus, exposure to 'country air', away from smoky cities, was initially believed to be the cure. It is now understood that exposure to sunlight results in

hydroxylation of vitamin D occurs in the liver and kidney, producing the active form. Therefore, renal and hepatic dysfunction may also be a cause of rickets. Additional roles for vitamin D in cellular metabolism have also been described.

Toxicity can result from overconsumption of dietary factors. Classic examples include:

• Vitamin A toxicity was recorded among northern polar explorers consuming livers from polar bears. Excessive intake of vitamin A has been shown to cause fetal malformations in early pregnancy.

• In the early 1950s, infants given excessive amounts of formula milk and cod liver oil supplements containing large amounts of vitamin D developed hypercalcaemia.

Once the link between a nutrient and a particular disease was established, public health measures were introduced to prevent or treat the disease, for example, prescribing folic acid to pregnant women for prevention of neural tube defects (NTD).

Several dietary factors implicated in disease

In some diseases, the role of individual dietary components is difficult to identify because people eat a range of foods that include many nutrients, some that may themselves interact with each other. While ongoing research adds to our understanding of the conditions, it also raises more questions. This is true for cardiovascular disease and cancer.

Other factors affecting susceptibility to disease

Dietary factors may not operate in isolation. Rather, their effects can be modified or amplified by fixed or changeable factors, including:

• Genetic susceptibility: nutrient–gene interactions
• Aspects of early life in the uterine environment
• Environmental factors
• Lifestyle

Even for a condition, such as being overweight, that has an apparently simple cause (excessive energy intake in relation to energy expenditure), the exact mechanisms involved and the ways to intervene for any one individual are not easy to find. They may include many other factors seemingly unrelated to energy intake, for example, psychological factors. Further, it should be recognised that in the diet–health–disease relationship, different factors may be involved in the *initiation, progression* and *treatment and/or prevention* of the disease. This complexity may make it especially difficult to identify precisely the role of dietary components in disease and to formulate policies intended to affect change.

Introduction to nutritional epidemiology

Nutritional epidemiology is the scientific study of the relationship between *exposure* to particular dietary factors and diseases (the *outcome*). Nutritional epidemiology can investigate the strength of such relationships and may establish causation.

Table 2.1 Examples of nutrition-related diseases predominantly associated with single dietary factors.

Disease/abnormality	Dietary factor responsible
Deficiency	
Scurvy	Vitamin C
Beriberi	Vitamin B_1
Goitre	Iodine
Rickets	Vitamin D
Anaemias	Iron/folate/vitamin B_{12}
Overconsumption	
Fetal abnormalities	Vitamin A
Infant hypercalcaemia	Vitamin D

Nutrition at a Glance, Second Edition. Edited by Sangita Sharma, Tony Sheehy and Fariba Kolahdooz.
© 2016 John Wiley & Sons, Ltd. Published 2016 by John Wiley & Sons, Ltd.

A number of standards must be fulfilled before any conclusions about causality can be drawn. The absence of any one of these standards does not necessarily preclude a relationship between exposure and outcome, but may imply that further information is needed.

Epidemiological evidence is usually collected when it is impossible or impractical to collect experimental evidence. However, once a potential causal relationship has been identified, experimental studies that can determine causality may be developed.

Simple measures to rectify deficiencies of individual nutrients

• Parboiling rice before it is milled ensures that some of the thiamin (vitamin B₁) in the husk is transferred into the grain.
• In iodine-deficient areas the addition of iodine to salt ensures that a frequently used commodity provides the missing nutrient.
• On the basis of evidence from experimental trials, women of childbearing age who might become pregnant are advised to take a folic acid supplement to reduce the risk of fetal NTD. In over 60 countries, frequently consumed grain products are now fortified with folic acid, and there has been a significant reduction in NTD cases as a consequence.

Examples of more complex conditions, with several dietary factors implicated

Cardiovascular disease

• Early studies showed that the type of the dietary fat was important in causality, with cholesterol intake and a high intake of saturated fats contributing to raised plasma cholesterol levels, increasing the risk of cardiovascular diseases.
• More recently, the benefits of monounsaturated fats, such as those consumed in a Mediterranean diet, have been recognised.
• The balance between different types of polyunsaturated fats is now considered relevant, including the importance of fish oils rich in omega-3 fatty acids.
• Other aspects of the diet are also implicated in cardiovascular diseases, including antioxidants (from fruit and vegetable intake) and dietary fibre known to be protective and salt, a high intake of which is known to raise blood pressure. High blood pressure serves as a contributing factor for cardiovascular diseases.

Cancer

The role of diet in the development of cancer is complicated because the disease develops over a long period of time and it is difficult to obtain reliable dietary intake information over many years prior to the diagnosis:
• Implicated dietary factors in the causalities include saturated fat, red meat, alcohol, salt, lack of dietary fibre, low fruit and vegetable intake, excessive energy intake, and dietary carcinogens such as heterocyclic aromatic amines (HAAs) formed from cooking meat at high temperature.
• Cancers at different sites appear to be associated with different dietary factors, such as high fat intake and increased risk of breast cancer versus high fibre intake and reduced risk of colorectal cancer.

Key standards that must be fulfilled before drawing conclusions about causality

• There is a dose–response relationship between exposure and outcome.
• The relationship is biologically plausible.
• Exposure to the dietary factor precedes the outcome.
• The relationship between exposure and outcome is strong.
• Biasing and/or confounding of both exposure and outcome by alternative factors is absent.
• Study design and methods are appropriate.

Summary

The relationship between diet and disease may be simple, involving single nutrient deficiencies that are readily treated. However, the majority of nutrition-related diseases have complex relationships with diet. In addition, variations in individual susceptibility are increasingly being recognised.

③ Energy intake: Food sources

Aim

1 To describe how energy intake from food is quantified

Energy is needed for all the functions performed by the body. These include:

- Metabolic activity at the cellular, tissue and organ level, which is largely outside of our conscious awareness and continues throughout life
- Voluntary actions performed as part of physical activity
- Tissue repair and replenishment of stores after physical activity
- Growth, during the early years of life, in adolescence and during pregnancy

Energy from food

The energy required by the body must be supplied by food. Macronutrients (carbohydrates, fats and proteins), together with alcohol, provide energy as they are broken down. Minerals and vitamins do not provide energy, but some are essential as cofactors in the biochemical pathways that release energy.

Methods for measuring food energy

The potential or *gross energy* content of a food can be measured using a *bomb calorimeter*. This is an apparatus in which a small sample of the food is combusted in the presence of pure oxygen under high pressure. The energy (heat) released from the food is absorbed by water, causing a small but measurable rise in temperature in the water from which, by a simple calculation, the gross energy content can be determined.

The breakdown of food in the body is not as efficient as when it is combusted in a bomb calorimeter. For example, cellulose and other forms of fibre will combust completely in a bomb calorimeter but are indigestible in humans. Therefore, the energy available to the body from a particular food is less than the gross energy content. This lower value is known as the *metabolisable energy* content.

The amount of metabolisable energy available from each macronutrient and from alcohol is known (Table 3.1). These *energy conversion factors* can be used to calculate the energy content of a food once its composition is known, and it is these values, rather than the gross energy content, that are found in food composition tables.

In calculating the energy content of foods and in diet planning, it is important to remember that assumptions made about the efficiency of digestion and absorption under normal circumstances may not be true in cases of illness involving diarrhoea or malabsorption syndromes or when laxatives are used.

Units used for measuring energy in nutrition

Traditionally, energy has been expressed in kilocalories (kcal), reflecting the observed generation of heat by metabolic reactions. More recently, the kilojoule (kJ), the SI unit for measurement of energy, has become the preferred unit among nutritionists. However, both units are still used, and members of the public generally recognise kilocalories better than kilojoules. It is therefore essential to know the conversion factor between the two units:

- 1 Kcal = 4.18 KJ

Larger amounts of energy may be expressed in terms of megajoules (MJ), where 1 MJ = 1000 kJ.

Energy conversion factors

The energy conversion factors for macronutrients and alcohol are:
- Carbohydrates (as monosaccharides): 3.75 kcal/g (=16 kJ/g)
- Fat: 9 kcal/g (=37 kJ/g)
- Protein: 4 kcal/g (=17 kJ/g)
- Alcohol: 7 kcal/g (=29 kJ/g)

Calculating the contribution of macronutrients to total energy intake

On the basis of the calculations illustrated in Table 3.1, it is also possible to calculate what percentage of the energy in a food is provided by which macronutrient.

So, taking white bread (which has a total energy content of 219 kcal/100 g) as an example,

- (172.9/219) × 100 = 79% of the energy comes from CHO
- (31.6/219) × 100 = 14.4% of the energy comes from protein
- (14.4/219) × 100 = 6.6% of the energy comes from fat

This type of calculation can also be applied to a whole meal, to a day's food intake for an individual, or to determine the major foods contributing to energy intake for an entire population.

Table 3.1 Example of use of energy conversion factors in calculating the total energy content of foods.

Food	CHO (g/100 g)	Energy from CHO/100 g (A)	Fat (g/100 g)	Energy from fat/100 g (B)	Protein (g/100 g)	Energy from protein/100 g (C)	Total energy/100 g of food (A + B + C)
		Factor used: 3.75 kcal/g		*Factor used: 9 kcal/g*		*Factor used: 4 kcal/g*	
White bread	46.1	172.9	1.6	14.4	7.9	31.6	219
Milk, semi-skimmed	4.7	17.6	1.7	15.3	3.4	13.6	46
Baked beans	15.3	57.4	0.6	5.4	5.2	20.8	84

Nutrition at a Glance, Second Edition. Edited by Sangita Sharma, Tony Sheehy and Fariba Kolahdooz.
© 2016 John Wiley & Sons, Ltd. Published 2016 by John Wiley & Sons, Ltd.

4 Energy: Control of food intake

Aims

1 To investigate the internal physiological mechanisms that control food intake
2 To discuss external influences on control of food intake

Control of food intake

Food intake is necessary to satisfy the energy needs of the body, although energy stores do provide a buffer against periods of starvation. Hunger and satiety are the sensations that indicate the need to start or stop eating, and these represent the internal *physiological control* of eating. However, humans are exposed to many *external influences* that affect food intake as well, which may modify or override these internal mechanisms.

Physiological control: Internal mechanisms

A number of physiological mechanisms have been identified that regulate food intake so as to ensure a sufficient energy supply but avoid excessive storage. These mechanisms are believed to operate as a feedback system.

Early work proposed that food intake was regulated by the need to control glucose, amino acid or temperature levels in the blood or to maintain a constant level of fat reserves. These mechanisms have not been totally discounted and probably play some role in short-term control of eating.

More recent work, performed mostly with animals, where feeding behaviour can more readily be controlled, has expanded this knowledge and revealed a wide range of **neurotransmitters**,

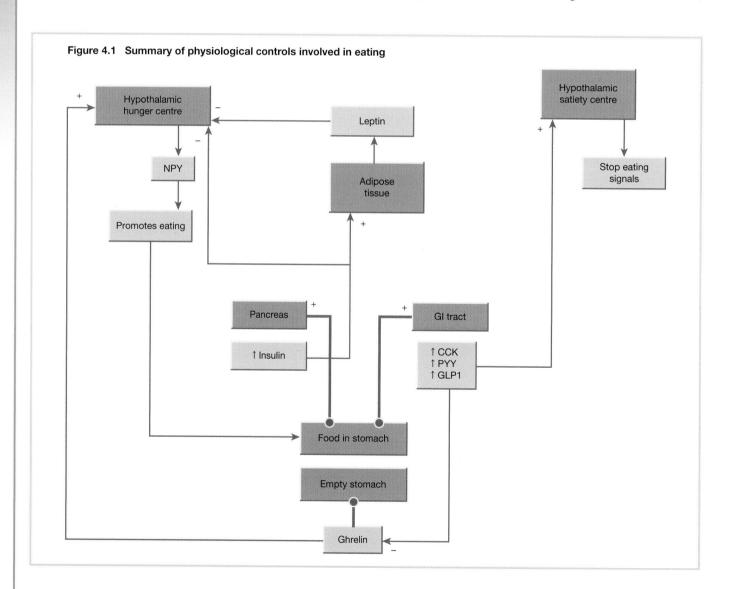

Figure 4.1 Summary of physiological controls involved in eating

Nutrition at a Glance, Second Edition. Edited by Sangita Sharma, Tony Sheehy and Fariba Kolahdooz.
© 2016 John Wiley & Sons, Ltd. Published 2016 by John Wiley & Sons, Ltd.

hormones and **brain peptides** that play a complex role in coordinating eating behaviour. Some of these factors appear to be involved in the drive to eat, whereas others are involved in the termination of eating. These factors are summarised in Figure 4.1.

Ghrelin is a peptide hormone released from the endocrine cells of the stomach that signals hunger. On reaching the arcuate nucleus in the hypothalamus, it stimulates the release of *neuropeptide Y* (NPY), which is a potent stimulant of food intake.

On eating, a number of gut hormones are released, including cholecystokinin (CCK), peptide YY (PYY 3–36) and glucagon-like peptide (GLP1). These hormones act both locally and centrally to inhibit the release of ghrelin, slow down stomach emptying and stimulate hunger-reducing neurones in the hypothalamus.

The effects of these hormones are modulated by insulin and leptin:
• Insulin begins to be secreted from the pancreas within minutes of starting to eat. It is believed to potentiate the satiating effects of CCK.
• Insulin also has a central effect to reduce the size of the meal consumed.
• Insulin is involved in the secretion of leptin, a hormone produced by adipose tissue, and eventually, leptin inhibits insulin secretion.
• An increase in leptin levels inhibits NPY and therefore food intake.
• Insulin also inhibits NPY, whereas fasting increases NPY synthesis, as insulin levels are low at this time.

Other neurotransmitter substances have been shown to have more specific associations with particular dietary constituents. For example:
• Serotonin is released following consumption of carbohydrate, leading to a feeling of satisfaction. This may be linked to carbohydrate cravings.
• Endorphins (endogenous opiates) have been linked to the hedonic response to sugar and fat; blocking their release may reduce the desire for high-fat or sugary foods.

External influences (see also Chapters 42 and 43)

In humans, the importance of these fundamental physiological mechanisms is difficult to establish, as they appear to be readily overridden by the **food environment** and **psychosocial factors**.

Food is constantly available in most Western environments, so people make their choices on the basis of taste (palatability), cost, convenience, social trends and peer pressure:

• *Palatability* – for most consumers, especially the younger age groups, intake is associated with high-fat, high-sugar, high-salt foods, often developed to enhance their taste. These foods have a high energy density.
• *Cost* – foods containing higher levels of fat and sugar are often cheaper than more nutrient-dense items. In addition, there has been a move towards selling foods in larger portion sizes, which appear financially economical. When there are financial constraints, people tend to look for maximum dietary energy for minimum cost and thus are more likely to choose the higher-fat/sugary foods that are high in calories.
• *Convenience* – the perceived busy lifestyle of many people has led to a desire for readily available foods that are easily consumed and with minimum levels of preparation being needed. The response of the food industry has been to produce an enormous range of prepared meals and fast foods that fulfil these requirements.
• *Snacking* – associated with the search for convenience is the move away from a 'three-meals-a-day' tradition and a pattern of eating that may include a much greater number of snacks during the day, of which none may be nutrient rich, but all of which may have a high energy density. In addition, soft drinks with a high energy density contribute energy, but have little or no satiety effect.
• *Social trends and peer pressure* – eating is a social activity, maintained and constrained by cultural factors. This can modify an individual's physiological eating controls by causing them to feel the need to comply with peer pressure (e.g. to eat fast food, to snack, to control body weight by restrained eating or by following a particular diet plan, to develop (positive or negative) attitudes to specific foods and to take exercise to increase physical activity). All of these make it more difficult for individuals to respond to their own food needs being signalled by the physiological control mechanisms.

Summary

Food intake is essential for survival, and there are physiological mechanisms to regulate it. However, the environmental factors encountered by many consumers result in poor regulation of food intake and, consequently, excessive consumption of energy in relation to needs. All of these factors make it challenging for public health policy-makers to address the rising incidence of overweight and obesity in most societies.

5 Energy: Measurement of requirements

Aim

1 To consider the ways in which energy requirements can be measured

Even when completely at rest, the human body requires energy constantly to carry out essential physiological functions including contraction of the heart and respiratory muscles, maintenance of transmembrane concentration gradients and normal cell turnover and repair. Energy usage increases when:

- Food needs to be digested.
- There is additional movement of some sort (e.g. physical activity).
- Infection (see Chapter 61) and burns (body needs more energy for physical repair)
- Body temperature needs to be increased (e.g. in a cold environment).
- Malabsorption

The body's energy requirement is met either from food intake or by drawing on stored reserves.

Principles of energy use

Energy is supplied by controlled combustion (i.e. oxidation) of macronutrients via a number of biochemical pathways including glycolysis, β-oxidation, the tricarboxylic acid (TCA) cycle and oxidative phosphorylation. The energy released is used mainly to synthesise adenosine triphosphate (ATP) from adenosine diphosphate (ADP) and inorganic phosphate. During periods of fasting, energy stores are mobilised by the action of hormones (including glucagon, growth hormone and cortisol) and oxidised to maintain the energy supply.

Measurement of energy expenditure

Direct calorimetry

Both the synthesis and utilisation of ATP are energetically inefficient processes, and heat is a major by-product. An individual's heat output is, therefore, an indicator of the energy transformations that are occurring in the body. This is the basis of direct calorimetry.

Direct calorimetry can be performed in a metabolic chamber (i.e. a specially adapted room where the subject can live). The subject's heat output is detected by sensors in the walls of the room, and this equates to their energy expenditure. The physical limitations of this environment make it impractical for routine use, but measurements made in this way have enabled other methods to be developed that are better at approximating real-life situations.

Indirect calorimetry

A more practical approach for measuring energy expenditure is to utilise information about gas exchanges that occur during metabolic reactions and the heat/energy output that is associated with them. These can be predicted from chemical formulae of the substrates and metabolic equations.

Table 5.1 Heat output per litre of oxygen consumed for different metabolic substrates.

Nutrient	Oxygen consumed (L/g)	Carbon dioxide produced (L/g)	RQ	Energy equivalent (kJ/L of O_2)
Glucose	0.746	0.746	1.0	20.7
Fats (mean)	1.975	1.402	0.71	19.8
Protein	0.962	0.775	0.81	19.25
Alcohol	1.429	0.966	0.663	20.4

The stoichiometric equation for the oxidation of glucose is given below; similar equations exist showing the oxidation of other substrates:

$$C_6H_{12}O_6 + 6O_2 = 6H_2O + 6CO_2 + 15.5\,kJ$$
(per g of glucose combusted)

Expressing these molar quantities as grams or litres,

$$(180\,g) + (6 \times 22.4\,L) = (6 \times 18\,g) + (6 \times 22.4\,L) + (2.78\,MJ)$$

Thus, combustion of 180 g of glucose requires 134.4 L of oxygen and produces 134.4 L of carbon dioxide and 2.78 MJ (i.e. 2780 kJ) of energy.

From this, it can be calculated that for every litre of oxygen consumed during glucose oxidation, the heat output is 20.7 kJ (i.e. 2780/134.4). Similar calculations can be performed to obtain the heat output per litre of oxygen consumed during the oxidation of fats, proteins and alcohol. These values are shown in Table 5.1.

Arising out of these calculations, if the amount of oxygen consumed by a subject during an activity or over a period of time can be measured, their corresponding heat production or energy expenditure can be calculated. Greater accuracy can be introduced by also measuring urinary nitrogen excretion, which allows incomplete metabolism of amino acids to be taken into account.

Various methods exist for obtaining information about *respiratory gas exchanges*. In principle, gases must be collected and analysed over a period of time. This can be achieved in:

- A closed system, such as a collecting bag (e.g. Douglas bag).
- A system where the flow of gases is continuously analysed, such as a ventilated hood, tent or canopy, which can also be attached to other respiratory equipment in the clinical setting.

When using these techniques, interference with normal respiratory patterns is a major obstacle, and care must be taken to allow subjects a period of equilibration. Fixed equipment also limits the range of activities that can be studied.

Nutrition at a Glance, Second Edition. Edited by Sangita Sharma, Tony Sheehy and Fariba Kolahdooz.
© 2016 John Wiley & Sons, Ltd. Published 2016 by John Wiley & Sons, Ltd.

The introduction of the *doubly labelled water* (DLW) technique has provided a means of obtaining energy expenditure data from free-living subjects in a non-invasive and non-intrusive manner. Measurements can be collected for periods of 7–14 days, in various real-life situations and in subjects of all ages. This method has become the 'gold standard' against which other methods are compared. However, the costs and availability of the labelled water make this technique unsuitable for large-scale studies.

The basic principle of the DLW technique is as follows:

1 The subject drinks a small amount of 'heavy' water, labelled with deuterium and oxygen-18 (^2H_2O and $H_2^{18}O$). These are naturally occurring nonradioactive isotopes of water.

2 The deuterium equilibrates with the body water and is washed out as part of body water turnover.

3 Oxygen-18 is also lost with body water but in addition is incorporated into carbon dioxide and lost in this way. Thus, oxygen-18 is lost faster than deuterium.

4 Samples of urine are collected over a period of up to 14 days and the rate of loss of the isotopes is monitored. The difference between them represents the carbon dioxide turnover.

Noncalorimetric methods

The use of heart rate monitoring equipment or motion sensors can provide information about physical activity. However, the validity of these techniques for accurate estimation of energy expenditure needs to be determined.

Respiratory quotient

The stoichiometric equations show the amount of carbon dioxide produced and oxygen consumed for a given amount of each substrate. This ratio ($CO_2:O_2$) is known as the respiratory quotient (RQ):

• If both oxygen consumption and carbon dioxide output are measured over a period of time, the RQ can be determined and the energy equivalent at the given RQ of oxygen consumed is computed.

• RQ varies with the substrate being metabolised; in practice, over a period of 24h, one can expect that the mixture of macronutrients used reflects their balance in a typical diet. Thus, for a Western diet with 35% energy from fat and 15% energy from protein, the RQ would be 0.87. This can be confirmed from concurrently kept dietary records.

• The energy yield per litre of oxygen is rounded to a mean of 20.3 kJ/L when details about RQ are not available.

6 Energy requirements: Components of energy expenditure

Aims

1 To identify the various components making up our total energy expenditure

2 To explore the determinants of energy expenditure and energy requirements

Components of energy expenditure

The energy expenditure of an individual can be broken down into three main components:

1 Basal (or resting) metabolic rate (BMR)

2 The thermic effect of food (TEF)

3 Energy expended during physical activity

In addition, growth during childhood and adolescence increases energy expenditure.

BMR

BMR is the energy expended by the body at rest. Energy expended at rest is sufficient only for maintaining vital functions, such as:

- Active transport across cellular membranes
- Contraction of fibres involved in essential mechanical work (e.g. respiration and the beating of the heart)
- Normal cell turnover

Because the concept does not make allowances for any internal processing of food or for muscular effort, measurement of BMR must be performed under strict conditions. The subject must be:

- Fasting
- In a state of mental and physical relaxation
- At a comfortable environmental temperature

These conditions can be difficult to achieve in practice, so resting metabolic rate (RMR) is often used instead to get a more realistic baseline measurement. RMR is estimated to be approximately 3% higher over 24 h than BMR. However, the two terms tend to be used interchangeably.

On average, BMR for an adult male is approximately 4.2 kJ (1 kcal)/min and remains relatively constant. Women in general have a metabolic rate about 5–10% lower than men. There is some variation between individuals, however. Major determinants of BMR include:

- Weight: Energy output is determined by cell mass. Therefore, body weight is a key determinant of BMR. Heavier individuals thus have a higher BMR.
- Gender: BMR is related to muscle mass, which is greater in males than females. Thus, males have a higher BMR for the same body weight. Women have a higher proportion of body fat, which has a lower BMR/kg than muscle.
- Age: BMR, expressed per kg body weight, declines from infancy to old age, as active cell mass decreases. The increment for growth is relatively small, averaging 21 kJ (5 kcal)/g of tissue gained. The additional requirement for growth is greatest at periods of growth spurts (in the first months of life and at the peak of puberty).

- Genetic factors: There are genetic differences in metabolic rate between people, but these have yet to be fully investigated. They probably account for less than 10% of the variability in BMR between individuals.
- Other factors: BMR is affected by certain drugs and pharmacological agents (e.g. nicotine, caffeine, amphetamines, capsaicin in chillies), disease states (e.g. fever, thyroid disease, cancers) and environmental conditions (extreme heat or cold). Fasting may result in a reduction in BMR, as the body attempts to adapt to a perceived life-threatening situation, even if this is brought about consciously by the individual in an attempt to lose weight.

For most sedentary individuals, BMR accounts for about 60–70% of the daily energy expenditure.

TEF

When a fasting subject consumes food, their heat production (i.e. heat output) goes up. This effect is called *diet-induced thermogenesis* (DIT) or *obligatory thermogenesis* and is due to the stimulation of metabolism caused by the need to process the food and store the macronutrients released.

Typically, TEF lasts for 3–6 h and is estimated to be equivalent to 10% of the energy content of the meal (or 10% of the total energy output for 24 h). TEF is greater with protein- and carbohydrate-containing meals than with fats.

Physical activity

This is the most variable component of daily energy expenditure, but the one over which individuals have most control.

The amount of energy expended during any type of physical activity is related to the subject's body size and, through this, to their BMR. Energy expended in physical activity can be calculated using factors known as *physical activity ratios* (PARs). The PAR value of an activity (e.g. walking, running, gardening, watching TV, or computer use) is the ratio by which the subject's energy output during that activity is increased above their BMR.

PAR values of a wide range of activities have been published, and these can be used to calculate the amount of energy expended during a period of time from records of activities undertaken at that time. It should be noted that PAR values are averages and do not accurately quantify the intensity of an activity or the amount of effort exerted. Thus, they should be used with caution in making judgements about a person's energy expenditure.

When intense physical activity is undertaken, BMR may be elevated for several hours afterwards and for up to 24 h after severe exercise. It is believed that this is associated with repair and recovery processes occurring in muscles.

Non-exercise activity thermogenesis (NEAT) is an additional component of energy expenditure due to small-scale movements that can be collectively described as 'fidgeting'. Although these appear to be minimal, their continuation throughout long periods of time suggests that they may account for substantial amounts of

Nutrition at a Glance, Second Edition. Edited by Sangita Sharma, Tony Sheehy and Fariba Kolahdooz.
© 2016 John Wiley & Sons, Ltd. Published 2016 by John Wiley & Sons, Ltd.

Table 6.1 Formulae for calculating BMR (MJ/day) (Schofield equations).

	Age range (years)	Regression formula for BMR (MJ/day)
Men	10–17	0.074 × weight (kg) + 2.754
	18–29	0.063 × weight (kg) + 2.896
	30–59	0.048 × weight (kg) + 3.653
	60–74	0.0499 × weight (kg) + 2.930
	75+	0.0350 × weight (kg) + 3.434
Women	10–17	0.056 × weight (kg) + 3.434
	18–29	0.062 × weight (kg) + 2.036
	30–59	0.034 × weight (kg) + 3.538
	60–74	0.0386 × weight (kg) + 2.875
	75+	0.0410 × weight (kg) + 2.610

energy expenditure and may explain the ability of some individuals to maintain a normal weight.

Equations for metabolic rate

In practical settings, the use of experimental methods to measure BMR or RMR may not be feasible. However, several equations have been developed based on measurements taken on large numbers of subjects that allow BMR to be calculated. These equations are based on a number of key indicators, including the subject's age, gender and body weight.

The most commonly used equations are the **Schofield** and **Harris–Benedict** equations. Although the latter were developed from limited data in the early 1900s, they are still in widespread use, especially in the USA. Schofield equations for calculating BMR are shown in Table 6.1.

Calculating total energy expenditure

This can be done by keeping records of 24-h periods of activity and using formulae for BMR and PAR values. An example is given in Table 6.2. Note that TEF is generally not included separately in these calculations, as it is considered to be subsumed within the PAR for eating.

In this example, the subject expended 11.07 MJ over the course of the day. As his BMR is 7.01 MJ, his overall *physical activity level* (PAL) for the day (i.e. the ratio by which his energy output was increased above BMR) was 1.58 (i.e. 11.07/7.01). In other words, he used almost 60% more energy than his BMR.

Compared with the typical population, whose PAL averages 1.4, this subject was relatively active, mainly because of his cycle ride after work.

Table 6.2 Example calculation of energy expenditure.

Activity	Duration (h)	PAR	BMR (kJ/h)	Energy used (kJ)
Energy used in an activity = duration of activity × PAR × BMR				
Sleeping	6	1.0	292	1752
Personal activities (washing, dressing, eating)	2	1.4	292	818
Driving to and from work	2	2.0	292	1168
Sitting at work (light office work)	9	1.5	292	3942
Cycle ride	2	4.0	292	2336
Watching TV	3	1.2	292	1051
Total for the day	24			11 067

The subject, a 45-year-old male weighing 70 kg, kept a record of his activities during one day. Using the Schofield equation, his BMR is therefore (0.048 × 70) + 3.653 = 7.01 MJ/day, or (7010/24) kJ/h = 292 kJ/h.

Adaptive thermogenesis

Research indicates that in certain individuals there exists a capacity for *adaptive thermogenesis*, which allows the body to dissipate excess energy intake as heat, using futile cycles that do not generate ATP.

This has been shown to be associated with uncoupling proteins (UCP), some of the genes for which have been identified. Varying levels of UCP activity in brown adipose tissue (BAT) have been demonstrated in animals that could resist weight gain consequent on overfeeding.

The importance of these mechanisms in humans remains unclear. It has been proposed that this was a mechanism of evolutionary advantage when nutrient-poor diets had to be consumed in large amounts, providing large amounts of energy with little nutritional content. The ability to dissipate the excessive energy allowed individuals to extract nutrients without becoming overweight. The prevalence of adequate food supplies makes this unnecessary in present times.

Summary

Energy expenditure is largely dependent on body size, which determines a person's BMR, and on the amount of energy used in physical activity. Physical activity has the greatest impact on energy expenditure, and even a relatively small increase in activity can make a meaningful difference to a person's daily energy output. For this reason, people are encouraged to include various forms of physical activity in their daily routines to help maintain energy balance.

7 Carbohydrates: Simple and complex carbohydrates

Aim

1 To describe the variety of carbohydrates found in the human diet and their sources

Carbohydrates (CHOs) typically provide somewhere between 40 and 80% of the energy consumed by humans, depending on the type of diet. In Western countries, CHOs usually provide about 45–50% of dietary energy, whereas in developing countries the figure can be much higher if traditional dietary patterns are still being followed. This situation is changing rapidly, however, as dietary patterns everywhere become more Westernised.

CHOs are classified as either **simple** or **complex**, depending on the number of monosaccharide units they contain. Three groups are recognised: *simple sugars* (monosaccharides and disaccharides), *oligosaccharides* and *polysaccharides* (see Table 7.1).

Monosaccharides

These are simple sugars consisting of 4–6 carbon atoms. The important ones in the diet are the 6-carbon sugars (*hexoses*), glucose, fructose and galactose.

Glucose is found in honey, table sugar and sugar-based confectionary, cakes, biscuits, vegetables, fruits and fruit juices.

Fructose is found in honey, table sugar, fruit and some vegetables. *High-fructose corn syrup* (derived from corn starch) is now used extensively as a replacement for sucrose in soft drinks, canned fruit, jams and jellies. It is cheaper than sucrose and has better freezing properties. This explains why fructose is now one of the major simple sugars in the Western diet. After absorption, fructose is metabolised in the liver, and the products are glucose, glycogen, lactic acid or fat, depending on the metabolic state of the individual.

Galactose is a component of the milk sugar, lactose, and is released by the action of the enzyme *lactase*. It is essential for neural tissue development in infants and can be transformed into either glucose or glycogen.

Disaccharides

Disaccharides are pairs of monosaccharides joined together by *glycosidic bonds*.

Sucrose is the most common disaccharide in the diet. It is formed by the condensation of glucose and fructose, which are joined together by an α 1–2 glycosidic bond. Sucrose can be extracted from sugar beet or sugar cane. By-products of sucrose extraction include molasses, golden syrup and brown sugar. Sucrose is also found in honey and maple syrup (in solution), as well as in fruit and vegetables (associated with the cellular structure).

Lactose is found in mammalian milk and consists of glucose and galactose joined together by a β 1,4-glycosidic bond. In the Western diet, lactose is obtained mainly from cow's milk and milk products (including foods containing milk powder or whey, such as milk chocolate, instant potatoes, biscuits and creamed soup). Lactose is widely used by the food industry as a food ingredient, and people who are *lactose-intolerant* need to be aware of its prevalence.

Maltose consists of two glucose units joined by an α 1,4-glycosidic bond. It is primarily found in germinating grains such as barley and wheat. The *malt* produced from sprouting grains is used in the production of fermented drinks including beer and whiskey. Small amounts of maltose are added to certain brands of biscuits, chocolate confectionary, breakfast cereals and malted drinks.

Oligosaccharides

Oligosaccharides contain up to 20 monosaccharide units. Some oligosaccharides (e.g. *stachyose*, *raffinose*, and *inulin*) occur naturally in plants such as leeks, onions, garlic, Jerusalem artichokes, lentils and beans. The sugars in these oligosaccharides are joined by β glycosidic bonds, which cannot be broken down by humans. Therefore, these oligosaccharides pass through the small intestine unchanged. However, on reaching the proximal colon, they undergo rapid fermentation by bacteria, resulting in the production of short-chain

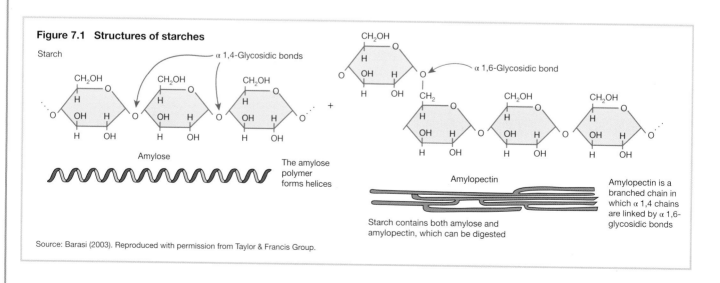

Figure 7.1 Structures of starches

Starch

α 1,4-Glycosidic bonds

α 1,6-Glycosidic bond

Amylose

The amylose polymer forms helices

Amylopectin

Amylopectin is a branched chain in which α 1,4 chains are linked by α 1,6-glycosidic bonds

Starch contains both amylose and amylopectin, which can be digested

Source: Barasi (2003). Reproduced with permission from Taylor & Francis Group.

Nutrition at a Glance, Second Edition. Edited by Sangita Sharma, Tony Sheehy and Fariba Kolahdooz.
© 2016 John Wiley & Sons, Ltd. Published 2016 by John Wiley & Sons, Ltd.

Table 7.1 Classes and products of CHOs in the digestive tract.

Class	Examples	Digestive products
Simple CHOs		
Monosaccharides	Glucose, fructose	Glucose, (some) fructose
Disaccharides	Sucrose	Glucose + fructose
	Lactose	Glucose + galactose
	Maltose	Glucose + glucose
Oligosaccharides	Raffinose	Fermented to short-chain fatty acids (SCFA), hydrogen, methane and carbon dioxide
	Inulin	
	FOS	
Complex CHOs		
Starch	Digestible starch	Glucose
	Resistant starch	Fermented to SCFA, hydrogen, methane and carbon dioxide
Non-starch polysaccharides	Cellulose	Some remain unchanged
	Non-cellulose polysaccharides, including hemicelluloses, pectins, gums and mucilages	Some fermented to SCFA, hydrogen, methane and carbon dioxide

fatty acids (SCFA) and gases, leading to flatulence. *Maltodextrins* are oligosaccharides that contain α-linked glucose units and are therefore digestible by humans. They are produced by partial hydrolysis of starch and are widely used by the food industry in the production of sweets, soft drinks, beer and other processed foods.

Polysaccharides

Polysaccharides consist of more than 20 monosaccharide units arranged in straight, branched or coiled chains. Traditionally, polysaccharides were classified as either *digestible* (available) forms, such as starches, or *non-digestible* (unavailable) forms, including cellulose and lignin. More recently, the convention has been to classify polysaccharides either as *starches* or *non-starch polysaccharides* (NSPs) (thus excluding lignin). The term '*dietary fibre*' is still widely used to encompass the full range of non-digestible CHOs, and this includes lignin.

Starch consists of a large number (typically thousands) of glucose molecules joined together in either straight or branched chains. In *amylose*, each glucose molecule is linked to the next one by an α 1,4-glycosidic bond. *Amylopectin* contains additional α 1,6-glycosidic bonds, resulting in a branched structure (see Figure 7.1). Many of the common starchy foods, such as potatoes,

cereals and beans, contain amylopectin and amylose in the approximate ratio of 3:1. The relatively high proportion of amylopectin allows starch to form stable gels with good water retention. Because of these properties, starches are widely used in the food industry as thickeners and stabilisers.

Dietary fibre, including NSPs

NSPs are long polymers of simple sugars and consist of both cellulose and non-cellulose components:

- Cellulose is the main component of plant cell walls and is made up of long chains (typically thousands) of glucose units joined together by β 1–4 linkages. This makes the molecule very resistant to digestion.
- Non-cellulose polysaccharides consist of hemicelluloses, pectins, β-glucans, gums and mucilages. Unlike cellulose, these contain mixtures of sugars (e.g. arabinose, xylose, mannose, fucose, glucose, galactose and rhamnose). They are more readily fermented as a food source for bacteria.

Energy plus a healthy bowel

Traditionally, it was thought that the major nutritional contribution of CHOs to health was as an energy source. However, it is now clear that CHOs also play a vital role in the healthy functioning of the bowel. The use of the terms 'glycaemic' and 'non-glycaemic' CHOs encapsulates this difference (see Chapter 8).

Other monosaccharides

Other monosaccharides are occasionally found in foods and include *xylose* and *arabinose* (white wine and beer), *mannose* (fruit) and *fucose* (in human breast milk).

Sorbitol, mannitol and *xylitol* are sugar alcohols that are used as sweetening agents in the food industry in foods such as diabetic foods, mints and sugar-free chewing gum. They have two valuable properties:

- They are absorbed from the gut and metabolised to glucose more slowly than other simple sugars. This delays the rise in blood glucose, which is of benefit to people with diabetes.
- They are not fermented by bacteria in the mouth and hence do not contribute to dental caries.

Fructo-oligosaccharides

Fructo-oligosaccharides (FOS) are prebiotics (i.e. non-digestible CHOs that act as food for probiotic bacteria in the colon). They consist of several fructose residues attached to glucose by β-glycosidic bonds. Because of their bond configuration, they are resistant to digestion by salivary and small intestinal enzymes. Thus, when used as sweeteners (e.g. in yogurts and other dairy foods), they reduce the energy content of the food while increasing its dietary fibre content. On entering the colon, however, they can be broken down by beneficial bacteria, such as *Bifidobacteria*, and used for energy.

8 Carbohydrates: Digestion and utilisation in the body

Aims

1 To describe how carbohydrates are digested
2 To introduce the concept of the glycaemic index

Digestion of carbohydrates

Monosaccharides do not require digestion before being absorbed. Absorption occurs mainly in the small intestine (SI).

Disaccharides are split by specific *disaccharidase* enzymes as they pass through the mucosal surface of the cells lining the SI. Deficiencies in these enzymes, especially *lactase*, result in an inability to break down the sugar, with consequent fermentation by bacteria lower down the intestine and associated gas production. Lactase commonly becomes unavailable in individuals who stop consuming milk after infancy, and *lactose intolerance* is widespread in many populations. Deficiencies of other disaccharidases may develop as a result of gastrointestinal disease or excess alcohol consumption.

Salivary *amylase* begins the digestion of cooked starch in the mouth. Low pH levels in the stomach prevent further digestion, but in the duodenum and jejunum, pH levels rise and amylase is released from the pancreas; this enzyme breaks alternate $\alpha 1$–4 linkages in both raw and cooked starches.

Amylose is degraded mostly to maltose and maltotriose (which consists of three glucose units), with small amounts of glucose being released.

Because of its more branched structure, *amylopectin* is initially broken down to oligosaccharides. These are subsequently degraded by specific *oligosaccharidases* situated on the mucosal brush border, producing glucose as the end product.

Resistant starch (in plant cell wall material or surrounded by fat in manufactured products) forms a physical barrier that slows the access of digestive enzymes to the starch.

Retrograded starches are starches that have been modified by temperature and/or the formation of a gel, so that on cooling, new bonds have formed, which are resistant to digestion by amylase.

Both resistant and retrograded starches may pass unchanged into the large intestine, where they can be fermented by bacteria to short-chain fatty acids (SCFA) and gases (see Table 8.1).

Glucose absorption

Glucose and galactose are transported from the SI across the apical membrane and into the bloodstream by a two-stage mechanism:

• A family of glucose transport proteins is located in cell membranes. Initially, the glucose moves down its concentration gradient from the SI lumen into the apical cells. The Na$^+$-linked transporter GLUT-1 facilitates this diffusion (Figure 8.1).
• Subsequently, sodium ions are actively transported out of the apical cell, and glucose molecules move from the apical cells into the bloodstream, using the second transport molecule GLUT-2 and facilitated diffusion.

Glycaemic effects of carbohydrates

Glycaemic index (Figure 8.2)

The glycaemic index (GI) provides an indication of how blood glucose levels change after ingesting different carbohydrates. A standard food (usually 50 g of glucose or white bread) is eaten, and changes in blood glucose are monitored over a period of time. The effect of a similar amount of a test food is then compared and the GI calculated. Although GI responses vary between individuals, the overall ranking of foods is similar. It is therefore possible to determine which foods have a low GI and which have a high GI (Table 8.2).

Lower GI foods may be preferred in circumstances where a prolonged glucose release is needed, such as in sporting performance, or to allow better blood glucose control in diabetics. Attention to the GI content of the diet has also been recommended for prevention of coronary heart disease, to achieve weight loss, and to protect against some cancers. However, the evidence for these effects is still not conclusive.

It should be remembered that GI values for single foods may not be replicated for whole meals and depend on the dietary mix.

Non-glycaemic effects of carbohydrates

Diets rich in NSP encourage chewing, which slows the process of eating and increases saliva flow. This contributes to satiety and promotes dental health.

As NSP moves down through the SI, divalent cations such as calcium, zinc and iron may bind to its surface, reducing their availability for absorption.

In the large intestine, *soluble fibre* is hydrolysed and fermented by the bacterial flora, resulting in the release of SCFA including acetic, propionic and butyric acids. Propionic and acetic acids are metabolised in the liver, but butyric acid is used locally by colon cells (colonocytes) as an essential source of energy. The multiplication of the bacterial flora increases bulk and water content of the stools.

Insoluble fibre reaches the colon largely unchanged and is not fermented by bacteria. The high water-holding characteristics of insoluble fibre together with the large bacterial mass result in an increase in total intracolonic mass. This stimulates peristalsis, increases the speed of movement of the colon contents, reduces transit time through the gastrointestinal tract and contributes to the overall laxation effect.

The wide range of CHOs consumed in the diet not only provides the body with glucose to maintain blood levels of this essential nutrient for brain and nervous system function but also with a food source for colonic bacteria, which enables a population of beneficial microorganisms to be maintained in the colon, thereby contributing to colon health.

Nutrition at a Glance, Second Edition. Edited by Sangita Sharma, Tony Sheehy and Fariba Kolahdooz.
© 2016 John Wiley & Sons, Ltd. Published 2016 by John Wiley & Sons, Ltd.

Figure 8.1   Transport of glucose (monosaccharide) from the small intestine (SI) lumen to the liver

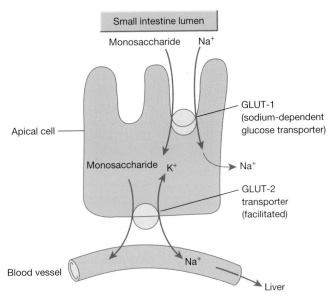

Figure 8.2   Calculation of glycaemic index

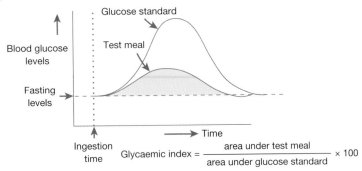

$$\text{Glycaemic index} = \frac{\text{area under test meal}}{\text{area under glucose standard}} \times 100$$

Table 8.1 Summary of starch digestibility.

Extent of digestion	Food sources
Readily and fully digested	Most cooked starches: sweet potatoes, tapioca
Slowly but completely digested	Flour-based products, for example, cakes, biscuits, raw cereals, coarsely ground grains
Not completely digested	Green bananas, seeds, cooked and cooled starches; some thickening agents

Table 8.2 Glycaemic index of some common foods.

Foods with high GI (>85)	Foods with moderate GI (60–85)	Foods with low GI (<60)
Bread (white or wholemeal)	Pasta and noodles	Apples, grapefruit, peaches, plums
Rice	Porridge	Beans, carrots
Raisins, bananas	Grapes, oranges	Milk, yogurt, ice cream
Potatoes, sweet corn	Crisps	Fructose
Glucose, sucrose, honey	Biscuits	Tomato soup
Soft drinks		

9 Fats: Types of fatty acids

Aims

1 To consider the major roles of fats in the body and the types of fats that are common in the diet
2 To describe specific nutritional characteristics of fatty acids

Major roles of fats

Fats (or *lipids*) have a number of important functions:
• They are a concentrated source of energy, providing approximately 9 kcal/g.
• They form an insulating layer under the skin that helps maintain body temperature.
• They form structural components in the body, such as cell membranes.
• They provide functional constituents for many metabolic processes.
• They are a vehicle for the intake and absorption of fat-soluble vitamins.
• They make an important contribution to flavour, texture and overall palatability of foods.

Types of fats

The most important lipids in nutrition are:
• *Triacylglycerols* (TAGs, also known as *triglycerides*): these contain three fatty acids attached (*esterified*) to a molecule of glycerol. TAGs comprise up to 95% of dietary lipids.
• *Phospholipids*: these consist of a glycerol backbone onto which is bonded two fatty acids (giving rise to a nonpolar region) and a polar 'head group' that contains a phosphoric acid residue joined to either sugars or amino acids. The most common example is phosphatidylcholine (lecithin). Because they are part hydrophilic and part hydrophobic (i.e. *amphipathic*), phospholipids can act at the interface between aqueous and lipid environments. This allows them to participate in cell membranes and to function as emulsifying agents.
• *Sterols*: contain carbon, hydrogen and oxygen arranged as ring structures, with associated side chains. Cholesterol is the main sterol found in animal tissues and is often bonded to fatty acids, forming cholesteryl esters. Plants contain phytosterols rather than cholesterol.

Fat-soluble vitamins are associated with these lipids.

Figure 9.1   Causes of variation between fatty acids

(a) Chain length
• From 2 to 24 carbons • Most common are 14-, 16-, 18-carbon chains

(b) Number of double bonds
• Determines saturation/unsaturation None = saturated fatty acid (SFA) One = monounsaturated fatty acid (MUFA) Several = polyunsaturated fatty acid (PUFA)

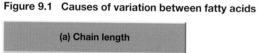

(c) Position of double bonds
• Distinguish fatty acid 'families' • Counted from CH_3 end of chain • First double bond on C-3, C-6 or C-9 represents *n-3*, *n-6* and *n-9* family, respectively (also known as omega, ω)

(d) *Cis/trans* isomers
Cis: predominant form – H atoms on same side of double bond; causes bending of chain *Trans*: H atoms on opposite sides of double bond; chains not bent, pack closely together

Figure 9.2   Interconversions between fatty acids within families

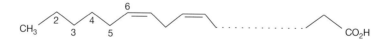

Diet → 18:2 (*n-6*) → 18:3 (*n-6*) → 20:3 (*n-6*) → 20:4 (*n-6*)
        Linoleic acid   γ-Linolenic acid   Dihomo-γ-   Arachidonic
                                           linolenic acid   acid

Diet → 18:3 (*n-3*) → 18:4 (*n-3*) → ......20:5 (*n-3*) → 22:6 (*n-3*)
        α-Linolenic acid   Eicosapentaenoic   Docosahexaenoic
                                      acid (EPA)   acid (DHA)

(Note: some intermediate products have been omitted from the *n-3* familiy for clarity)

Nutrition at a Glance, Second Edition. Edited by Sangita Sharma, Tony Sheehy and Fariba Kolahdooz.
© 2016 John Wiley & Sons, Ltd. Published 2016 by John Wiley & Sons, Ltd.

Fatty acids

Fatty acids are the main components of dietary lipids. A fatty acid consists of a hydrocarbon chain, with a carboxyl (–COOH) group at one end and a methyl (–CH$_3$) group at the other end. Fatty acids differ from one another in a number of ways, including their chain length, number of double bonds, position of double bonds along the chain and isomeric (i.e. *cis* or *trans*) configuration around the double bonds (Figure 9.1). These structural variations cause the physical properties of fatty acids (and of lipids containing them) to be quite diverse, and this, in turn, affects their metabolic role and consequences for health.

Saturated fatty acids

Saturated fatty acids (SFAs) contain the maximum number of hydrogen atoms attached to each carbon (i.e. there are no double bonds) and tend to be solid at room temperature:
- Fat from cows' milk contains SFAs synthesised by rumen bacteria and is the main dietary source of short- and medium-chain SFAs (4–10 C chain length). Butter is rich in these fatty acids.
- The majority of SFAs in the diet contain 14, 16 and 18 carbons and come from coconut oil (C14), palm oil (C16) and animal and hydrogenated fats (predominantly C18).
- Longer-chain SFAs, up to 24 carbons in length, are synthesised within brain tissue membranes.

Monounsaturated fatty acids

- Monounsaturated fatty acids (MUFAs) contain one double bond, the main example being oleic acid (18:1, *n*-9), derived primarily from olive and rapeseed oils.
- Meats provide MUFAs in varying amounts, depending on the fat content. Oily fish provide MUFAs in small amounts.
- In India, mustard seed oil provides a longer-chain MUFA called erucic acid (22:1, *n*-9).

Polyunsaturated fatty acids

Because of their greater content of double bonds, polyunsaturated fatty acids (PUFAs) have the lowest melting point of all types of fatty acids and are liquid at room temperature. When used in the manufacture of spreading fats, emulsification is used to produce a firmer spread:
- The major PUFAs contain 18, 20 or 22 carbons; have up to six double bonds; and belong to either the *n*-3 or *n*-6 families.
- PUFAs and their derivatives regulate membrane fluidity and other membrane properties. The *n*-3 PUFAs have a particularly important role in the brain, nervous system and retina.
- PUFAs are also used in the formation of metabolic regulators called *eicosanoids*. This category of compounds includes prostaglandins, prostacyclins, thromboxanes and leukotrienes. Eicosanoids derived from the *n*-3 and *n*-6 families of fatty acids differ in their biological potency and functions, and an altered balance between them can affect physiological processes such as haemostasis and inflammation.

The body is unable to insert a double bond any closer than 7 carbons from the methyl (CH$_3$) end of a fatty acid. Thus, humans cannot synthesise linoleic acid (18:2 *n*-6) and α-linolenic acid (18:3 *n*-3), the parent compounds of the *n*-6 and *n*-3 families. Therefore, these are *essential fatty acids* that must be supplied in the diet. Once provided and inside the cell, they can be built up into longer *n*-3 and *n*-6 fatty acids by a sequence of desaturation and elongation reactions involving the formation of new double bonds and the addition of 2-C units, respectively (Figure 9.2).

Trans fatty acids

Unsaturated fatty acids can contain one or more double bonds arranged in the *trans* position. Within the body, trans fatty acids (TFAs) have similar characteristics to SFAs because they can pack closer together than *cis* fatty acids. TFAs have been associated with detrimental effects on plasma lipids, including raised levels of low-density lipoproteins (LDLs) and lowered high-density lipoproteins (HDLs). Because of this, it is now widely accepted that TFAs increase the risk of coronary heart disease. The US Centers for Disease Control and Prevention (CDC) estimates that elimination of partially hydrogenated vegetable oils (PHOs, the major source of industrially produced TFAs) from the food supply could prevent 10 000–20 000 coronary events and 3 000–7 000 coronary deaths annually in the USA.

Fats and disease

Because of the involvement of fats in the aetiology of cardiovascular disease and certain cancers, as well as their potential role in the development of obesity, the intake and composition of dietary fats continue to be the subject of extensive research.

Shorthand notation for fatty acids

Differences in fatty acid structure can be summarised in shorthand notation, as illustrated by two examples:

C18:2, *n*-6 is linoleic acid, with 18 carbons and two double bonds, the first of which starts on the sixth carbon from the methyl (CH$_3$) end of the molecule.

C18:3, *n*-3 is α-linolenic acid, with 18 carbons and three double bonds, the first of which starts on the third carbon from the methyl end of the acid.

Falling intakes of SFAs

The intake of SFAs has fallen in the West over the last 20–30 years, from around 20% of total energy to 11–12%. This has resulted from:
- A general reduction in the consumption of meat and animal products, as energy expenditure has decreased.
- Healthy eating advice, which has promoted a reduction in both total fat intake and specifically SFAs. The rationale for this advice is based on the association between SFA intake and plasma cholesterol levels and the increased cardiovascular disease risk.

The 'Mediterranean diet'

Oleic acid is the main fatty acid in the 'Mediterranean diet', which has been associated with cardiovascular health benefits. Consumption of MUFAs has been promoted as part of healthy eating advice.

n-3 and *n*-6 PUFAs

PUFAs of the *n*-6 family are recommended as partial substitutes for SFAs in diets to help prevent cardiovascular disease, through a reduction of LDL cholesterol levels. Advantages of *n*-3 PUFAs include effects on lipaemia and on haemostatic factors.

The intake of *n*-6 PUFAs has increased since the 1970s, mainly due to the widespread usage of vegetable oils in food processing, and in Western countries now stands at roughly 6% of dietary energy. However, the resulting increase in the ratio of *n*-6 to *n*-3 PUFAs, to levels averaging 8:1, is causing concern, and efforts are being made to re-establish a ratio closer to 1:1, which is believed to have existed prior to the growth of the food processing industry.

Reducing TFAs

TFAs occur naturally in meat and dairy products from ruminant animals and thus are difficult to avoid in ordinary, non-vegan diets. However, the other major source of TFAs is PHOs, which are added to a variety of food products including baked goods, deep fried foods, snacks, sweets and margarines. Because of the mounting evidence of harm caused by trans fats, Denmark, Austria, Iceland and Switzerland have enacted legislation banning industrially produced TFAs from the food supply. Brazil, Argentina, Chile, South Africa and the USA have also taken steps to reduce or eliminate trans fats from food, while the UK government has asked major food chains to remove industrially produced trans fats from their products on a voluntary basis. Labelling regulations in some countries have also been updated and now require that any TFAs present in foods must be declared.

10 Fats: Compound lipids (triglycerides, phospholipids, cholesterol, and phytosterols)

Aims

1 To consider the structure of compound lipids including triglycerides, phospholipids and important dietary sterols
2 To summarise the nutritional significance of these lipids

Up to 95% of the total fat intake in the diet is in the form of triglycerides, with the remainder being present as free fatty acids, phospholipids, cholesterol and plant sterols (*phytosterols*).

Triglycerides

Triglycerides consist of a glycerol molecule onto which are bonded three fatty acids (Figure 10.1). Food triglycerides differ greatly in the types of fatty acids they contain, and this variation greatly affects their physical properties. In humans and animals, triglycerides tend to contain mainly saturated fatty acids, whereas fish triglycerides tend to have more polyunsaturated fatty acids, such as 20:5 *n*-3 (eicosapentaenoic acid, EPA) and 22:6 *n*-3 (docosahexaenoic acid, DHA). Polyunsaturated fatty acids have lower melting points than saturated fatty acids, and it is this adaptation that allows adipose tissue triglycerides in fish to remain liquid at low water temperatures.

Triglycerides are the main storage form of **energy** in the body, providing about 9 kcal/g.

Phospholipids

Phospholipids consist of a glycerol backbone onto which are bonded two fatty acids, one each at C1 and C2, and a phosphate group at C3. Attached to the phosphate group is a *functional group*, which can be serine, choline, ethanolamine or inositol (Figure 10.1). Phospholipids are named according to their functional group.

Phospholipids are widely distributed in the diet, though in small amounts, as they are an essential component of all cell membranes. Liver and eggs are important animal food sources of phospholipids, while soya bean and wheat germ are rich plant sources (Table 10.1).

Within the body, phospholipids contribute to the structural integrity of cell membranes by forming a **lipid bilayer**, with the polar (phosphate-containing) end of the molecule facing towards aqueous environments (i.e. the intracellular or extracellular fluid) and the fatty acid tails pointing away from these regions. Membrane phospholipids are also an important source of essential fatty acids

Figure 10.1 Structures of compound lipids found in the diet: triglycerides, phospholipids, cholesterol and some common phytosterols

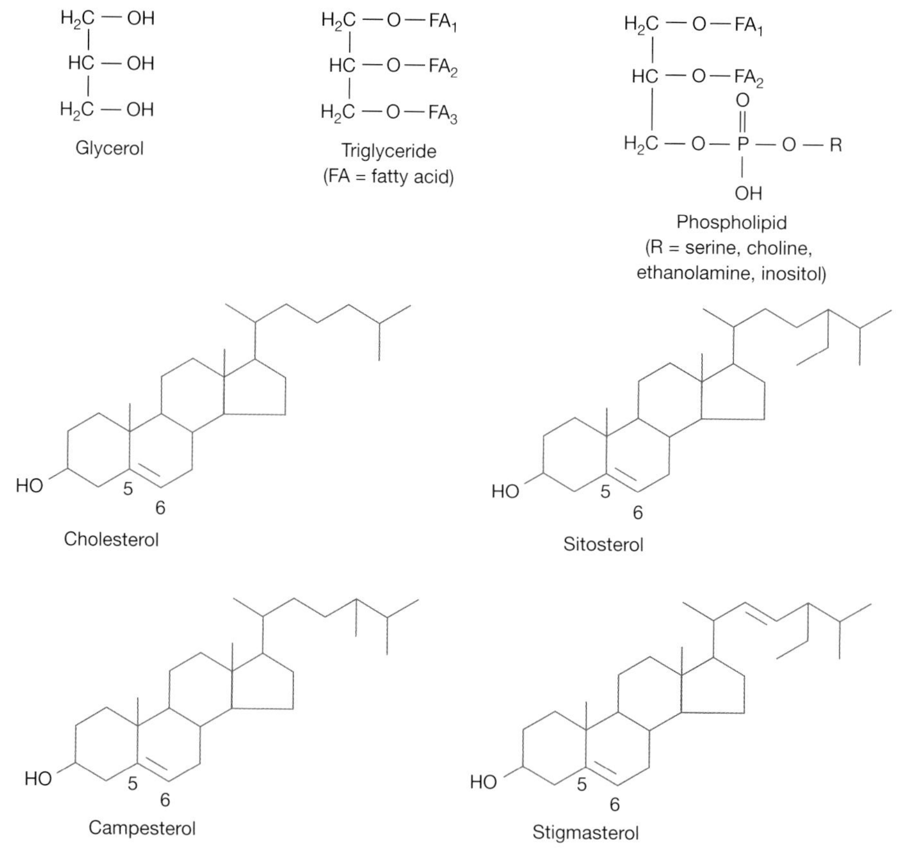

Glycerol

Triglyceride (FA = fatty acid)

Phospholipid (R = serine, choline, ethanolamine, inositol)

Cholesterol

Sitosterol

Campesterol

Stigmasterol

Nutrition at a Glance, Second Edition. Edited by Sangita Sharma, Tony Sheehy and Fariba Kolahdooz.
© 2016 John Wiley & Sons, Ltd. Published 2016 by John Wiley & Sons, Ltd.

Table 10.1 Summary of the occurrence of main types of fat in the diet.

Type of fat	Main dietary sources
Short-chain SFA (C4–C10)	Milk and milk products, including butter
SFAs with 14–18 carbons	Meat, animal foods and fats Coconut and palm oils
MUFAs, especially C18:1	Olive and rapeseed oils Meat fats (moderate amounts)
PUFAs, *n*-6	Specific fatty acids from this family occur as follows: Linoleic acid (C18:2, *n*-6): seed oils (sunflower, soya bean and corn), meat, eggs and nuts γ-Linolenic acid (C18:3, *n*-6): borage, blackcurrant and evening primrose oil Arachidonic acid (C20:4, *n*-6): small amounts in meat and egg yolks
PUFAs, *n*-3	Specific fatty acids from this family occur as follows: α-Linolenic acid (C18:3, *n*-3): dark-green vegetables, meat from grass-fed ruminants, seed oils (flaxseed, soya bean and rapeseed) Eicosapentaenoic acid (EPA) (C20:5, *n*-3) and docosahexaenoic acid (DHA) (C22:6, *n*-3): oily fish and fish oils
Triglycerides	Butter, vegetable spreads and oils, nuts, full-fat dairy products, fatty meats and fish, some snack foods and confectionary
Phospholipids	Small amounts in soya bean, wheat germ oils; animal foods, eggs
Cholesterol	Foods of animal origin: eggs, organ meats, shellfish
TFAs	Products from ruminant animals, hydrogenated fats in manufactured goods

for the production of **eicosanoids**, which act as local chemical messengers. Phosphatidyl choline (lecithin) is widely used in the food processing industry as an **emulsifier**.

Cholesterol

Cholesterol is the principal sterol found in the body and is synthesised from the metabolic intermediate **acetyl coenzyme A** in all tissues but mainly in the liver.

In the diet, cholesterol is obtained from animal foods, with eggs and liver being the richest sources. Cholesterol intakes in Western diets are typically between 250 and 700 mg/day. Absorption of cholesterol between individuals is variable, but is generally less than 50%.

Cholesterol plays an essential role in **membrane structure** and in facilitating transport across membranes. It is also the starting point for the synthesis of **bile acids** and certain **hormones** (e.g. corticosteroids, progesterone, oestrogen, testosterone, and vitamin D). Elevated plasma cholesterol levels, principally carried in the low-density lipoprotein (LDL) fraction, are a major determinant of the risk of atherosclerosis.

Phytosterols

Plants do not produce cholesterol but instead produce *phytosterols*, the main dietary forms of which are β-sitosterol, campesterol and stigmasterol (Figure 10.1). These compounds differ from cholesterol in having extra substituents and/or double bonds on the hydrocarbon side chain. Saturation of the double bond between C5 and C6 on the ring structure converts phytosterols to *phytostanols*.

Typical sources of phytosterols include vegetable oils, nuts and cereals. Intakes in Western diets are thought to be about 250 mg/day, with vegetarian diets containing considerably more.

Both phytosterol and phytostanol esters have been marketed in recent years as **functional food ingredients** (typically in dairy spreads and yogurts) to help reduce plasma cholesterol. In the gastrointestinal tract, they reduce cholesterol absorption and promote its excretion in the faeces by a number of mechanisms including co-precipitation, competitive inhibition for space on micelles and increased cholesterol efflux from enterocytes. Optimal intake of these compounds for plasma cholesterol reduction appears to be about 2 g/day.

Lowering dietary cholesterol

Healthy eating advice has principally been focused on dietary modification to reduce plasma LDL levels. However, there is genetic variability between people in LDL levels and in the way they respond to cholesterol intake. Because of this, reductions in dietary cholesterol are no longer considered a major part of dietary advice for most people.

Low-fat diets

Fat is perceived by many people as the component of the diet that should be reduced as much as possible. However, a certain amount of fat is required to fulfil the important roles that fat has in the body. Diets that are low in fat can be very bulky, as the energy density of the diet is reduced, and more food has to be consumed to achieve an adequate energy intake.

When consumers wish to reduce their energy consumption, reducing their fat intake can be helpful, but under these circumstances, it is important to ensure that essential fatty acids and fat-soluble vitamins are still being supplied to meet nutritional requirements.

Fats: Digestion and utilisation in the body

Aims

1 To consider how fats are digested and transported in the body
2 To study fat storage and utilisation

Fat digestion and absorption

In order for dietary fat to be effectively digested and absorbed, a number of obstacles must be overcome. These obstacles and the body's mechanisms for overcoming them are summarised in Table 11.1.

Transport of fats in the body: Lipoproteins

Because fats are hydrophobic, they cannot circulate freely in the blood. Instead, they are transported around the body in a variety of aggregate particles known as lipoproteins. The composition of lipoproteins is not constant, as constituents are continually being taken up and released (Table 11.2).

The main function of lipoproteins is to transport triacylglycerol (TAG) and cholesterol originating from the diet or endogenous synthesis. However, lipoproteins also carry other fat-soluble materials, including vitamins. Proteins, known as *apolipoproteins*, serve as 'identifiers' for the particles and determine their uptake by receptor sites.

Chylomicrons

Chylomicrons are the largest and lightest of the lipoproteins. Their function is to transport dietary TAG to the circulation via the **lymph system**. Chylomicron concentrations peak in the circulation 2–4 h after a fat-containing meal, but they may continue to enter for up to 14 h after a particularly high-fat meal.

As they travel through the body, chylomicrons release fatty acids under the action of *lipoprotein lipase* (LPL), an enzyme at the endothelial surface of capillaries. After delivery, the *chylomicron remnants* are taken up by the liver. The current needs of the body for immediate energy (in the muscle) or storage (in the adipose tissues) determine at which sites LPL is most active (Figure 11.1).

Very-low-density lipoproteins

Very-low-density lipoproteins (VLDLs) are made in the liver by the re-synthesis of TAG from fatty acids delivered to the liver. Peak release of VLDLs from the liver occurs 2–3 h after a meal, but if chylomicrons are still present, these are preferentially metabolised.

As VLDL lose TAG, their cholesterol concentration rises, and they become low-density lipoproteins (LDLs).

LDLs

The principal function of LDLs is to transport cholesterol to tissues where it is needed for cell membrane structure and function and for synthesis of metabolites, such as steroid hormones.

LDL receptors on the cell surface recognise the **apoB100** protein on the outer surface of LDLs and mediate the uptake of LDL particles into the cells. LDL receptor activity is regulated by intracellular free cholesterol levels. Thus, LDL uptake can be varied to meet cellular needs for cholesterol (Figure 11.2).

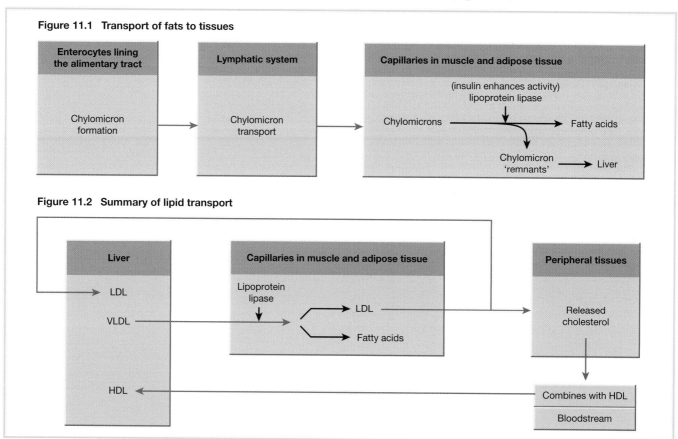

Figure 11.1 Transport of fats to tissues

Figure 11.2 Summary of lipid transport

Nutrition at a Glance, Second Edition. Edited by Sangita Sharma, Tony Sheehy and Fariba Kolahdooz.
© 2016 John Wiley & Sons, Ltd. Published 2016 by John Wiley & Sons, Ltd.

Table 11.1 Obstacles to fat digestion and their physiological solutions.

Problem	Solution	Consequences
Dietary fat is not miscible with aqueous digestive juices	Large fat particles are broken down in the stomach by a churning action	A coarse emulsion reaches the duodenum Hormones (e.g. cholecystokinin) released to slow down stomach emptying and promote release of bile
Digestive enzymes cannot process large lipids	Bile is released from the liver via the gall bladder. It reduces the coarse emulsion to small micelles, which can be acted on by pancreatic lipase	Lipase splits fatty acids from TAGs to yield glycerol, fatty acids and some monoacylglycerols
Some digestion products are too large to enter the circulation directly. Short- and medium-chain fatty acids can be absorbed directly	They are packaged into chylomicrons, where hydrophilic constituents form the outer coat and hydrophobic products are in the interior. Bile acids are reabsorbed from the ileum and recirculated	Chylomicrons pass into the lymphatic system draining the digestive tract and are carried to the peripheral circulation, in which they enter at the thoracic duct

Table 11.2 Typical composition of lipoprotein particles (as %).

Particle	TAG	Cholesterol	Phospholipid	Protein
Chylomicron	90	5	3	2
(VLDL)	60	12	18	10
(LDL)	10	50	15	25
(HDL)	5	20	25	50

High-density lipoproteins

High-density lipoproteins (HDLs) are synthesised in the intestines and the liver. Their role is to collect free cholesterol and other lipids from the peripheral tissues. During this process, the cholesterol is esterified by a plasma enzyme called *lecithin–cholesterol acyltransferase* (LCAT) to form cholesterol esters (CE), which are then sequestered in the core of the particle, thereby maintaining a concentration gradient of free cholesterol into the HDL.

CE may be taken directly to the liver and excreted in bile or exchanged for TAG from VLDLs and chylomicrons. If this happens to excess, TAG-rich HDLs (*small dense HDLs*) become a substrate for hepatic lipase and are rapidly catabolised; this may lead to lower circulating levels of HDLs. This then reduces the normal *reverse cholesterol transport* process, and cholesterol levels in the tissues may increase.

Because LDLs and HDLs are intimately involved with cholesterol transport, they are believed to be critical in the development of atherosclerosis and heart disease.

Adipose tissue

Fat is stored as an energy reserve in adipocytes, which are found in adipose tissue. These cells make up only about half of the total cell numbers within the tissue, with fibroblasts, macrophages and vascular tissue making up the remainder. Adipose tissue itself contains approximately 79% fat, 18% water and 3% protein:
• *White adipose tissue* is the predominant form. These cells store fat as a single droplet, which almost fills the entire cell. The type of fat present reflects the type of dietary fat consumed. However, on a low-fat diet, the fat is mainly that synthesised in the body and contains mostly palmitic (C16:0), stearic (C18:0) and oleic (C18:1 *n-9*) acids.
• There are also small amounts of *brown adipose tissue* (BAT), mostly found in young children but also in adults. BAT has many more mitochondria, blood capillaries and nerve fibres than white adipose tissue. In young children and animals, BAT is a means of generating heat. It may play some role in energy-wasting mechanisms in adults and so help in maintaining energy balance.

The healthy adult male contains about 17% of his body weight as fat, while for healthy females the figure is approximately 27%. Most of this fat is found subcutaneously. Deposits within the chest cavity and abdomen increase with fatness and are associated with increased health risks.

Mobilisation of stored fat

There are differences between abdominal fat and the fat stored in the thighs and buttocks:
• Intra-abdominal fat is more sensitive to lipolytic stimuli, and the fat released from this region is carried directly to the liver via the portal vein, triggering metabolic responses.
• Subcutaneous fat is more resistant to lipolysis and is more likely to be protected from daily fluctuations.
• Fat adjacent to lymph nodes is thought to support the immune system and may expand in chronic inflammatory states at the expense of fat in other regions.

Metabolism of stored fat

Fat storage and release is under the control of hormones, principally insulin and noradrenaline. There is a continuous flux of fats into and out of the adipocytes. Fat storage occurs principally in the *postprandial phase* under the influence of insulin, when there are increased numbers of chylomicrons and VLDLs in the circulation.

In theory, fat can be synthesised from carbohydrates for storage also, but this rarely happens, except in circumstances of very high carbohydrate intake. Thus, most fat stored in adipose tissue is derived from dietary and endogenous fats.

Fat utilisation occurs under the influence of noradrenaline, which causes the release of fatty acids and their oxidation to yield adenosine triphosphate (ATP). Some fat oxidation occurs most of the time in the human body to fuel metabolic and physical activity.

Adipose tissue also has other functions including:
• Secretion of *leptin*, a hormone that acts on receptors in the hypothalamus to regulate food intake and energy expenditure
• Production of numerous other cytokines, called *adipokines*, which are involved in regulating insulin sensitivity, blood pressure and inflammatory responses

Loss of control

As body fat levels increase, there is a reduced ability of adipose tissue to respond to regulatory signals, with an increase in circulating lipid levels and the risk of fat depositing in the liver and skeletal muscle.

Insulin resistance is a feature of obesity, and the disposal of glucose is also affected. Type 2 diabetes may result and be accompanied by a range of complications, including hypertension, damage to peripheral blood vessels, hyperlipidaemia and elevated risk of cardiovascular disease.

12 Proteins: Chemistry and digestion

Aims

1 To describe the basic chemical structure of amino acids and proteins
2 To consider how proteins are digested

Proteins form the basic building blocks of all living cells. They are present in cell membranes and organelles, as well as in the form of enzymes and chemical messengers (e.g. hormones and cytokines) that integrate body functions. In contrast to carbohydrates and fats, which only contain carbon, hydrogen and oxygen, proteins also contain nitrogen and are the most abundant nitrogen-containing molecules in the body.

Structure of proteins

Proteins are made up of one or more chains of *amino acids*, joined together by *peptide bonds* (Figure 12.1). The sequence of amino acids in a protein is called its *primary* structure. As the chain grows, interactions occur between amino acids that come to lie adjacent to each other. These interactions include hydrogen bonding between oxygen and nitrogen atoms, electrostatic or hydrophobic interactions or the formation of disulphide (S–S) bridges within or between side chains. As a result, the protein becomes folded and cross-linked in various ways, giving rise to what are called its *secondary*, *tertiary* and *quaternary* features. Folding and cross-linking:

• Contribute great strength and elasticity to particular structural proteins, such as collagen in tendons or elastin in blood vessels
• Create reactive sites for receptors or enzymic activity

Amino acids

Apart from proline, amino acids have a common basic structure, as shown in Figure 12.1. They contain a central α-carbon atom, onto which is bonded a carboxyl (COOH) group, an amino (NH_2) group, a hydrogen atom and an aliphatic, aromatic, acidic or basic side chain (called the *functional group*) (Table 12.1). Functional groups may be hydrophilic or hydrophobic in nature, which results in the amino acids themselves having these properties.

The sequence in which the amino acids are present in a protein is what determines both its identity and function. Body protein is made up of 20 different amino acids, in combinations ranging from approximately 50 to well over 1000 in any one protein. Thus, there is enormous diversity in composition between proteins in the body.

Digestion and absorption of proteins

In their native form, most proteins are very resistant to digestion, with only the superficial bonds being susceptible to protein-digesting (*proteolytic*) activity. However, once a protein has been denatured by exposure to either heat or acid, the forces holding the structure together become weakened, and digestion can occur. Cooking of foods and the acidity of the stomach contents both contribute to increasing the digestibility of proteins.

Protein-digesting enzymes are synthesised as inactive *proenzymes* or *zymogens* and become activated only after secretion into the stomach or duodenum. This feature serves to protect these organs from autodigestion.

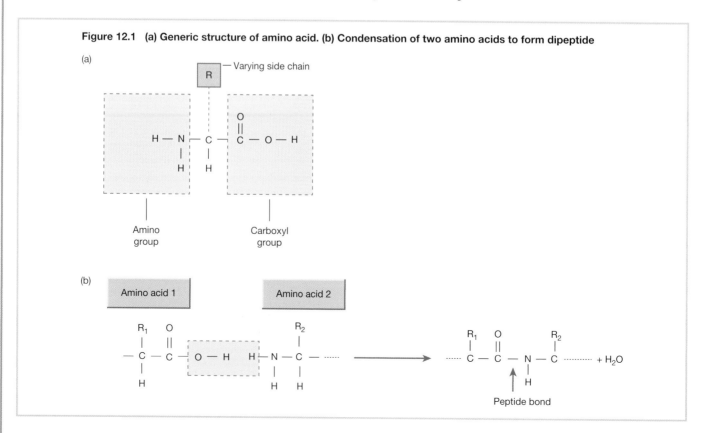

Figure 12.1 (a) Generic structure of amino acid. (b) Condensation of two amino acids to form dipeptide

Nutrition at a Glance, Second Edition. Edited by Sangita Sharma, Tony Sheehy and Fariba Kolahdooz.
© 2016 John Wiley & Sons, Ltd. Published 2016 by John Wiley & Sons, Ltd.

During protein digestion, polypeptide chains are hydrolysed at specific sites, exposing more terminal sites for further cleavage. In this way, progressively shorter peptide chains are produced.

Table 12.1 Classification of amino acids.

Aromatic	Aliphatic	Acidic	Basic
Phenylalanine	Glycine	Aspartic acid	Lysine
Tyrosine	Alanine	Asparagine	Arginine
Tryptophan	Valine*	Glutamic acid	Histidine
	Leucine*	Glutamine	
	Isoleucine*		
	Serine		
	Threonine		
	Cysteine†		
	Cystine†,‡		
	Methionine†		
	Proline		

*Branched-chain amino acids.
†Sulphur-containing amino acids.
‡Cystine is two cysteine residues linked together via a disulphide (S–S) bond.

Overall, this results in the liberation of free amino acids as well as small peptides, which are themselves further split during the process of absorption by *aminopeptidases* located within the intestinal mucosa. The sequence of events in protein digestion is summarised in Table 12.2.

Normally, dietary protein is almost completely digested. However, the presence of indigestible cell wall material and trypsin inhibitors (in raw beans) will interfere with the process. In general, legumes are considered the least effectively digested form of dietary protein source.

Absorption of amino acids occurs both by passive diffusion and by sodium-dependent active transport mechanisms. Absorbed amino acids enter the circulation via the hepatic portal vein. Some intact protein may be absorbed in very young infants, which is beneficial as it confers some immunity. However, this also means that exposure to inappropriate dietary proteins at this stage of life can give rise to allergic reactions.

In addition to the dietary amino acids presented for absorption, the intestinal mucosa also absorbs considerable amounts of endogenous amino acids (~80 g/day). These amino acids are derived from secretions into the small intestine and from cells sloughed off the mucosal surface.

Table 12.2 Sequence of events in protein digestion.

Organ/site	Secretion(s)	Action and products
Mouth/teeth/chewing action	Saliva	Lubricates food, allows breakdown to smaller pieces
Stomach	Hydrochloric acid (HCl)	HCl • Denatures proteins • Activates pepsinogen to pepsin at pH <4
	Pepsinogen	Pepsin • Breaks polypeptide chains to smaller units → shorter polypeptides
Pancreas	Bicarbonate	Bicarbonate • Increases pH (to ~7.5) to allow enzymes to work
	Pancreatic enzymes • Trypsinogen*	Trypsin (formed from trypsinogen) • Cleaves polypeptides with basic terminal amino acid • Activates other proteolytic enzymes
	• Chymotrypsinogen	Chymotrypsin • Cleaves polypeptides with a neutral terminal amino acid
	• Carboxypeptidases	Carboxypeptidases • Remove successive amino acids from carboxy terminal of peptide chain
	• Endopeptidases*	Endopeptidases • Attack bonds within the peptide chain
Small intestine	Enterokinase (also called enteropeptidase)	Enterokinase • Activates trypsin and endopeptidases
	Aminopeptidases	Aminopeptidases • Complete the breakdown of small peptide chains (tri- and dipeptides) as they pass through the intestinal mucosa

*Activated by enterokinase from the small intestine.

13 Proteins: Functions and utilisation in the body

Aims

1 To identify the main functions of proteins in the body
2 To recognise the critical role played by essential amino acids in protein function and metabolism

After digestion and absorption, amino acids enter what is conceptualised as the cellular *amino acid pool* and are used to synthesise proteins required for various functions in the body. These include structural proteins (e.g. keratin, collagen), contractile proteins (e.g. actin, and myosin), certain hormones (e.g. insulin, growth hormone) and transport proteins (e.g. haemoglobin, transferrin), as well as enzymes, blood clotting factors, antibodies and receptors. The metabolism and functions of proteins are summarised in Figure 13.1.

Metabolism of amino acids

Protein synthesis and breakdown

There is a continuous turnover of protein in the body, amounting to some 3–6 g/kg body weight per day.

In healthy adults, synthesis and breakdown are in balance, while during growth, there is an excess of synthesis over breakdown.

In wasting conditions (e.g. starvation, cancer or following surgery or trauma), breakdown exceeds synthesis.

Protein synthesis is regulated principally by **insulin**, while protein catabolism is mainly under the control of **glucocorticoids**, which are hormones secreted by the adrenal cortex in response to adrenocorticotrophic hormone from the anterior pituitary.

At the cellular level, DNA transcription into messenger RNA (mRNA) forms the template along which protein synthesis can occur on the ribosome.

Essential and non-essential amino acids (see Table 13.1)

• The body is unable to make nine of the amino acids used in protein synthesis, so these must be supplied by the diet or derived from the breakdown of other proteins. These are known as the *essential* or *indispensable* amino acids. Lack of any one of these will limit the synthesis of protein even if all the other required amino acids are present in adequate amounts.

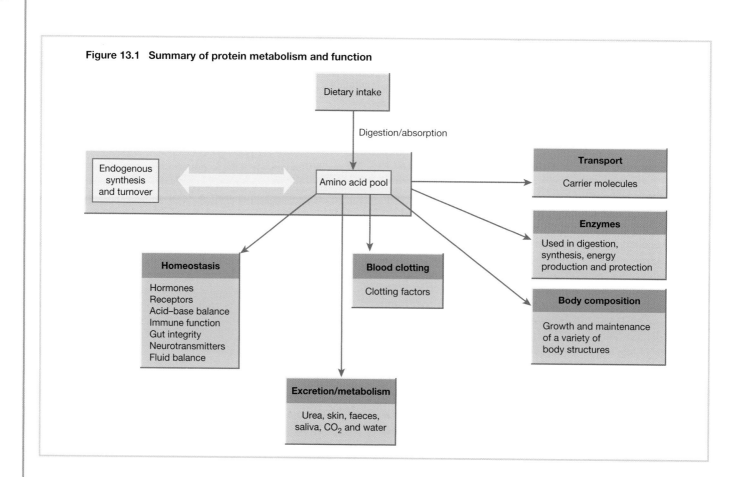

Figure 13.1 Summary of protein metabolism and function

Nutrition at a Glance, Second Edition. Edited by Sangita Sharma, Tony Sheehy and Fariba Kolahdooz.
© 2016 John Wiley & Sons, Ltd. Published 2016 by John Wiley & Sons, Ltd.

- In addition, there are a number of other amino acids that can be synthesised in the body under normal conditions as long as the necessary precursor molecules are available. For example, cysteine can be made from methionine and tyrosine from phenylalanine. However, these amino acids too become *conditionally essential* in the absence of these precursors. This is also the case in prematurity and in disease or physiological stress, where the capacity for synthesis is outstripped by the need for the amino acid.
- The remaining amino acids can be made from metabolic intermediates that are not limiting and so do not have to be supplied as such by the diet. These are referred to as the *non-essential* or *dispensable* amino acids.

Utilisation of amino acids

Protein synthesis is an energy-demanding process; it has been calculated that for every gram of protein synthesised, the energy requirement is 4.2 kJ (1 kcal). Protein synthesis occurs more rapidly after a meal than in the fasting state, due to the greater supply of amino acids available to the cells. On average, the energy used in protein synthesis accounts for about 12% of the basal metabolic rate.

In addition to protein synthesis, some amino acids are used to synthesise other important molecules such as nitric oxide, haem, creatine, glutathione, nucleotides, hormones and neurotransmitters (Table 13.2). These molecules regulate vital functions in the body and represent a substantial proportion of the daily turnover of specific amino acids.

Oxidation of amino acids

The body cannot store excess amino acids, so those that are not used either directly or indirectly (by conversion to another amino acid where possible) are oxidised. This process can be considered in two parts:

1 Removal of the amino group initially yields ammonia, which is converted to urea in the liver. Some of this is excreted via the kidneys, but the remainder is reabsorbed into the colon from the bloodstream and recycled by the bacteria to carbon dioxide and ammonia, which can be used for the synthesis of nitrogenous compounds. This cycle is termed *urea salvage*.

2 The carbon skeleton of the amino acid is ultimately converted to carbon dioxide and water, with the release of energy in the form of ATP. This occurs particularly in the liver, which obtains a major part of its fuel requirements from this oxidation. Glutamine breakdown is a major source of fuel for the gut and white blood cells. The final pathway by which the carbon skeletons of amino acids are utilised depends on their structure. The majority are metabolised to glucose and are termed *glucogenic*. *Ketogenic* amino acids (including leucine and lysine) give rise to acetoacetic acid and ultimately yield acetyl coenzyme A (acetyl CoA). Some amino acids can be both glucogenic and ketogenic, including tryptophan, methionine, cysteine, phenylalanine, tyrosine and isoleucine.

Table 13.1 Essential and non-essential amino acids.

Indispensable (essential) amino acids	Conditionally indispensable (essential) amino acids	Dispensable (non-essential) amino acids
Histidine	Arginine	Alanine
Isoleucine	Cysteine	Aspartate
Leucine	Glutamine	Asparagine
Lysine	Glycine	Glutamate
Methionine	Proline	Serine
Phenylalanine	Tyrosine	
Threonine		
Tryptophan		
Valine		

Table 13.2 Use of amino acid for synthesis of derived products.

Amino acid	Product	Function
Arginine	Nitric oxide	Leukocyte function, vascular tone, neurotransmitter
	Creatine	Energy production
Glycine	Haem	Oxygen transport
	Creatine	Energy production
Tyrosine	Hormones: thyroid, and melanin	Homeostasis
	Neurotransmitters (adrenaline, noradrenaline, and dopamine)	Neuronal integration
Tryptophan	Nicotinic acid	Vitamin function
	Serotonin (5-hydroxytryptamine)	Neurotransmitter function
Histidine	Histamine	Neurotransmitter, inflammatory response
Lysine	Carnitine	Lipid metabolism
Cysteine, glutamate and glycine	Glutathione	Antioxidant role
Methionine	Creatine	Energy production
Glutamine	Nucleotides	Cell division
	Glutathione	Antioxidant role

Summary

Proteins are essential for life, but it is the amino acids they contain that are the key to their functions. Amino acids are efficiently released from food and are utilised in the body to fulfil a broad range of functions.

14 Proteins: Needs, sources, protein quality and complementation

Aims

1 To quantify the body's need for protein
2 To identify food sources of protein and evaluate how these fulfil protein needs

The need for protein

Protein is required at all times for maintenance of the body's structure and functions. Extra protein may be required during growth, in pregnancy and for tissue repair after injury. Establishing how much protein is required by individuals is difficult, for three reasons:

• Protein deficiency, which would be used as a basis for quantifying the requirement, is a nonspecific condition that affects many processes and thus is difficult to define.
• The body is able to adapt to varying levels of protein intake, and protein metabolism is affected by levels of energy intake.
• The methods available are imprecise and rely on balance studies, which rarely include all constituents of protein flux.

Nitrogen balance

Protein metabolism in the body has traditionally been extrapolated from nitrogen intake and excretion, using the concept of 'nitrogen balance'.

Nitrogen balance is the difference between a person's intake and losses of nitrogen:

• When a person is in *positive nitrogen balance*, this implies that protein is being utilised and retained in the body, in the form of growth or major tissue repair. Nitrogen balance does not become positive simply because a person has a high protein intake, because if it is not needed, the extra protein consumed will simply be used for energy and the excess nitrogen (from amino groups) excreted as urea.
• A *negative nitrogen balance* is where losses from the body exceed intake. This is indicative of protein breakdown and may arise because of injury or a catabolic state (e.g. severe infection, major surgery, or cancer cachexia). It may also occur with low energy intakes or outright starvation, where the body is forced to use protein for energy rather than for maintenance and repair.

The use of nitrogen measurement to assess protein balance is based on the assumption that proteins contain about 16% nitrogen. Values for nitrogen flux can therefore be converted to protein flux by multiplying by 6.25 (i.e. 100/16).

Nitrogen is lost in:

• Urine (as urea, uric acid, creatinine, and ammonium compounds)
• Faeces (unabsorbed nitrogen and bacterial protein)
• Skin, hair, nails, saliva, sweat, breath and colonic gases (all of which are difficult to quantify)

Despite the inherent difficulties in measuring nitrogen loss, it has been calculated that when the diet is totally devoid of protein, the daily nitrogen losses amount to 55 mg/kg body weight. Multiplying this value by 6.25 gives us an equivalent protein loss

of 0.34 g/kg body weight, which is termed as the *obligatory loss*. When the efficiency of utilisation of protein is then taken into account, a daily maintenance requirement of 0.66 g/kg body weight is obtained.

Assessing protein quality

Dietary proteins must be converted into body proteins to fulfil an individual's physiological needs. However, proteins can differ quite dramatically from each other in their amino acid composition depending on the types of foods they come from. *Protein quality* can be defined as *the efficiency with which a protein can be utilised by the body*.

Various methods exist for evaluating the quality of different dietary proteins, including digestibility, biological value (BV), net protein utilisation (NPU) and amino acid score. None of these methods are completely satisfactory, however, and new methods continue to be developed.

Amino acid score

The fundamental determinant of protein quality is that the protein supplies amino acids in correct proportion to the body's needs. For a protein to be useful, therefore, it must provide the *essential amino acids* in the appropriate amounts (non-essential amino acids can be synthesised from other amino acids as required).

Synthesis of any new protein can only occur up to the limit of the essential amino acid that is present in the least amount relative to the body's needs. This is termed the *limiting amino acid*. Thus, for all of the essential amino acids in a protein, an 'amino acid score' can be calculated, with the lowest score indicating the limiting amino acid.

A variation of this method called the *protein digestibility–corrected amino acid score* (PDCAAS) was developed by the FAO, and this gives more accurate results as it takes protein digestibility into account.

Protein complementation

Typically, lysine is the limiting amino acid in cereals, while sulphur amino acids (methionine and cysteine) are limiting in legumes and occasionally tryptophan or threonine may be limiting in certain foods. When people consume mixed diets, however, the fact that they are eating different classes of foods at the same time helps to balance out or compensate for shortages of amino acids in certain specific food groups. For example, rice is deficient in lysine, whereas lentils are deficient in methionine. Eating the two foods together, in the form of lentil curry and rice, gives a better balance of amino acids overall than is present in either of the individual two foods themselves. This is called *protein complementation*.

Recommended intakes for protein

Recommendations for protein intake in adults among different countries are broadly similar: for example, the US RDA is 0.8 g/Kg body weight per day (National Research Council, 2005). The EU

Nutrition at a Glance, Second Edition. Edited by Sangita Sharma, Tony Sheehy and Fariba Kolahdooz.
© 2016 John Wiley & Sons, Ltd. Published 2016 by John Wiley & Sons, Ltd.

population reference intake (PRI) is slightly higher at 0.83 g/kg body weight per day (EFSA, 2012). The UK's Department of Health (1991) recommendations used the safe level of intake of 0.75 g/kg body weight to establish the reference nutrient intake (RNI) for protein. This is equivalent to about 56 g/day for an adult male and 45 g/day for a female. These values represent approximately 8–9% of total energy intake and are lower than the amounts of protein actually being consumed in the UK at the present time (~67 g/day or about 15% of the energy intake).

Protein requirements are higher in:
• Patients recovering from major disease
• Athletes in training, who may require a larger amount of protein per kilogram body weight

Excessively high protein intakes may contribute to kidney disease or bone demineralisation, but evidence for this is equivocal. Intakes at 1.5 g/kg body weight are considered to be the safe upper limit.

Dietary protein sources

Worldwide, the availability of plant proteins is relatively consistent, at about 50 g/person/day. However, the availability of animal protein sources varies widely, from <5 to ≥50 g/person/day, highest in most developed countries. The supply of protein in relation to energy is generally 10–12%, with some exceptions in countries where protein-poor staples, such as cassava and plantain, are eaten.

Deficiency of protein

Inadequate protein intakes rarely occur alone and are generally found within a wider picture of undernutrition. Insufficient caloric intake causes protein to be used for energy, making it unavailable for tissue maintenance or growth.

In *children*, protein deficiency causes stunted growth, muscle wasting, poor wound healing and increased risk of infection. Plasma albumin levels are also reduced, resulting in oedema. The classical description of this syndrome is *kwashiorkor*, although it is considered that other deficiencies (e.g. fatty acids and minerals) contribute to the overall picture (see Chapter 37).

In *hospital malnutrition syndrome*, patients may have increased needs for protein due to injury, trauma and the need for tissue repair but may be unable to consume sufficient amounts. In a process driven by cytokines, muscle protein is broken down to provide amino acids for the immune system and the synthesis of acute-phase proteins in the liver. The synthesis of normal transport proteins in the liver may be reduced. There is an overall negative nitrogen balance, which may represent protein losses of 5–70 g/day, depending on the magnitude of the trauma.

There are a number of implications of hospital malnutrition syndrome that affect the outcome for patients. These include:
• Increased risk of complications and poor wound healing
• Poor immune status and risk of infection
• Reduced muscle strength and inability to swallow and cough
• Apathy, depression and reduced quality of life
Attention to nutritional support is vital to minimise these risks.

Methods of assessing protein quality

Digestibility (expressed as N)

Protein digestibility is calculated as the proportion of N intake that is absorbed across the GIT. In equation form, % digestibility can be expressed as

$$\% \text{ Digestibility} = \frac{100 \times (\text{N intake} - \text{faecal N})}{\text{N intake}}$$

(Note: the amount excreted in faeces also includes *endogenous nitrogen* from intestinal secretions, intestinal cells and bacteria, and for accuracy, these should be taken into account. Measurements using radioactively labelled nitrogen suggest that up to 50% of faecal N may be of endogenous origin.)

• Protein digestibility from animal sources is much greater than from plant sources. Digestibility for egg is given as 97%.
• Poor digestibility, of between 60 and 80%, is found in legumes and cereals with tough cell walls, particularly when uncooked, and is a factor in diets that are low in protein.

NPU

NPU is the proportion of *consumed* N that is *retained* in the body. It can be measured in human volunteers fed specific sources of protein over test periods. In equation form, NPU is expressed as

$$\% \text{ NPU} = \frac{100 \times [\text{N intake} - (\text{faecal N} + \text{urinary N})]}{\text{N intake}}$$

(Note: for accuracy, faecal and urinary loss should be adjusted for endogenous losses.)

Individual proteins give a range of NPU values when tested separately.

Maize	36
Wheat	49
Rice	63
Soya	67
Cow's milk	81
Egg	87

In practice, however, unless these sources represent the only protein in the diet, combinations of protein sources can increase the amount of N retained due to the process of protein complementation.

BV

BV measures the proportion of *absorbed* N that is *retained* in the body. The calculation is

$$\% \text{ BV} = \frac{100 \times [\text{N intake} - (\text{faecal N} + \text{urinary N})]}{(\text{N intake} - \text{faecal N})}$$

(Again, faecal and urinary N should be adjusted for endogenous losses.)

BV is 100 for egg protein and 75 for beef and fish; values above 70 are considered to reflect protein quality sufficient to maintain growth.

15 Dietary supplements

Aims

1 To define dietary supplements and introduce different forms and types
2 To describe benefits and risks of dietary supplements

Definition of dietary supplements

Currently, there is no consensus definition of dietary supplements. The definition varies in different countries.

In Europe, the European Union Food Supplements Directive defines food supplements as 'foodstuffs the purpose of which is to supplement the normal diet and which are concentrated sources of nutrients or other substances with a nutritional or physiological effect, alone or in combination, marketed in a dose form, namely forms such as capsules, pastilles, tablets, pills and other similar forms, sachets of powder, ampoules of liquids, drop dispensing bottles, and other similar forms of liquids and powders designed to be taken in measured small unit quantities where "nutrients" means the following substances: (i) vitamins, (ii) minerals'.

In India, dietary supplements are nutraceutical products containing ingredients specified by the Food Safety and Security Act 2006.

In the USA, the Dietary Supplement Health and Education Act of 1994 defines dietary supplement as 'a product (other than tobacco) intended to supplement the diet that bears or contains one or more of the following dietary ingredients:

(a) A vitamin;
(b) A mineral;
(c) An herb or other botanical;
(d) An amino acid;
(e) A dietary substance for use by man to supplement the diet by increasing the total dietary intake; or
(f) A concentrate, metabolite, constituent, extract, or combination of any ingredient described in clause (a), (b), (c), (d), or (e)'.

Therefore, a certain product claimed to be a dietary supplement may not be one in another country. For example, green tea extract may be considered as a dietary supplement in the USA, but not in the UK.

Examining the prevalence of supplement use may be difficult as surveys may not capture seasonal and occasional users and consumers may define dietary supplements differently from information collectors.

Benefits of dietary supplements

Nutritional needs among children, the elderly, athletes and pregnant and lactating women may be higher than the general population. Also, medical conditions such as acute or chronic diseases may alter the requirement for a certain nutrient. Conscious consumption of dietary supplements by the aforementioned population may benefit their nutritional status.

Herbs have been used as medicine in some cultures and as naturopathic and homeopathic medicines. Scientific evidence supports the effects of some herbs on improving overall health and stimulating healing for certain conditions, however, such evidence is not yet available for other herbs.

Risks of using dietary supplements

Depending on dosage and frequency of consumption, dietary supplements may cause toxicity of some nutrients that may accumulate in the body, such as vitamin A. The safe range of nutrient intake may differ among subgroups depending on physiological state and environmental factors. Two intervention studies that investigated β-carotene and reduced cancer risk, the Alpha-Tocopherol, Beta-Carotene Cancer Prevention Study and the Beta-Carotene and Retinol Efficacy Trial, were closed down when supplementation of β-carotene increased the incidence of lung cancer among smokers. Several hypotheses have been proposed:
• Smokers may be more vulnerable to disruption of normal homeostasis due to excess nutrient intake than non-smokers through an unexplained mechanism.
• High β-carotene intake may inhibit absorption of other antioxidative nutrients.
• Large doses of β-carotene may cause prooxidant damage to lungs already damaged by cigarette smoking.

Dietary supplements may interact with either prescription or over-the-counter medications (increase or decrease drug activity) or trigger side effects or allergic reactions. For instance, vitamin E may interact with an anticoagulant, warfarin, and increase the risk for bleeding.

Nutrient–nutrient interactions are also possible for minerals of the same valence such as iron and zinc, which share transporters across the intestinal lumen, and some vitamins such as folic acid and vitamin B_{12}. For example, excessive iron intake may impair absorption of zinc.

Pregnant (or planning to become pregnant) and lactating women and children need to be more careful, since many dietary supplements have not been tested in these populations.

Existing medical conditions may prohibit a person from taking dietary supplements. For example, people with haemochromatosis, which is a genetic disease causing storage of excessive iron in the body, should avoid iron supplementation to prevent further increase of iron and potential complications such as liver disease.

Many dietary supplements claim to be 'natural', which does not necessarily imply 'safe' or 'stable'. Claims on the label do not always guarantee the product quality. Dietary supplements may contain compounds or ingredients that are not listed on the label, and desired dietary ingredients may be below or above the stated amount. Contamination with other herbs, pesticides, metals or unnecessary compounds also may be possible.

For safe use of dietary supplements

Prior to deciding to take any dietary supplement, it is recommended to:
- Consider that many dietary supplements are never meant to treat or prevent disease.
- Consult healthcare providers for possible interactions with medications or allergic reactions.
- Seek science-based information regarding safety and efficacy of the supplement from credible organisations.
- Read instructions and recommended dosage on the label carefully.
- Be aware of recommended dosage and duration of consumption and benefits and risks related to the dietary supplements.
- Contact the product manufacturer if further information is required.
- Be aware that products available online may not be strictly regulated.

16 Micronutrients: Fat-soluble vitamins

Aims

1 To identify the fat-soluble vitamins
2 To consider their dietary sources, biological functions and key structural features

The fat-soluble vitamins are vitamins A, D, E and K. Although we typically refer to them as if they were single compounds, they do in fact exist in more than one form, as *vitamers*.

The structures of the fat-soluble vitamins are shown in Appendix A1. Typical dietary sources are shown in Table 16.1. Biological functions are described briefly in this chapter, while their roles and interactions with other nutrients in the functioning of various systems are explained in greater detail in Chapters 20, 21, 22, 23, 24, 25 and 26.

Vitamin A

The term 'vitamin A' refers to all compounds that possess *retinol activity* and includes:

Retinol, retinal and retinoic acid
β-Carotene and other provitamin A carotenoids

a Retinol consists of a hydrocarbon chain with a *β-ionone* ring at one end and an alcohol group at the other. The usual form is *all-trans* retinol. Retinol is found in animal foods only; sources include liver, eggs, meat, milk, other dairy products, oily fish and fish oils.

b The carotenoids include:

- α- and β-carotene
- α- and β-cryptoxanthin
- Lutein, zeaxanthin, lycopene and astaxanthin

Carotenoids are responsible for the yellow, red, orange and pink colours of various fruits, vegetables and marine foods (e.g. corn, tomatoes, carrots, oranges, pumpkins, salmon and shrimp).

Although there are hundreds of carotenoids in the food supply, only a few (most notably β-carotene) have retinol activity. During digestion, β-carotene is split by a mucosal enzyme, *15,15′-dioxygenase*, yielding two molecules of retinol. Other provitamin A carotenoids are split into retinal and *apo-carotenoids*; the retinal is then converted into retinol.

Vitamin A plays an essential role in **cell differentiation** (especially in epithelia and bone cells) and therefore growth, red blood cell formation and the immune system and as part of the **visual pigment** in the retina.

Vitamin D

Vitamin D is produced on exposure of precursors (*ergosterol* in plants and *7-dehydrocholesterol* in the skin of animals, including humans) to sunlight or artificial UV-B light of approximately 290–320 nm wavelength.

Upon irradiation, these compounds are converted to:

Ergocalciferol (vitamin D_2)
Cholecalciferol (vitamin D_3)

Further metabolism (hydroxylation) in the liver and kidney is required to give the fully active forms:

- *1,25-Dihydroxyvitamin D_2*
- *1,25-Dihydroxyvitamin D_3* (calcitriol)

Table 16.1 Food sources of fat-soluble vitamins.

Vitamin	Food sources
Vitamin A	As retinol: in animal foods, including liver, meat, milk and dairy products, eggs, oily fish and fish oils
	As carotenoids: in plant foods, including green, red and orange vegetables, and orange/red fruit
Vitamin D	Synthesised in skin on exposure to UV light
	Dietary sources important when UV exposure limited: oily fish and fish oils, liver, eggs and dairy products
	Fortified products: margarine, breakfast cereals, milk-based drinks, and baby foods
Vitamin E	Vegetable oils, whole cereals and their products, green leafy vegetables, nuts and seeds
	Poultry, fish and eggs
Vitamin K	Vegetable oils and their products, green leafy vegetables, non-green leafy vegetables (e.g. spring onion and broccoli) and liver

Although synthesis in the skin is the major route of vitamin D acquisition, dietary sources become extremely important when sunlight exposure is limited, as is the case for at least half the year for populations living at higher northern and southern latitudes or when there are cultural or lifestyle factors that cause inadequate sunlight exposure. Natural food sources are quite limited and include oily fish and fish oils, liver, eggs, butter and cream. Some food products may be fortified with vitamin D, including margarine, milk, orange juice and breakfast cereals.

Vitamin D, as calcitriol, **maintains plasma calcium** by increasing calcium absorption from the gut, reducing calcium excretion via the kidneys and mobilising calcium from the bone. Calcitriol acts by binding to, and activating, nuclear receptors that modulate gene expression. More than 50 genes are regulated by calcitriol, including genes involved in calcium metabolism, insulin secretion and immune function. It also plays a role – by a non-genomic mechanism – in the regulation of **cell proliferation and differentiation**.

Vitamin E

Vitamin E consists of two families of compounds, *tocopherols* and *tocotrienols*.

There are four forms of each:

- α-, β-, γ- and δ-tocopherol
- α-, β-, γ- and δ-tocotrienol

All consist of a *chromanol* ring joined to a *phytyl* tail. The ring contains a hydroxyl (OH group) from which the H is easily removed by free radicals, giving it **antioxidant properties**. The other positions on the ring are occupied by either methyl (CH_3) groups or H. The phytyl tail of tocopherols is *saturated*, while in tocotrienols it is *unsaturated*, having three double bonds.

Tocopherols can exist in eight stereoisomeric forms. This is because the CH_3 groups that are attached at C2, C4′ and C8′ on the tail are asymmetrical. In other words, there is no corresponding CH_3 group on the opposite side. Natural α-tocopherol (e.g. found in vegetable oils, wholegrain cereals, nuts, seeds, meats, etc.) is in the *RRR* form, whereas synthetic α-tocopherol is an equal mixture of all eight possible stereoisomers. This mixture is called *all-rac-*α*-tocopherol* and only has about half the biological activity of the *RRR* form.

Vitamin E may exist as the free alcohol or in the form of esters (e.g. α-tocopheryl acetate and α-tocopheryl succinate). Esters are more stable and are used for vitamin E fortification. The free vitamin is released by *hydrolyse* enzymes in the small intestine prior to absorption.

Vitamin E is the body's **major antioxidant in lipid environments** such as cell membranes and lipoproteins. By virtue of its structure and lipid solubility, it plays a major role in maintaining the integrity, stability and function of cellular membranes.

Vitamin K

Vitamin K refers to the compound 2-methyl-1,4-naphthoquinone (menadione) and those of its derivatives that possess *anti-haemorrhagic activity*.

The vitamin K family consists of:
• *Phylloquinones* (K1 series) – These are produced by plants and contain a 20-carbon (or longer) tail, which is made up of 4 or more 5-carbon (*isoprene*) units. Phylloquinones have one double bond on the tail, situated on the proximal isoprene unit.
• *Menaquinones* (K2 series) – These are produced by bacteria. The side chain is made up of 4–13 isoprene units, and there is a double bond on each of the isoprene units.
• *Menadione* (K3) – This is the synthetic form of the vitamin. It has no anti-haemorrhagic activity until at least four isoprene units are attached to it. This series of reactions can occur in the body, so menadione can be regarded as a **provitamin**. Biologically, it is about twice as potent as the natural forms.

Vitamin K, as phylloquinone, is obtained from vegetable oils and their products, green leafy vegetables and non-leafy green vegetables. Beef liver contains menaquinone produced by rumen microorganisms, while cheese and yogurts contain small amounts of menaquinone derived from the starter cultures used in manufacture.

Vitamin K is essential for **post-translation modification** (also known as γ-*glutamylation*) of proteins involved in **blood clotting** (prothrombin, factor VII, IX and X) and **bone formation** (osteocalcin). This process involves the addition of extra COOH groups onto specific glutamic acid residues on the proteins after they have been synthesised, which has the effect of increasing their calcium binding properties.

17 Micronutrients: Water-soluble vitamins

Aims

1 To identify the water-soluble vitamins
2 To consider their dietary sources, biological functions and key structural features

The water-soluble vitamins are vitamin B_1, B_2, B_6, niacin, biotin, pantothenic acid, folate, B_{12} and vitamin C. Typically, the B vitamins act as **coenzymes** (or cofactors) for specific enzymes by donating or accepting chemical groups as part of biochemical reactions. Vitamin C has an antioxidant role in aqueous environments.

The structures of the water-soluble vitamins are shown in Appendix A2. Typical dietary sources are shown in Table 17.1. Biological functions are described briefly in this chapter, while their roles and interactions with other nutrients in the functioning of various systems are explained in greater detail in Chapters 20, 21, 22, 23, 24, 25 and 26.

Vitamin B_1 (thiamin)

Thiamin consists of a substituted *pyrimidine ring* and a *thiazole* (thio = 'sulphur containing') nucleus that are joined together by a methylene (CH_2) bridge. After absorption, thiamin is converted to its coenzyme form by the addition of two phosphate groups to form **thiamin diphosphate** (**TDP**) (or cocarboxylase). As TDP, thiamin plays an essential role in carbohydrate metabolism and nerve function.

Vitamin B_2 (riboflavin)

Riboflavin consists of the 5-carbon sugar, *ribose*, linked to an *isoalloxazine* ring. Its coenzyme forms are **flavin mononucleotide** (FMN) and **flavin adenine dinucleotide** (FAD). FMN is formed by the addition of a phosphate group onto the CH_2OH group of the ribose unit, while FAD contains an adenine unit linked to riboflavin through two phosphate groups.

Riboflavin is essential for oxidation–reduction reactions as part of the metabolism of amino acids, fats and carbohydrates. It also supports antioxidant function in the cell by acting as a coenzyme for the enzyme *glutathione reductase*.

Vitamin B_6 (pyridoxine)

The vitamin B_6 family consists of *pyridoxine*, *pyridoxal* and *pyridoxamine*, along with their phosphorylated derivatives. The most important biologically active form is **pyridoxal phosphate** (PLP).

PLP functions as a coenzyme for enzymes involved in amino acid metabolism, haem synthesis, release of glucose from glycogen (glycogenolysis) and synthesis of certain neurotransmitters.

Niacin

Niacin is the generic name for *nicotinic acid* and *nicotinamide*. Niacin can be synthesised from the amino acid tryptophan; however, the process is inefficient, and about 60 mg of tryptophan is required to synthesise 1 mg of niacin. The active forms are **nicotinamide adenine dinucleotide** (NAD+) and **nicotinamide adenine dinucleotide phosphate** (NADP+).

Like riboflavin, niacin participates in a wide variety of oxidation–reduction reactions in the metabolism of amino acids, fats and carbohydrates. It also plays a role in second messenger activity and DNA repair mechanisms.

Vitamin B_7 (biotin)

Biotin is a sulphur-containing compound that functions as a coenzyme for a small number of enzymes that catalyse **carboxylation reactions**. These enzymes are involved in gluconeogenesis, fatty acid synthesis and the breakdown of branched-chain amino acids. The biotin is attached as a prosthetic group to the enzyme at a lysine residue and can donate or accept a carboxyl (COOH) group in exchange for a hydrogen atom on its ring.

Table 17.1 Food sources of water-soluble vitamins.

Vitamin	Food sources
Thiamin (vitamin B_1)	Whole grain cereals, fortified breakfast cereals, enriched flour, beans, seeds and nuts, pork, and liver
Riboflavin (vitamin B_2)	Milk and milk products, liver, eggs, fortified breakfast cereals, cereal products containing milk or eggs, and dark-green vegetables
Pyridoxine (vitamin B_6)	Fortified breakfast cereals, wholegrain cereals, peanuts, walnuts, pulses, meat (including liver and poultry), fish, potatoes and vegetables
Niacin	Can also be synthesised from tryptophan, so obtained from protein-containing foods. Main sources are meat (including poultry and liver), legumes, cereals, milk and dairy products, seafood, vegetables and peanuts
Biotin	Widely distributed: liver, eggs, peanuts, yeast, bran, vegetables, meat, fish, cereals and milk
Pantothenic acid	Widely distributed: meat (especially organ meats), eggs, peanuts, milk, potatoes and green leafy vegetables
Folate	Green leafy vegetables, other vegetables, liver, fortified cereal products (including breakfast cereals), wholegrain cereal products, some bread, peanuts, citrus fruit and juices, and potatoes
Vitamin B_{12}	Found only in foods of animal origin: useful sources are liver, meat, eggs, milk, and fish
Vitamin C	Fruits (citrus and blackcurrants especially rich), green vegetables (also peppers, tomatoes), and potatoes (varies with season)

Nutrition at a Glance, Second Edition. Edited by Sangita Sharma, Tony Sheehy and Fariba Kolahdooz.
© 2016 John Wiley & Sons, Ltd. Published 2016 by John Wiley & Sons, Ltd.

Pantothenic acid

Pantothenic acid consists of *dimethyl, dihydroxybutyric acid* (pantoic acid) joined to the amino acid *beta-alanine*. There are two coenzyme forms: **coenzyme A** (CoA), in which pantothenic acid is linked via a phosphodiester group with adenosine diphosphate, and **acyl carrier protein** (ACP), in which it is joined to a serine residue of the protein. In its coenzyme forms, pantothenic acid plays a central role in the metabolism of proteins, fats and carbohydrates.

Folate

Folic acid consists of a *pteridine ring* joined through a methylene bridge to *para-aminobenzoic acid* (PABA) and one *glutamic acid* residue. Folic acid is a synthetic compound and is only found in fortified foods and vitamin supplements. Natural folates have several extra glutamates attached and are called **polyglutamates**. During digestion, the extra glutamates are removed by the enzyme *γ-glutamyl hydrolase* (conjugase) to yield mainly **monoglutamates**.

Within cells, folic acid is reduced to **tetrahydrofolate** (THF) through the action of *dihydrofolate reductase*. Further metabolism involves the attachment of **one-carbon units** – either methyl (CH$_3$), methylene (CH$_2$), methenyl (CH), formyl (CHO) or formimino (CHNH) groups – to N$_5$ and/or N$_{10}$ on the molecule.

These one-carbon units are required in the biosynthesis of serine, methionine, glycine, choline, purine nucleotides (adenine and cytosine) and deoxythymidine monophosphate (dTMP). Because of this, folate plays a critical role in cell division, growth and development.

Vitamin B$_{12}$ (cobalamin)

Vitamin B$_{12}$ consists of a tetrapyrrole ring structure (*corrin ring*) with a cobalt ion in the centre. The synthetic compound is called **cyanocobalamin**, while vitamin B$_{12}$ in the liver and tissues of animals occurs as **methylcobalamin** or **5′-deoxyadenosylcobalamin**.

Vitamin B$_{12}$ acts as a coenzyme for the conversion of homocysteine to methionine (a reaction that also requires folate), as well as for the breakdown of odd-chain fatty acids and the amino acids valine, isoleucine and threonine. Vitamin B$_{12}$ is critical for normal nerve myelination.

Vitamin C (ascorbic acid)

Most animals can make vitamin C from glucose, but in humans, the enzyme L-*gulonolactone oxidase*, which is responsible for the conversion of gulonolactone to ascorbic acid, is absent, so it must be obtained from the diet. The active form of vitamin C is **ascorbic acid**, and during metabolism, the oxidised form, **dehydroascorbate**, is formed.

The main function of vitamin C is as a **reducing agent**. It promotes iron absorption and is required for the hydroxylation of proline in collagen to form hydroxyproline, which is necessary for normal connective tissue formation, wound healing and bone remodelling. It also plays a role in the breakdown of tyrosine; in the synthesis of epinephrine, bile acids and steroid hormones; and in the regeneration of oxidised vitamin E.

Choline

Choline (*2-hydroxy-N,N,N-trimethylethanolamine*) is an essential nutrient that is sometimes included in the water-soluble vitamins group. It plays a structural role in cell membranes as a component of **phosphatidylcholine** and **sphingomyelin**. It is also a precursor of the neurotransmitter **acetylcholine**. Choline is required for lipid transport and metabolism and is an important methyl donor. Methylation of cytosine in CpG sites in DNA by choline can influence gene expression.

Choline can be synthesised in the body from ethanolamine using S-adenosylmethionine (SAM) as a coenzyme. However, it is mainly obtained from the breakdown of phospholipids in the diet.

Features of B vitamins

Apart from vitamin B$_{12}$, which is unique in that it is only obtained from animal foods and requires intrinsic factor for absorption, the B vitamins in general share a number of features:
- Widely distributed in both plant and animal sources.
- Cereals generally constitute the main source.
- Water soluble and readily absorbed, with the excess excreted in urine.
- Affected by cooking processes and lost into cooking water.

18 Micronutrients: Major minerals

Aims

1 To identify the major minerals required by the body and key biological functions
2 To consider their dietary sources

Minerals are *inorganic* substances required by the body in small amounts. Depending on their dietary requirements, they are classified either as **major minerals** (*macrominerals*) or **trace elements**.

The major minerals are calcium, phosphorus, magnesium, sodium, potassium, chloride and sulphur.

Calcium

Calcium is the most abundant mineral in the body, representing about 1.5–2% of body weight and accounting for almost 40% of the total mineral mass:

• More than 99% of calcium is present in the bones and teeth, mainly in the form of hydroxyapatite crystals deposited onto an organic framework of collagen and non-collagenous proteins. About 60% of the weight of the bone is due to the presence of these calcium-rich deposits, which provide strength and density to the bone.

• In addition to its structural role, calcium (as Ca^{2+}) acts as a signalling agent (or 'on–off switch') for a wide variety of physiological processes including skeletal and smooth muscle contraction, neurotransmitter function and cell proliferation and differentiation. Stimulation of cell membrane receptor proteins by nerve impulses, hormones or neurotransmitters causes a transient rise in intracellular Ca^{2+} concentrations, either by allowing calcium to enter through the cell membrane or by releasing it from intracellular stores. The increased cytosolic Ca^{2+} binds to a calcium receptor (calmodulin), which, in turn, causes various kinases to phosphorylate specific proteins, allowing them to carry out their biological function. The high intracellular Ca^{2+} concentrations are quickly brought back to normal again by the action of a membrane Ca^{2+}–Mg^{2+} ATPase pump, allowing the cycle to repeat again as necessary.

• Calcium also stabilises or activates many enzymes, including several in the blood coagulation cascade, and is needed for the release of some hormones.

Because of calcium's crucial role as an intracellular signalling agent, plasma Ca^{2+} concentrations are kept under strict hormonal regulation. Parathyroid hormone (acting through $1,25(OH)_2$ vitamin D) increases plasma calcium, whereas calcitonin (in infants and children at least) lowers it.

Major dietary sources of calcium are milk and dairy products (Table 18.1). Other sources include calcium-enriched soya milk, flour and bread (if fortified), other cereal products, green vegetables and fish with bones (e.g. canned salmon or sardines). Phytic acid in unrefined cereals and especially oxalates in some green leafy vegetables such as spinach and rhubarb reduce calcium bioavailability.

Rickets can occur with calcium deficiency although the usual cause is vitamin D deficiency. Children and adolescents need sufficient calcium so that they can achieve optimal bone mass by their early 20s. In mature and older adults, having an adequate calcium intake can slow the rate of bone loss and reduce the risk of *osteoporosis*.

Phosphorus

Phosphorus is the second most abundant mineral in the body, comprising about 1% of body weight. Approximately 85% of body phosphorus is present in the bones and teeth, as part of hydroxyapatite. The remaining 15% is distributed throughout the body, where it is found in both **organic** and **inorganic** form.

Organic phosphate is present in:

• Membrane phospholipids – phosphate group attached to the glycerol backbone.
• Phosphorylated sugars – glucose-6-phosphate, fructose-1,6-diphosphate, etc.
• High-energy compounds – ATP, ADP, creatine phosphate, etc.
• DNA and RNA – phosphate groups link the sugars along the backbone of these molecules.
• Phosphoproteins (e.g. casein in human milk and other phosphoproteins involved in intracellular signalling).
• Lipoproteins – contain phospholipids as part of their structure.

Inorganic phosphate (predominantly $H_2PO_4^-$ and HPO_4^{2-}) is important for buffering pH changes in the blood and for whole-body regulation of acid–base balance.

Hypophosphataemia and phosphorus deficiency are common in severely ill, hospitalised patients, but phosphorus deficiency is extremely rare in normal healthy individuals because of its widespread distribution in foods. Animal products are better sources of *available phosphorus* than plant sources because plants, especially cereals, contain much of their phosphorus as phytic acid (inositol hexaphosphate), which is difficult to break down due to the absence of *phytase* in the human digestive system.

The widespread use of phosphate additives in highly processed foods, such as polyphosphate water binders in processed meats and phosphoric acid in some soft drinks, may be contributing to a growing imbalance between phosphorus and calcium intakes, and there is concern about the potentially detrimental effects that a high P:Ca intake ratio could have on bone and renal health.

Magnesium

Magnesium is the second most abundant intracellular cation in the body (after potassium) and plays an essential role in many processes including energy metabolism, nucleic acid and protein synthesis, intracellular signalling, blood clotting and muscle contraction.

About 60% of the total body magnesium is present in the bone, of which roughly two-thirds is present in the hydroxyapatite crystal structure. The rest is present on the surface of the bone, where it forms a labile pool that can be exchanged with plasma.

Nutrition at a Glance, Second Edition. Edited by Sangita Sharma, Tony Sheehy and Fariba Kolahdooz.
© 2016 John Wiley & Sons, Ltd. Published 2016 by John Wiley & Sons, Ltd.

Table 18.1 Food sources of the major minerals.

Mineral	Food sources
Calcium	Milk and dairy products. Fortified soya milk, green leafy vegetables, fish with small bones, nuts and seeds. Dried fruit. Fortified flour and its products. Fortified orange juice. Hard water
Phosphorus	Meat, poultry, fish, eggs, nuts and dairy products are useful sources. Also used as an additive in bakery goods, processed meats and soft drinks
Magnesium	High levels of magnesium found in whole grains, legumes, nuts, seafood and green leafy vegetables. Moderate levels occur in fruit and dairy products. Refined and processed foods are low in magnesium
Sodium	Natural food sources, especially plant foods, contain low levels of sodium. Food preparation and processing add sodium to the diet, during cooking, as preservatives, flavouring agents and texture enhancers. Inclusion of processed foods, for example, cheese in the diet raises sodium intakes by varying amounts
Potassium	Widely distributed in food, especially of plant origin; rich sources include bananas, kiwi fruit, avocado, potato and spinach. Meat and fish are important dietary sources. Cereals and dairy products may be useful if eaten regularly. Processed foods are often low in potassium
Sulphur	Eggs and milk proteins are particularly rich in methionine (which contains sulphur). Sulphur is also present in food additives and preservatives such as magnesium sulphate, sodium sulphate, potassium sulphate and metabisulphites

Magnesium is required for more than 300 enzymatic reactions. Two mechanisms are proposed to explain its action:

1 By binding directly to an enzyme as its ionic form, Mg^{2+}, magnesium may alter the structure and activity of the enzyme or provide a catalytic function.

2 Mg^{2+} also binds to nucleotide tri- and diphosphates (e.g. ATP^{4-}, ADP^{3-}), and it has been found that all enzymes using these types of substrates (e.g. *Ca-ATPase, Na–K ATPase*) also require magnesium for product formation.

Specific magnesium-requiring enzymes include:
- Hexokinase and phosphofructokinase (glycolysis)
- Thiokinases (fatty acid oxidation)
- Pyruvate carboxylase (gluconeogenesis)
- Transketolase (hexose monophosphate shunt)
- Creatine kinase (formation of creatine phosphate)
- Adenylate and guanylate cyclase (intracellular signalling)
- DNA and RNA polymerases

Magnesium deficiency may occur in hospital patients (due to surgery, drug therapies, etc.), as well as in individuals with conditions that affect magnesium intake, absorption or retention (e.g. protein–energy malnutrition, diarrhoea, coeliac disease, Crohn's disease, ulcerative colitis, chronic renal disease, cirrhosis, and alcoholism). There are also a small number of genetic diseases that affect magnesium metabolism. Symptoms of magnesium deficiency include low serum calcium and potassium levels, altered bone metabolism and neuromuscular and cardiovascular abnormalities.

Electrolytes: Sodium, chloride and potassium

Sodium plays a critical role in maintaining normal fluid balance in the body. It is also essential for nerve impulse propagation, muscle contraction and active transport across cell membranes. About 50% of sodium is found in the extracellular fluid, where it is the major positively charged ion (cation); the rest is found in the bone (40%) and intracellular fluid (10%).

Dietary sodium is essentially fully absorbed in the small intestine, so control of body sodium occurs via excretion. More than 90% of sodium excretion takes place through the kidneys. Losses in faeces are small, except from diarrhoea, and little is lost through the skin except as a result of excessive sweating. Regulation of body sodium involves a complex interplay of intra- and extra-renal factors including enzymes, hormones and neurotransmitters.

Sodium retention is linked to elevated blood pressure. Many individuals can consume a high sodium diet without affecting blood pressure because they excrete it adequately. However, some individuals excrete sodium more slowly and are said to be salt sensitive. For these individuals, as well as people with kidney disease, a low-sodium diet is recommended.

Chloride is the major negatively charged ion (anion) in the extracellular fluid. Along with sodium, chloride affects body fluid distribution. It is also required for the production of HCl in the stomach.

Potassium is the major cation in the intracellular fluid, where it is predominantly bound to protein and phosphate. Like sodium, potassium is essential for body fluid and acid–base balance, nerve impulse propagation and muscle contraction. Numerous studies have shown that a high potassium intake lowers arterial blood pressure.

Sulphur

Sulphur is present in the amino acids methionine and cysteine and thus plays an essential role in protein structure. Disulphide (S–S) bonds between sulphur amino acids are important features of proteins that protect the body, such as skin, hair and nails. Sulphur is also involved in reactions of energy metabolism as a component of thiamin, biotin, coenzyme A, acyl carrier protein and lipoic acid.

Other functions include:
- Chondroitin sulphate – a major component of cartilage, providing much of its resistance to compression
- Glutathione – a sulphur-containing tripeptide that participates in the body's antioxidant defence system
- Sulphur (as sulphate) – participates in drug-detoxifying pathways in the liver and helps buffer changes in body pH.

Since sulphur is obtained mainly from dietary proteins, a mixed diet is unlikely to be deficient.

19 Micronutrients: Trace elements

Aims

1 To identify the trace elements required by the body
2 To consider their dietary sources and key biological functions
    The trace elements include iron, zinc, copper, iodine, selenium, manganese, fluoride and chromium (Table 19.1).

Iron

Iron in the forms in which it mostly occurs (as iron oxide complexes and metallic iron) is virtually insoluble and difficult to absorb, making it biologically limiting. In aqueous environments, iron can be found in its oxidised (ferric, Fe^{3+}) or reduced (ferrous, Fe^{2+}) state. Ferric iron is more stable, but conversion to ferrous iron is necessary for absorption as well as for its biological functions. The fact that iron switches easily between these two states is a key property of iron-containing enzymes and other proteins, including:

• *Aconitase* – this mitochondrial enzyme contains an iron–sulphur cluster and catalyses the conversion of citrate to isocitrate in the TCA cycle.
• *Haem* – haem contains an iron atom at the centre of a porphyrin ring. Haem iron is found in red blood cells (as haemoglobin) and in muscle (as myoglobin) and is essential for oxygen transport and utilisation. Haem iron is also present in peroxidases (e.g. catalase, myeloperoxidase, and lactoperoxidase), which have defence functions, and cytochromes, which are primarily responsible for the generation of ATP via the electron transport chain.
• *Metalloenzymes* – various other enzymes, including monooxygenases (involved in amino acid metabolism) and dioxygenases (needed for leukotriene synthesis), contain iron in a non-haem form.

    Iron stores are controlled almost entirely by regulating absorption. Iron absorption from food is generally low but increases when stores are depleted and when needs are greatest, as in growing children or menstruating or pregnant women.

    Forms of dietary iron, factors influencing absorption, the role of iron in red blood cells and the consequences of iron deficiency are discussed in Chapter 22.

Zinc

Zinc carries out a wide range of catalytic, structural and regulatory functions in the body. Certain enzymes (known as Zn metalloenzymes) require zinc for catalytic activity. Removal of zinc causes a reduction in activity without affecting the enzyme protein irreversibly, and reconstitution with zinc restores activity. Examples of zinc metalloenzymes include:

• *Carbonic anhydrase* – produces bicarbonate and is essential for acid–base balance and release of CO_2 in lungs
• *Alkaline phosphatase* – important for phosphorus homeostasis and bone mineralisation
• *Carboxypeptidase A* – a proteolytic enzyme produced by the pancreas, hydrolyses peptide bonds at C-terminal
• *RNA polymerases* – carry out RNA transcription from DNA

    Zinc is a structural component of *Zn finger transcription factors*. These are proteins that bind to DNA and help increase or decrease the transcription of genes into mRNA. Through the action of transcription factors, different cells in the body, which all have the same genome, can be made to express different proteins and thus perform different functions. Examples of Zn finger transcription factors include the retinoic acid and calcitriol receptors. In the antioxidant enzyme *Cu–Zn superoxide dismutase*, zinc appears to stabilise the complex structure of the enzyme.

    Zinc plays a regulatory role in immunity, signal transduction and programmed cell death (*apoptosis*).

Table 19.1 Food sources of the trace elements.

Trace element	Food sources
Iron	Found in meat, fish and eggs; liver is a very rich source. Haemoglobin and myoglobin in these provide haem iron, which is well absorbed. Non-haem iron occurs principally in foods of plant origin: cereals, legumes and vegetables. Absorption is poorer from these sources and strongly affected by other dietary components
Zinc	Found in protein-containing foods, such as meat, seafoods, eggs and dairy products. Cereals and legumes are potentially good sources, but bioavailability may be low due to the presence of phytate. Fruit and leafy vegetables are low in zinc
Copper	Main contributors in the diet are meat, meat products and cereal products. Rich sources include liver, shellfish, nuts and seeds, legumes and whole cereal grains. Bananas, potatoes, tomatoes and mushrooms are intermediate sources
Iodine	Seafoods, including seaweed, are a rich source; milk is a source from iodide compounds in the dairy industry. Bakery goods contain iodide from flour improvers. For example, salt may be iodised
Selenium	Selenium content of foods varies with the soil levels and is related to the protein content. Brazil nuts are a rich source; meat, eggs, cereals, dairy products and fish contribute selenium in the overall diet
Manganese	Manganese is obtained primarily from wholegrain cereals, legumes, nuts and tea
Fluoride	Present in water at varying concentrations. May be added in fluoridation. Also found in tea and seafoods
Chromium	Content is very variable: rich sources are spices, yeast, beef, whole grains, legumes, dried fruit and nuts. Refined foods have a low content

Many of the world's population may be at risk of zinc deficiency due to low intakes and/or low bioavailability of zinc from the diet. In general, zinc is better supplied and more efficiently absorbed from animal foods than from plants. Phytate in plant foods (especially cereals and legumes) irreversibly binds zinc in the intestinal lumen.

Groups at greatest risk include infants, children, adolescents and pregnant and lactating women. Symptoms include growth retardation, delayed sexual maturation, diarrhoea, dermatitis, impaired wound healing and depressed immune response. In developing countries, zinc supplementation trials in infants and children have shown promising results in reducing morbidity and mortality from infectious diseases.

Nutrition at a Glance, Second Edition. Edited by Sangita Sharma, Tony Sheehy and Fariba Kolahdooz.
© 2016 John Wiley & Sons, Ltd. Published 2016 by John Wiley & Sons, Ltd.

Copper

Copper is a component of many enzymes and other proteins and plays an essential role in iron metabolism, neurotransmitter synthesis, connective tissue formation, energy metabolism and antioxidant protection.

The following enzymes all contain copper:
• *Ceruloplasmin* – helps in the transfer of iron from storage sites to sites of haemoglobin synthesis
• *Dopamine-β-hydroxylase* – converts dopamine to norepinephrine in the brain
• *Cytochrome c oxidase* – reduces oxygen to water in the electron transport chain, allowing ATP production
• *Lysyl oxidase* – acts on lysine and hydroxylysine during cross-link formation in collagen and elastin
• *Superoxide dismutase* – converts superoxide anion to hydrogen peroxide as part of antioxidant defence
• *Tyrosinase* – plays a role in melanin formation, responsible for hair, skin and eye colour

Copper also appears to play a role in the immune system, blood clotting and myelin formation in the central nervous system.

Dietary sources of copper include meats (especially organ meats), shellfish, whole grains, legumes, nuts and seeds. Milk is a poor source. Absorption is regulated, and the efficiency of absorption increases when dietary copper intake is low. Copper is delivered from the liver to the tissues bound to ceruloplasmin.

> Copper deficiency is rare in humans. Reported symptoms include reduced red and white blood cell numbers (*anaemia*, *leukopenia* and *neutropenia*) and osteoporosis.
>
> A number of genetic defects in copper metabolism have been reported, including:
> • Menkes disease – this is a fatal disorder in which impaired copper release from intestinal mucosal cells leads to low levels of copper in the liver and brain, progressive nerve degeneration and death within the first few years of life.
> • Wilson disease – this disease is characterised by impaired copper efflux from tissues, leading to copper accumulation in the liver, brain and cornea. It is treated by *chelation therapy* (e.g. D-penicillamine).

Iodine

Iodine is a component of the thyroid hormones *tri-iodothyronine* (T3) and *thyroxine* (T4). These hormones play a major role in controlling the body's basal metabolic rate. T4 acts largely as a precursor to T3, which is the biologically active form. T3 interacts with nuclear receptors in target organs – particularly the liver, kidneys, muscle, heart and developing brain – to promote the synthesis of hormones, enzymes and other key proteins and thereby increase metabolic activity in tissues.

T3 and T4 are synthesised in the thyroid gland by iodination of tyrosine residues attached to a glycoprotein called *thyroglobulin*. Synthesis is regulated by the action of *thyroid-stimulating hormone* (TSH), produced by the pituitary gland in response to low circulating levels of T4. TSH causes the thyroid gland to enlarge (goitre) and stimulates all the major steps in thyroid hormone production.

> Thyroid hormone synthesis can be inhibited by **goitrogens** in certain foods (e.g. brassicas, cassava, and some varieties of millet), as well as by tobacco smoke and certain drugs.

Iodine deficiency gives rise to *hypothyroidism*. Symptoms include goitre, extreme fatigue, mental impairment, depression, weight gain and low basal body temperatures.

In pregnancy, maternal iodine deficiency increases the risk of miscarriages, other pregnancy complications, low birth weights and decreased child survival. There is also a greatly increased risk of infants being born with *cretinism* (a severe and permanent form of cognitive delay), as well as additional developmental defects such as deaf mutism, short stature and other neuromuscular abnormalities.

> **Salt iodisation** has largely eliminated the problem of iodine deficiency in developed countries. However, it remains a serious public health problem in developing countries and is the leading cause of preventable cognitive delay in children. In communities where iodine deficiency is endemic, a large proportion of the population may have some degree of intellectual impairment. This reduces people's educational potential and adversely affects economic productivity in the entire community.

Selenium

Selenium replaces sulphur in the amino acids *selenocysteine* and *selenomethionine*, which are found in certain *selenoproteins*, including:
• *Glutathione peroxidases* – these enzymes break down hydrogen peroxide and fatty acid-derived hydroperoxides as part of the antioxidant defence system. They may also play a regulatory role in metabolism.
• *Thioredoxins* – these enzymes play a role in oxidant defence, DNA synthesis and cell signalling.
• *Iodothyronine deiodinases* – remove iodine and so regulate the concentration of active thyroid hormones, T3 and T4.

Dietary sources of selenium include organ and other meats, seafood, dairy products and vegetables. Cereals can be important sources but this depends on the selenium concentration of the soil where they are grown.

> Two deficiency diseases, Keshan disease, a form of cardiomyopathy, and Kashin–Beck disease, which causes dwarfism and joint deformities in children and adolescents, have been reported in low-selenium areas of China.
>
> In animal studies, some viruses (including a strain of influenza) became more virulent on passing through selenium-deficient hosts. This suggests that selenium could be a key nutrient in counteracting viral infections in humans.
>
> Epidemiological and *in vitro* studies have suggested a role for selenium in the prevention of prostate cancer. However, evidence is conflicting, as a recent randomised, double-blind, placebo-controlled clinical trial found that selenium supplementation did not benefit men with low selenium status and increased the risk of high-grade prostate cancer among men with high selenium status.

Other trace elements: Manganese, fluoride and chromium

• Manganese is an essential cofactor for a number of metalloenzymes, including superoxide dismutase, pyruvate carboxylase, xanthine oxidase, arginase and galactosyltransferase.
• Fluoride is associated with the structure of the bones and teeth. It is incorporated into apatite, forming *fluorapatite*, which increases hardness of teeth and resistance to dental caries.
• Chromium, as a component of glucose tolerance factor, potentiates the action of insulin. It may also be involved in lipid metabolism.

20 Micronutrients: Role in metabolism

Aims

1 To identify the micronutrients involved in energy-producing metabolic pathways
2 To consider other roles of these micronutrients

Overview of metabolism

Central to metabolism is the tricarboxylic acid (TCA) cycle, as products from the breakdown of all three macronutrients ultimately enter this pathway (Figure 20.1).

Energy release in metabolic pathways occurs as a result of oxidation and involves the removal of hydrogen atoms and their transfer to hydrogen acceptor molecules. These acceptor molecules are nicotinamide adenine dinucleotide (NAD), flavin mononucleotide (FMN), flavin adenine dinucleotide (FAD) and cytochromes. The acceptor molecules form the *electron transport chain* in oxidative phosphorylation, producing ATP, and ultimately carbon dioxide and water.

The *B vitamins act as essential cofactors in metabolism* (Table 20.1). In general, they:
- Facilitate the release of energy
- Are involved in the electron transport chain
- Act as cofactors in the synthesis of metabolic derivatives

Thiamin (vitamin B_1) in its active form, thiamin diphosphate (TDP), has a central role in the TCA cycle and carbohydrate metabolism as a coenzyme for the following enzymes:

- Pyruvate dehydrogenase: this enzyme converts pyruvate to acetyl coenzyme A (CoA) at the start of the TCA cycle.
- α-Ketoglutarate dehydrogenase: catalyses the conversion of α-ketoglutarate to succinyl-CoA within the TCA cycle.
- Branched-chain keto acid dehydrogenase: completes the metabolism of the branched-chain amino acids valine, leucine and isoleucine, whose products can also enter the TCA cycle
- Transketolase: as part of the pentose phosphate pathway, this enzyme metabolises glucose and is a source of reduced nicotinamide adenine dinucleotide phosphate (NADPH) required for fatty acid synthesis and 5-carbon sugars for DNA synthesis.

Thiamin deficiency (beriberi) mainly affects the brain and nervous system, with resulting neuropathy and central neurological changes. Heart failure may occur due to raised lactate levels, formed from pyruvate. Early treatment with thiamin can be effective, except in the most severe neurological damage, when effects are likely to be permanent. Traditionally associated with rice-eating communities, the deficiency now occurs in individuals who are chronically malnourished or affected by alcoholism, drug abuse, HIV and AIDS.

Riboflavin (vitamin B_2), as part of FMN and FAD, plays an essential role in:
- Fatty acid oxidation
- Purine catabolism (with the enzyme xanthine oxidase)
- Neurotransmitter synthesis (with monoamine oxidases)

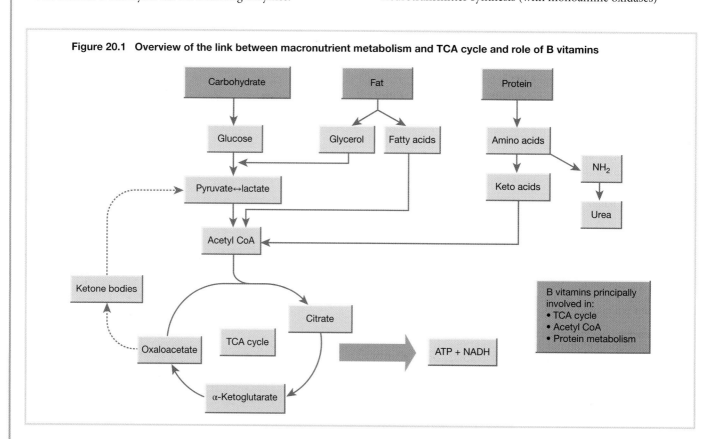

Figure 20.1 Overview of the link between macronutrient metabolism and TCA cycle and role of B vitamins

Nutrition at a Glance, Second Edition. Edited by Sangita Sharma, Tony Sheehy and Fariba Kolahdooz.
© 2016 John Wiley & Sons, Ltd. Published 2016 by John Wiley & Sons, Ltd.

Table 20.1 Principal roles of B vitamins in metabolism.

Vitamin	CHO	Fats	Proteins	Others
Thiamin	✓			
Riboflavin	✓	✓	✓	Purine catabolism
				Neurotransmitter synthesis
				Antioxidant role
				Metabolism of other minerals/vitamins
Niacin	✓	✓	✓	Steroid hormone synthesis
				Cholesterol synthesis
Vitamin B$_6$	✓		✓	Steroid hormone activity
Pantothenic acid	✓	✓	✓	Acetylcholine synthesis
				Joint structure and lubrication
Biotin	✓	✓		Gluconeogenesis, fatty acid synthesis
Folate			✓	Purine and thymidylate synthesis
				DNA methylation
Vitamin B$_{12}$		✓	✓	Amino acid metabolism, breakdown of odd-chain fatty acids, nerve myelination

- Drug metabolism (with mixed function oxidases)
- Glutathione reductase (an antioxidant role, in conjunction with selenium)

In addition, riboflavin interacts with other nutrients in the metabolism of folate, pyridoxine and vitamin A; in the conversion of tryptophan to niacin; and in the absorption of iron from the digestive tract.

Riboflavin is very efficiently recycled in the body, so that deficiency is not fatal. However, marginal deficiency appears to be relatively widespread. Requirements are increased during growth and tissue repair, and turnover is higher in catabolic states.

Pathological changes associated with riboflavin deficiency affect:
- The mouth – resulting in lesions to the lips (cheilosis), corners of the mouth (angular stomatitis) and tongue (glossitis);
- The eyes – causing conjunctivitis, photosensitivity and vascularisation of the cornea
- The skin – leading to dermatitis, especially of the nose, cheeks and forehead

Vitamin B$_6$ in its active form, pyridoxal phosphate (PLP), has many metabolic roles, including:
- Amino acid metabolism: over 100 enzymes use PLP as a coenzyme in various types of reactions including transamination, deamination, decarboxylation and transsulphuration.
- Glycogenolysis: release of glucose from glycogen stores requires PLP as a coenzyme for the enzyme glycogen phosphorylase.
- Regulation of steroid hormone activity: PLP terminates the action of steroid hormones on the nuclear receptor.

Deficiency of vitamin B$_6$ is rare and nonspecific. Signs include:
- Anaemia
- Changes to the mouth and tongue (similar to riboflavin deficiency)
- Dermatitis (as in riboflavin and niacin deficiencies)
- Muscular/neurological signs, including muscle twitching, numbness, difficulty in walking, fatigue, headache and convulsions.
   Depressed immune status, with poor lymphocyte responsiveness and depressed cytokine production, has been reported.

Niacin, as its coenzyme forms, NAD and nicotinamide adenine dinucleotide phosphate (NADP), acts as a coenzyme for more than 200 enzymes involved in the metabolism of carbohydrates, fatty acids and amino acids:
- NAD mainly acts as a hydrogen acceptor in oxidative reactions including glycolysis, β-oxidation of fatty acids, TCA cycle and oxidation of alcohol. The NADH formed can be used to produce ATP through oxidative phosphorylation and for glucose synthesis (gluconeogenesis).
- NADP is mainly used as NADPH (generated by the pentose phosphate pathway) in energy-requiring reactions such as synthesis of fatty acids, cholesterol and glutamate.

Deficiency of niacin results in *pellagra*, characterised by dermatitis, diarrhoea, dementia and (ultimately) death.
- The dermatitis occurs in areas of the skin exposed to sunlight.
- Inflammation also extends to the whole of the digestive tract, resulting in acute discomfort on eating, heartburn, indigestion, diarrhoea and rectal burning.
- The dementia resembles a psychosis.
   Niacin in cereals is often present in a bound form, which reduces bioavailability. Diets based on maize, in which tryptophan levels are also low, are characteristically associated with pellagra. Alcoholics and cancer patients may exhibit the deficiency.

Pantothenic acid is a part of CoA and acyl carrier protein (ACP) and is central to metabolism:
- CoA is involved in the TCA cycle (e.g. as acetyl-CoA, succinyl-CoA).
- Oxidation of carbohydrates and ketogenic amino acids.
- Synthesis of fatty acids (e.g. malonyl-CoA).

In addition, it is needed for the synthesis of acetylcholine, cholesterol, hyaluronic acid and chondroitin sulphate found in joints:
- ACP is involved in fatty acid synthesis as a carrier for the growing fatty acid chains.

Biotin is a cofactor for carboxylase enzymes, which carry carbon dioxide units in many metabolic pathways:
- Pyruvate carboxylase: catalyses the conversion of pyruvate to oxaloacetate during gluconeogenesis
- Acetyl-CoA carboxylase: converts acetyl-CoA to malonyl-CoA as the first step of fatty acid synthesis
- Propionyl-CoA carboxylase: catabolises isoleucine, valine, threonine, methionine and odd-chain fatty acids
- β-methylcrotonyl-CoA carboxylase: catalyses an essential step in the breakdown of leucine

Folate is required for the interconversion of certain amino acids (e.g. serine to glycine and homocysteine to methionine); however, its major roles are in the synthesis of DNA and RNA and in DNA methylation.

Vitamin B$_{12}$ is also required for the conversion of homocysteine to methionine and for the production of succinyl-CoA from methylmalonyl-CoA during the breakdown of isoleucine, valine, threonine, methionine and odd-chain fatty acids.

The metabolic roles of folate and vitamin B$_{12}$ are considered in more detail in Chapter 22.

21 Micronutrients and circulatory system I

Aims

1 To consider the micronutrients of importance in maintaining cardiac function
2 To identify the micronutrients that may affect blood pressure
3 To consider how blood clotting is affected by micronutrients

A number of micronutrients interact to maintain the heart and circulatory system, including the production of the formed elements of the blood. Figure 21.1 gives an overview.

Cardiac function

To sustain the heart in maintaining the circulation, cardiac muscle must be supplied with adequate nutrition. In addition to needing the macronutrients for its normal energy supply, the heart is especially vulnerable to deficiencies in certain micronutrients.

Thiamin is critical for the release of energy through glycolysis and the TCA cycle. Thiamin deficiency symptoms include cardiac enlargement and oedema. These symptoms are associated with impaired conversion of pyruvate to acetyl CoA, causing increased levels of pyruvate and lactate in the blood and resulting in vasodilation and increased workload for the heart. Thiamin may improve cardiac function in patients with chronic heart failure.

Selenium is a structural component of the enzyme *glutathione peroxidase* and thus has an antioxidant function. Selenium deficiency has been associated with a cardiomyopathy, first discovered in China (*Keshan disease*), which in severe cases is associated with multiple areas of necrosis throughout the heart muscle. However, this condition is rare.

Plasma **sodium**, **potassium**, **calcium** and **magnesium** concentrations must be kept within strict limits for the normal electrical activity of the heart. Abnormal levels, which can result in cardiac arrhythmias, are likely to reflect pathological processes or the effects of drug action rather than dietary inadequacies.

Blood pressure (refer to Chapter 18)

Sodium is the main cation found in the blood and extracellular fluid, where it accounts for 95% of the cations present. As such, it plays a major role in the regulation of body fluids, including blood pressure and acid–base balance.

Plasma sodium concentration depends on the balance between sodium excretion and absorption via the kidneys. This is regulated by neural and hormonal mechanisms, including the hormones renin, angiotensin and aldosterone, which regulate sodium levels, and antidiuretic hormone and atrial natriuretic peptide, which balance the water levels in response.

Changes in sodium levels can affect blood pressure, but are not in themselves necessarily the cause of high blood pressure. Nevertheless, there is considerable evidence to support the proposition that reducing sodium intakes can bring about a reduction in blood pressure.

> Sodium is mainly consumed as an ingredient of processed foods, including meat products, cereal products, cheese and snack foods. Sodium intakes from natural sources would be only about 10% of the total amount currently being consumed.

Potassium is predominantly an intracellular ion and is associated in exchange mechanisms with sodium. Increased dietary intakes of potassium have been associated with a reduction in blood pressure, as it promotes natriuresis (loss of sodium in the

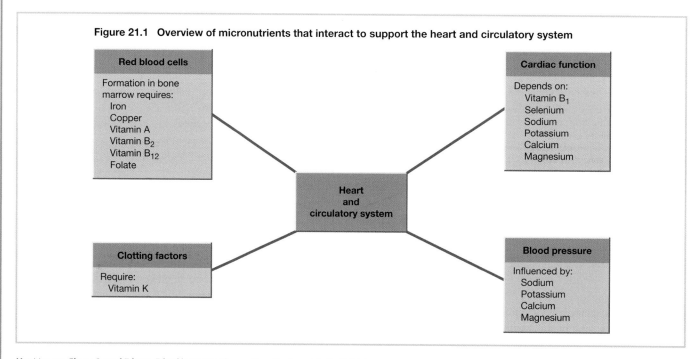

Figure 21.1 Overview of micronutrients that interact to support the heart and circulatory system

Red blood cells

Formation in bone marrow requires:
Iron
Copper
Vitamin A
Vitamin B_2
Vitamin B_{12}
Folate

Cardiac function

Depends on:
Vitamin B_1
Selenium
Sodium
Potassium
Calcium
Magnesium

Clotting factors

Require:
Vitamin K

Heart and circulatory system

Blood pressure

Influenced by:
Sodium
Potassium
Calcium
Magnesium

Nutrition at a Glance, Second Edition. Edited by Sangita Sharma, Tony Sheehy and Fariba Kolahdooz.
© 2016 John Wiley & Sons, Ltd. Published 2016 by John Wiley & Sons, Ltd.

urine). It is proposed that an increase in potassium intakes to offset some of the sodium in the diet would be beneficial for cardiovascular health.

> Potassium-rich foods are chiefly vegetables, bananas, potatoes and nuts; moderate amounts of potassium can be obtained from cereals and meat.

Calcium is also important in blood pressure regulation, and diets rich in calcium, especially from dairy products, have been found to be effective in reducing blood pressure.

Normal **magnesium** levels maintain smooth muscle tone and are implicated in control of blood pressure. Magnesium may also protect cardiac muscle from injury during ischaemia.

Food sources of magnesium include wholegrain cereals, nuts, legumes and green leafy vegetables.

Clotting factors

Four of the proteins involved in the blood clotting cascade, namely, *prothrombin* and *factors VII, IX* and *X*, require the addition of an extra carboxyl (COOH) group onto the γ-carbon of certain glutamic acid residues after the proteins themselves have been synthesised. This *post-translational modification* increases the calcium binding properties of the proteins and is essential for normal blood clotting ability. The enzyme that catalyses this step, *γ-glutamyl carboxylase*, requires **vitamin K** as an essential cofactor. Therefore, deficiency of vitamin K, or interference with its recycling, has a major impact on blood clotting and can lead to haemorrhaging.

Warfarin, which is used extensively as an anticoagulant drug in patients with deep vein thrombosis, prevents the recycling of vitamin K by blocking the enzyme *vitamin K epoxide reductase*. Thus, there is less γ-carboxyglutamate formation and therefore a reduced tendency for clots to form.

Dietary deficiency of vitamin K is rare because the vitamin is widespread in food. The richest sources are dark-green vegetables, vegetable oils and spreads (including products containing these).

Vitamin K is also synthesised by bacteria in the colon, but there are situations in which this synthesis is inhibited, such as prolonged antibiotic therapy, use of mineral oil laxatives and in fat malabsorption syndromes.

22 Micronutrients and circulatory system II

Aim

1 To identify and describe the micronutrients that are important in the formation and function of red blood cells

Red blood cells

Red blood cells (RBCs) transport oxygen from the lungs to the tissues and bring back carbon dioxide to the lungs so it can be exhaled. Oxygen transport occurs by incorporation into haemoglobin, which is a ferrous iron-containing molecule. Therefore, **iron** is critical in the function of RBCs.

Iron in the body

Approximately 60% of the body's iron content (total ~4 g) is found in haemoglobin and 15% is present in the bone marrow, where RBC production occurs. The remainder is:

• Stored as ferritin in the liver, bone marrow and spleen (ferritin is a protein containing up to 4000 atoms of iron in its interior to minimise toxic effects; plasma ferritin levels reflect the body's iron stores)
• In functional enzymes (such as cytochromes) throughout cells
• In myoglobin in muscle (myoglobin is a pigment with a high affinity for oxygen)
• In small amounts in the circulation, attached to transferrin, the iron transport protein

Iron intake and absorption

Two forms of iron occur in the diet: haem (organic) and non-haem (inorganic). Foods rich in haem iron are animal foods including meat, liver, fish and eggs, while sources of non-haem iron include cereals (e.g. fortified breakfast cereals, and bread), legumes, green vegetables, nuts and dried fruit.

The absorption of haem iron is greater than that of non-haem iron. The latter is very susceptible to factors that can act as either promoters or inhibitors, which can make up to a tenfold difference to the efficiency of absorption (Table 22.1). Advising people to enhance promoting factors and reduce inhibitors can make a substantial difference to their iron status.

Iron is potentially toxic to cells because of its pro-oxidant properties, and therefore iron absorption is tightly controlled to match the body's needs. Ingested iron that is not immediately required remains in the enterocytes and is shed at the end of their life cycle in the faeces. Conditions that result in excessive iron deposition (e.g. haemochromatosis) can cause damage to the liver, heart and endocrine glands.

There is no capacity for excretion of absorbed iron, other than by loss of blood or the shedding of cells.

Breakdown of RBCs in the reticuloendothelial system provides the endogenous source of iron. Up to 25–30 mg of iron is

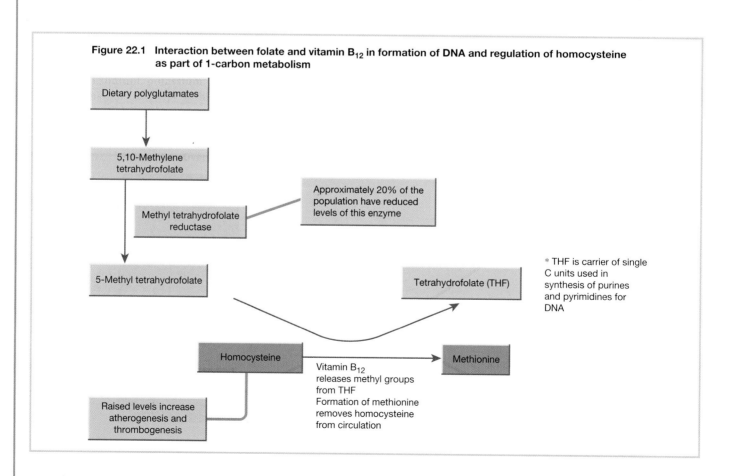

Figure 22.1 Interaction between folate and vitamin B$_{12}$ in formation of DNA and regulation of homocysteine as part of 1-carbon metabolism

Nutrition at a Glance, Second Edition. Edited by Sangita Sharma, Tony Sheehy and Fariba Kolahdooz.
© 2016 John Wiley & Sons, Ltd. Published 2016 by John Wiley & Sons, Ltd.

Table 22.1 Factors affecting absorption of non-haem iron.

Factors promoting absorption	Factors inhibiting absorption
Vitamin C	Phytate (in whole cereal grains)
Citric acid	Polyphenols (in tea, coffee and nuts)
Lactic acid	Oxalic acid (in tea, spinach)
Fructose	Phosphates (in egg yolk)
Peptides from protein sources, especially meat	Calcium
	Zinc
These enhance the solubility of iron, facilitating absorption	These either bind with iron, making it less soluble, or compete for binding sites

transported in the body per day from sites of absorption or release for either storage or utilisation.

Failure to supply sufficient iron to meet the body's needs results in a depletion, which passes through several stages:
1 Normal status: serum ferritin >15 μg/L and haemoglobin >120/135 g/L (women/men).
2 Ferritin stores depleted (<15 μg/L), but sufficient iron recycled to maintain normal RBC production.
3 Depletion of functional iron: transferrin saturation begins to fall (critical value <16%), as less iron is transported.
4 Haemoglobin concentration falls <120/135 g/L (women/men), and microcytic (<80 fL), hypochromic RBCs are produced, typical of iron deficiency anaemia (IDA).

IDA is the most common nutritional deficiency in the world, with a range of pathological consequences, including changes to the digestive tract, loss of appetite, reduced work capacity and eventually heart failure.

IDA can also affect the function of white blood cells, reducing their ability to destroy invading organisms.

Addressing IDA involves a number of measures, including:
- Fortification of widely consumed foods
- Home fortification of semi-liquid foods using Sprinkles
- Use of supplements
- Education to improve dietary practices to enhance the bioavailability of iron consumed
- Introduction of greater diversity of iron sources into the diet

Other nutrients affecting RBCs

Copper is also found in RBCs and is present in the plasma in the enzyme *caeruloplasmin*. This enzyme converts ferrous (Fe^{2+}) iron to the ferric (Fe^{3+}) form, which binds to transferrin for transport to sites of either synthesis or storage. Copper deficiency can result in hypochromic anaemia. Dietary copper deficiency is rare in humans, although there is a rare congenital condition, Menkes disease, which affects copper absorption.

Vitamin A facilitates the use of storage iron for haemopoiesis (blood cell formation), and IDA can be a consequence of vitamin A deficiency; both vitamin A deficiency and IDA are important causes of perinatal morbidity and mortality.

Folate and vitamin B$_{12}$ are essential for the formation of purines and pyrimidines for the synthesis of DNA and RNA and as such are crucial for cell division, including the formation of red and white blood cells:

- Folate (as tetrahydrofolate, THF) carries 1-carbon units that are used in this biosynthesis.
- Vitamin B$_{12}$ is required to release the methyl (CH_3) group from 5-methyltetrahydrofolate and regenerate THF to enable it to receive further 1-carbon units. This dependence of folate metabolism on vitamin B$_{12}$ is termed the 'methyl folate trap'. Without B$_{12}$, the methylation of DNA may become inadequate to sustain gene transcription.
- The methyl group removed during this reaction is used in the formation of methionine from homocysteine and helps to lower plasma homocysteine levels (see Figure 22.1). Elevated homocysteine may be a contributory factor in atherosclerosis.
- Both folate and B$_{12}$ deficiencies result in an inability of developing cells to increase their DNA prior to division. Under these circumstances, newly synthesised RBCs are large (megaloblastic), have a reduced density and are fewer in number. This results in reduced oxygen-carrying capacity of the blood and an anaemia that in the case of B$_{12}$ deficiency prior to the discovery of effective treatment was invariably fatal, hence the term 'pernicious anaemia'.

Folate deficiency may arise due to inadequate intake, increased needs (e.g. in pregnancy), malabsorption syndromes (e.g. in alcoholics) or interference in metabolism by drugs. Folate deficiency in pregnancy must be treated with supplements to avoid anaemia affecting the fetus. The role of periconceptional folic acid supplementation in the prevention of neural tube defects is considered in Chapter 45.

Dietary sources of folate include green leafy vegetables, other vegetables, fortified cereals, citrus fruits and fruit juices. Cooking losses can be high, especially if foods are kept hot or reheated.

Vitamin B$_{12}$ deficiency is most commonly due to a failure of absorption consequent on a lack of intrinsic factor. An autoimmune reaction destroys the gastric cells that produce intrinsic factor, or an antibody prevents the B$_{12}$ from binding with the intrinsic factor because of an autoimmune disease, causing pernicious anaemia. Older people, as well as having lower intrinsic factor production, may also have a reduced ability to release free vitamin B$_{12}$ from food proteins due to gastric atrophy. A dietary lack of vitamin B$_{12}$ can occur in individuals, such as vegans, who consume no animal products in their diet, as these are the only dietary sources of the vitamin.

In addition to megaloblastic anaemia, neurological complications (including short-term memory loss, chronic fatigue, depression, paraesthesia and irreversible paralysis) are also associated with vitamin B$_{12}$ deficiency, resulting from a progressive demyelination of nerve cells. High intakes of folic acid can 'mask' the diagnosis of vitamin B$_{12}$ deficiency because the anaemia responds to folic acid. This could allow the accompanying nerve demyelination to continue until it becomes irreversible.

Riboflavin is a coenzyme for the enzyme *5,10-methylenetetrahydrofolate reductase*, which produces 5-methyltetrahydrofolate as part of the 1-carbon metabolic pathways. Riboflavin deficiency may also impair iron absorption, resulting in hypochromic anaemia.

Pyridoxine (vitamin B$_6$) is required for the incorporation of iron into haem and thus has a role in RBC formation. The enzyme *cystathionine-β-synthase*, which breaks down homocysteine, also has a requirement for vitamin B$_6$ as a coenzyme.

Overall, the nutrients involved in maintaining the blood and circulatory system can be obtained from a varied diet.

23 Micronutrients: Protective and defence roles I

Aim

1 To identify the nutrients involved in sustaining the functions of the immune system

Physiological systems are continually being challenged by changes in the *internal* environment from metabolic or defence reactions, as well as by *external* factors, such as microorganisms or chemical substances that enter the body.

Various defence mechanisms exist to maintain homeostasis, the majority of which depend on micronutrients for their operation (Figure 23.1). Inadequate levels of certain micronutrients can compromise this protection and increase the risk of disease. Conversely, adequate or enhanced levels may be actively protective.

Immune system defences

The immune system plays a crucial role in protecting the body against the dangers posed by infection, inflammation and trauma. To function optimally, the cells of the immune system require an appropriate nutrient supply:

• Formation of the cellular components of the immune system requires normal cell division to be sustained.
• Macronutrients are needed to provide energy for the metabolic activity of the cells, and many micronutrients are needed to release this energy (see Chapter 20).
• When the immune system is responding to a challenge, energy requirements are increased.
• The immune defence system includes a number of proteins (e.g. *immunoglobulins*, *cytokines*, and *acute-phase proteins*) and lipid-derived substances (such as *prostaglandins*), which are synthesised from the appropriate amino acid and lipid precursors.
• Invading organisms are killed by an oxidative burst, which uses *superoxide radicals* and can result in oxidative damage to the host cells. Appropriate antioxidant mechanisms must be in place as protection against this.

Nutritional inadequacy compromises the immune system and its ability to respond to a challenge. This can be seen in malnourished individuals, especially children, who are exceptionally vulnerable to infections and are unable to recover swiftly from them. The condition is aggravated by a loss of appetite, possible malabsorption, increased loss of nutrients and higher requirements.

Specific micronutrients play particular roles in the immune system (Table 23.1). It should not, however, be assumed that high levels of these nutrients are necessarily ideal, as in some cases they may have a detrimental effect.

Vitamin A is important for:
• Integrity of epidermal and mucosal surfaces and thus the physical barrier against the environment
• Activation of macrophages and differentiation of monocytes in the immune response

Deficiency is associated with increased incidence and severity of infectious diseases, especially respiratory and diarrhoeal diseases and measles. Supplementation with vitamin A significantly reduces mortality from infection. However, very high doses of vitamin A can depress immune function. In many developing countries, vitamin A intake is low, and single large doses of the vitamin can be given as a supplement to help reduce maternal mortality and protect children from infection.

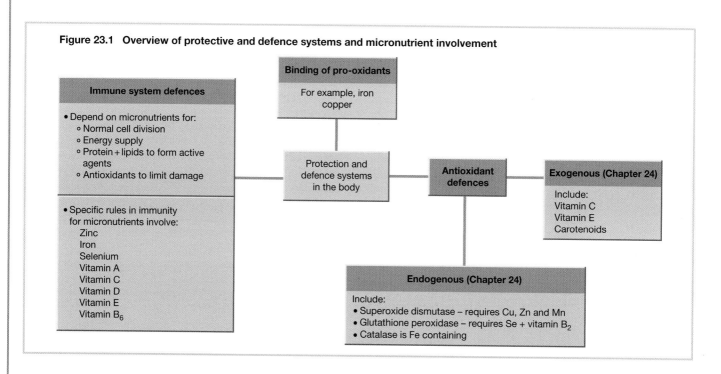

Figure 23.1 Overview of protective and defence systems and micronutrient involvement

Table 23.1 Summary of principal micronutrients involved in the maintenance of the immune system.

Nutrient	Role in immune system	Evidence of importance
Vitamin A	Maintains epithelial surface; physical barrier Activates macrophages	Deficiency associated with increased incidence and severity of infectious disease
Vitamin B$_6$	DNA and RNA formation for lymphocytes and cytokine production	Impaired immune response in older subjects, reversed on supplementation
Vitamin C	Concentrated in white blood cells. As an antioxidant, it protects against free radical damage of phagocytosis	May reduce severity of cold symptoms
Vitamin D	Present in immune cells, may be immunosuppressive	
Vitamin E	Enhances humoral and cellular immunity	Supplementation improves immune responses in older adults
Zinc	Development of T-lymphocytes Activity of immune cells	Effectively used in treatment for diarrhoea associated with poor nutrition
Iron	Low status inhibits phagocytic activity Improved status may encourage pathogen growth	
Selenium	Deficiency associated with reduced ability to kill pathogens	

Vitamin B$_6$ is used in the synthesis of nucleic acids for DNA and RNA formation. Impairment of this process affects lymphocyte proliferation and cytokine production and hence impacts on immune function in deficiency states. Supplementation reverses this impairment.

Folate and **vitamin B$_{12}$** are also involved in the synthesis of DNA and RNA. However, their effects on the function of the immune system are less obvious than might be expected.

Vitamin C concentration in leucocytes is high, and decreases during the course of an infection, due to dilution by newly released cells with lower vitamin content. Neutrophils contain high levels of vitamin C to protect against the *oxidative burst*. However, excessively high intakes of vitamin C (>600 mg/day) can inhibit the formation of superoxide and reduce the effectiveness of neutrophils.

> The balance of evidence in relation to vitamin C giving protection against the common cold points to a reduced severity of symptoms, but no reduction in the risk of infection.

There are receptors for **vitamin D** in most immune cells, implying a regulatory role. Most evidence suggests an immunosuppressant role, although further work is needed.

Supplementation with **vitamin E** enhances both humoral and cellular immunity, possibly by reducing the potential immunosuppressive effects of free radicals and lipid peroxides. However, doses above 800 mg/day may be counterproductive.

Zinc is important for the development of many of the cellular components of the immune system, especially the T-lymphocytes, and the activity of the cells. This includes chemotaxis, phagocytic activity and the oxidative burst. There is a fall in plasma zinc levels on infection, which may deprive the pathogens of essential zinc, and is an important protective response against potential prooxidant effects. Zinc is taken up at this time by the liver and lymphocytes.

> Zinc in the diet tends to accompany protein, so low-protein diets are likely to be low in zinc. Good sources are lean meat, seafoods and dairy products. Pulses and wholegrain cereals are important for non-meat eaters. Absorption of zinc is affected by promoters (animal products, and amino acids) and inhibitors (binding to insoluble salts, such as phytate, phosphate and the presence of large amounts of iron or calcium in the diet).

Zinc supplementation at an appropriate dose has been found to be an effective treatment in diarrhoea associated with poor nutrition, especially in children.

Decreased lymphocyte numbers are also a feature of **copper** deficiency, which is reversible on repletion. Excess amounts of copper have an immunosuppressive effect.

The role of **iron** in the immune system is complex. Low iron status impairs the ability of neutrophils to kill pathogens and proliferation of lymphocytes.

Treatment of iron-deficient individuals is frequently associated with an exacerbation of infection, possibly due to enhancement of the growth of the pathogen by the additional iron.

Selenium deficiency is associated with reduced immunocompetence, in particular the ability of cells to kill pathogens. Animal studies have demonstrated that in tissues that are experiencing oxidative stress, due to impaired antioxidant status, viruses may mutate to more virulent forms. This has been proposed in selenium deficiency but may be exacerbated by concurrent vitamin E deficiency and excess intakes of polyunsaturated fats.

Summary

Having an adequate level of a range of micronutrients is important to support normal immune function. The question of supplementation with micronutrients remains unresolved, as high levels of some may be counterproductive, suppressing immune function. In addition, an imbalance may increase the requirements for other components. A balanced diet, following healthy eating guidelines, is the better alternative. It also provides phytochemicals, which may have important, as yet unrecognised, roles.

24 Micronutrients: Protective and defence roles II

Aims

1 To explain the potential risks from free radicals in the body
2 To consider the role of micronutrients in antioxidant defence systems

Free radicals

A free radical is any species capable of independent existence that contains one or more unpaired electrons. An unpaired electron is one that occupies an atomic or molecular orbital by itself. Examples

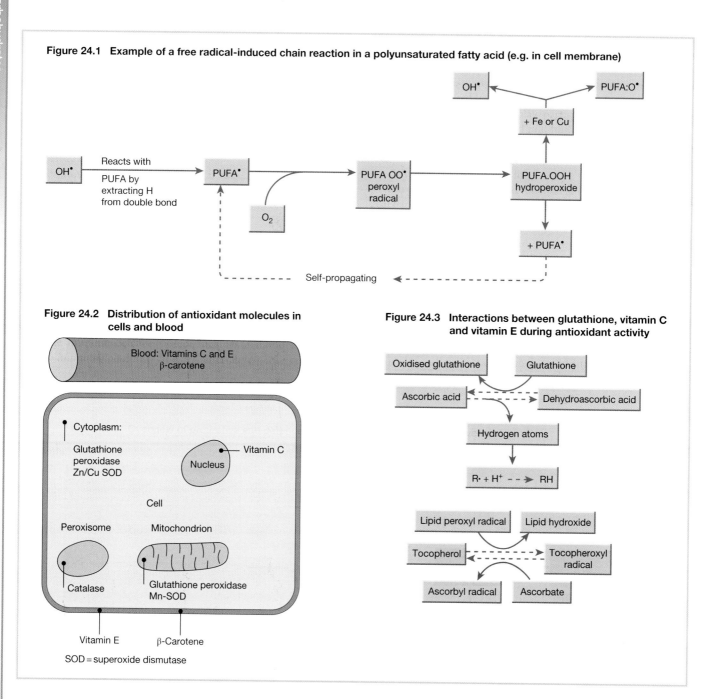

Figure 24.1 Example of a free radical-induced chain reaction in a polyunsaturated fatty acid (e.g. in cell membrane)

Figure 24.2 Distribution of antioxidant molecules in cells and blood

SOD = superoxide dismutase

Figure 24.3 Interactions between glutathione, vitamin C and vitamin E during antioxidant activity

Nutrition at a Glance, Second Edition. Edited by Sangita Sharma, Tony Sheehy and Fariba Kolahdooz.
© 2016 John Wiley & Sons, Ltd. Published 2016 by John Wiley & Sons, Ltd.

include the hydrogen radical (H·), hydroxyl radical (OH·), superoxide radical (O_2^-) and nitric oxide (NO·).

Generation of free radicals

Free radicals can be formed by the loss or gain of a single electron from a non-radical compound. They can also be formed when a covalent bond is broken, if one electron from the shared pair remains with each atom. Free radicals are generated continuously in the body by several processes:
• Metabolic processes in the electron transport chain, catalysed by metal ions (such as copper and iron).
• Defence mechanisms of the inflammatory process; white cells generate free radicals to kill ingested bacteria in phagocytosis or secrete free radicals into the surrounding tissues to destroy damaged tissue. Areas of ischaemic or damaged tissue may contain high levels of free radicals.
• Dissociation of oxygen from haemoglobin.
• Exposure to cigarette smoke, sunlight, certain chemicals and high oxygen tension (e.g. incubators).

Stabilisation of free radicals

The presence of unpaired electrons makes free radicals unstable, and some, in particular the hydroxyl radical, are highly reactive. Free radicals can be stabilised in a number of ways. They can:
• Join together with another free radical
• Remove an electron from a non-radical, leaving that molecule with an unpaired electron and turning it into a free radical
• Donate an electron to a non-radical, creating a recipient that is a free radical
• Remove a hydrogen atom from a C–H bond, leaving the C with an unpaired electron (these commonly react with oxygen to form a peroxyl radical, as happens in lipid peroxidation; see Figure 24.1)

Most of the above events initiate a chain reaction, which can be damaging to the cell unless prevented or terminated. Damage can occur to a variety of targets, including DNA, cellular and subcellular membranes, enzymes and lipoproteins.

Contributory factors

Iron and copper are potential catalysts for free radical formation and are therefore found in the body in a *bound state*, generally attached to proteins, to limit their availability. Trauma and inflammatory states cause a reduction in binding, releasing free ions and forming free radicals. However, plasma iron binding capacity increases at this time, to minimise the consequences.

Defence mechanisms

There are many antioxidants present in various compartments within the body that fulfil a protective role. Their distribution is shown in Figure 24.2. In general, an antioxidant is any substance that significantly delays or prevents the oxidation of a target substrate, usually by becoming oxidised itself.

Endogenous antioxidants include a number of enzymes, which require minerals for their action. These include:
• **Superoxide dismutase**, which requires *zinc, copper* and *manganese* for activation (depending on the location) and converts the superoxide radical to hydrogen peroxide and oxygen.
• **Glutathione peroxidase**, which is a *selenium-* and *glutathione-* requiring enzyme and reduces peroxides to water. The reduced glutathione needed for this reaction is generated by the enzyme *glutathione reductase* in a reaction requiring NADPH and FAD.
• **Catalase**, which removes hydrogen peroxide and is a haem-containing protein, therefore requiring *iron*.

In addition, there are *exogenously* derived antioxidants, of which vitamin C, vitamin E and the carotenoids are the most important.

Vitamin C is present in the *aqueous environment* of the cell and plasma and is an effective scavenger of a wide range of free radicals. It donates an electron to the free radical, deactivating it, and itself becomes an ascorbyl radical. This is regenerated back to ascorbate, using glutathione, without causing oxidative damage itself.

Particularly high concentrations of vitamin C are found in white blood cells, the eye and in lung tissue, where its antioxidant effects are critical against high levels of free radicals, oxygen and pollutants, respectively.

Vitamin C is mainly obtained in the diet from plant foods, with rich sources among both fruits (citrus fruits, berries, and summer fruits) and vegetables (peppers, broccoli, cauliflower, and tomatoes). If potatoes are eaten regularly, they can provide a consistent intake. While cooking losses can be high, consuming at least five servings of fruits and vegetables per day (400 g) is an effective way of achieving adequate vitamin C status, especially if some are eaten raw.

Vitamin E is the major antioxidant found in the *lipid environment*, especially in the lipid bilayers of biological membranes. Particularly large concentrations occur in organs exposed to highly oxygenated blood, such as the lungs and heart:
• The vitamin (as α-tocopherol) is able to donate hydrogen from its chromanol ring to a lipid peroxyl radical, producing a lipid hydroperoxide and a tocopheroxyl radical.
• The tocopheroxyl radical has low reactivity, thus breaking the chain reaction of lipid oxidation. It can be regenerated to α-tocopherol by ubiquinone, vitamin C or glutathione (which also requires glutathione peroxidase and therefore selenium; Figure 24.3).

Signs of vitamin E deficiency include neurological and muscular damage and may be attributable to the effects of free radicals on membranes.

Vitamin E is supplied by vegetable oils and from wholegrain cereals, which contain the vitamin in the germ of the grain.
Green leafy vegetables, some fruits and nuts also supply vitamin E. Manufactured foods, such as potato or cereal products, may provide some vitamin E, due to the fat used in the recipe. Animal foods are not important sources of vitamin E, although eggs, fish and poultry may contain small amounts.

Carotenoids have been shown to quench singlet oxygen (a more reactive form of oxygen than ground state oxygen, though not a free radical) by absorbing the excitation energy. The major carotenoid normally considered in this respect is β-carotene. However, there are many other carotenoids with antioxidant properties, including lycopene and lutein.

Carotenoids are found in plant foods as red or yellow pigments. Rich sources include carrots, dark-green leafy vegetables, broccoli, red peppers, tomatoes, apricots, peaches and mangoes.

25 Micronutrients: Structural role in bone I

Aims

1 To study the factors involved in the formation of bone
2 To identify the role of calcium in the formation and maintenance of the skeleton

The human skeleton

The skeleton serves several key roles:
- Provides the framework to which is attached the musculature of the body
- Provides protection for the more delicate organs, such as the brain and organs of the chest
- Acts as a reservoir for some minerals and is important in acid–base regulation
- Is a site of blood cell synthesis

Composition of bone

Bone can be classified as cortical (compact) or trabecular (spongy), with corresponding structural and metabolic characteristics (Table 25.1). Bones comprise an extracellular organic matrix made up of proteins (predominantly *collagen*), on which inorganic substances are deposited:
- The **proteins** play important roles in regulating the mineralisation of bone and include *alkaline phosphatase*, which is **zinc** containing, and *γ-carboxylated proteins*, which are dependent on **vitamin K**.
- The major mineral constituents of bone are **calcium** and **phosphate**, combined as *hydroxyapatite*, laid down around collagen fibres to form a rigid structure.
- Other minerals such as **magnesium**, **fluoride** or **strontium** may occasionally replace calcium in the crystalline structure, changing the size of the crystals and affecting strength and solubility.

Table 25.1 The main types of bone found in the human body.

Type of bone	Amount and main locations	Main characteristics
Cortical (or compact)	80–85% of total bone; in long bones	Very dense, slowly metabolised
Trabecular (or spongy)	15–20% of total bone; in vertebrae, flat bones and ends of long bones	More readily metabolised and therefore more susceptible to fracture Forms a mesh of calcified trabeculae (a scaffold), blood cells formed within the spaces, which are filled with marrow

Nutrient involvement in bone health

See Figure 25.1 for an overview.

Calcium

Calcium is the most prevalent mineral, with approximately 1 kg being present in the bones of an adult. Bones act as a source of ionised calcium for nerve and muscle function and for blood clotting. Plasma calcium levels are maintained within narrow limits by an efficient feedback control system.

The body's requirement for calcium varies with the rate of bone development, rather than metabolic needs. The daily need is at its highest during the peak growth spurt of adolescence, reaching 1300 mg/day. Therefore, calcium intakes are especially critical at this time, to ensure adequate mineralisation of the bone.

Calcium absorption is influenced by a number of promoting and inhibitory factors. Factors that promote calcium absorption

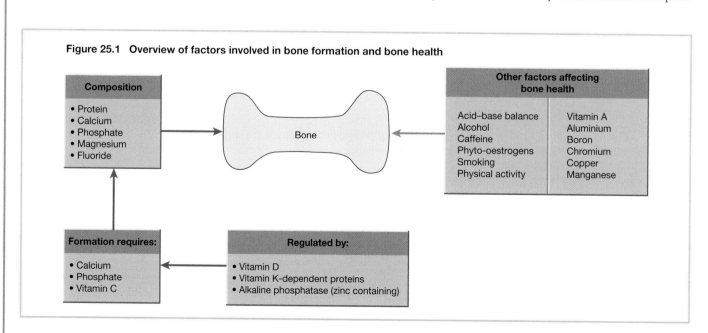

Figure 25.1 Overview of factors involved in bone formation and bone health

Composition
- Protein
- Calcium
- Phosphate
- Magnesium
- Fluoride

Bone

Other factors affecting bone health

Acid–base balance	Vitamin A
Alcohol	Aluminium
Caffeine	Boron
Phyto-oestrogens	Chromium
Smoking	Copper
Physical activity	Manganese

Formation requires:
- Calcium
- Phosphate
- Vitamin C

Regulated by:
- Vitamin D
- Vitamin K-dependent proteins
- Alkaline phosphatase (zinc containing)

Nutrition at a Glance, Second Edition. Edited by Sangita Sharma, Tony Sheehy and Fariba Kolahdooz.
© 2016 John Wiley & Sons, Ltd. Published 2016 by John Wiley & Sons, Ltd.

include vitamin D, lactose, dietary protein, non-digestible oligo-saccharides and acidic conditions in the jejunum. Factors that inhibit calcium absorption include phytate (e.g. in wholegrain cereals, and chapattis), oxalate (e.g. from spinach, beetroot, and chocolate), use of antacids, unabsorbed dietary fats, excessive intakes of dietary fibre and large intakes of phosphoric acid (e.g. in carbonated drinks).

Unabsorbed calcium, together with calcium secreted into the digestive tract, is lost in the faeces. This calcium can bind to fats in the digestive tract, forming soaps, and reduce fat absorption. Equally, fat malabsorption can remove calcium from the large intestine.

Calcium balance can be achieved at a variety of levels of calcium intake, which demonstrates that calcium absorption is well controlled to match the needs of the body. Even at low intakes, calcium balance remains neutral. Only in the adolescent, where needs are increased, is there a positive balance; this is achieved by increasing the efficiency of absorption and reducing urinary loss.

Calcium balance is regulated by activity at:
- The gut (absorption)
- The kidney (excretion)
- The bone (mobilisation and deposition)

These sites are controlled by feedback mechanisms involving the interaction of several calcium-regulating hormones (parathyroid hormone, calcitonin and the active form of vitamin D, 1,25-dihydroxycholecalciferol). Serum calcium levels only become abnormal if there is a failure of this homeostatic mechanism and not as a result of changes in dietary calcium intakes.

Bone formation, resorption and remodelling

- **Bone formation** is carried out by *osteoblasts*. It continues throughout life but takes place predominantly until the late teens and then at a reduced rate up to the age of 25–30.
- **Bone resorption** is carried out by *osteoclasts*. It continues throughout life, increasing after the age of 30 and accelerating in the 10–15-year period after the menopause in women. In men, bone loss continues gradually into old age. This loss of bone mass results in osteoporosis. When the loss of bone mass reaches a critical point, the bone may fracture on stress or impact.
- **Osteocytes** are the most numerous cells, embedded throughout the bone. They play a role in regulating bone metabolism, for growth, repair and supplying calcium to plasma.
- Variations in the remodelling process can result in changes to bone density and mass. The process of remodelling is under hormonal control by parathyroid hormone, calcitonin and active vitamin D. Growth hormone, glucocorticoids and oestrogen are also involved.

Main sources of calcium in Western diets

- Milk and dairy products (alternative sources for vegetarians include tofu set with calcium and calcium-enriched soya milk).
- Cereals and cereal products (may be fortified with calcium).
- Green leafy vegetables.
- Small fish (eaten with their bones).
- Some seeds and nuts are additional sources, but their importance depends on the amounts eaten, as levels are lower than in dairy products.
- Hard water may provide an important source of calcium in some geographical locations.

26 Micronutrients: Structural role in bone II

Aim

1 To identify the role of other micronutrients in the formation and maintenance of the skeleton and their interaction with calcium

Concerns about the increasing prevalence of osteoporosis have focused attention on the role of nutritional and non-nutritional factors in bone health.

Vitamin D

Vitamin D is essential in the regulation of calcium balance, and a deficiency will result in inadequate bone mineralisation, as seen in rickets (in children) and osteomalacia (in adults). Although the amounts of structural proteins (i.e. the collagen matrix) are normal in these deficiency states, the bone is softer, particularly at the growth points, and is susceptible to deformation. This results in the characteristic bow legs or knock-knees and deformed spine seen in children with rickets and causes back and joint pain in adults, with difficulty in walking.

Metabolic role

The active form of vitamin D is 1,25-dihydroxycholecalciferol (calcitriol), which is produced in two stages by the addition of hydroxyl groups.

The first stage occurs in the liver, yielding 25-hydroxycholecalciferol, which is the form commonly measured in the blood.

The second stage of activation occurs in the kidney. This step is regulated by parathyroid hormone secreted in response to falling plasma calcium levels.

Overall, the effect of active vitamin D is to raise plasma calcium levels by:
- Increasing absorption of calcium at the gut by promoting the synthesis of a calcium-binding protein (calbindin-D)
- Increasing reabsorption of calcium at the kidneys
- Modulating the mobilisation and deposition of calcium and phosphorus in the bones

A summary of the main interactions between vitamin D and calcium balance is shown in Figure 26.1.

Sources of vitamin D

Vitamin D is supplied in a number of foods, including dairy products (levels may be lower in low-fat versions, unless fortified), spreading fats, oily fish, liver, meat and eggs and fortified breakfast cereals. However, dietary vitamin D intake in general tends to be low, so for most people, the major source is by synthesis in the skin from 7-dehydrocholesterol on exposure to ultraviolet light (290–320 nm wavelength). At high northern and southern latitudes, sunlight of this wavelength reaches the earth only during the summer months.

Populations living in arctic or subarctic regions are especially at risk of vitamin D insufficiency because of limited solar ultraviolet (UVB) exposure (e.g. as a result of protective clothing, high geographic latitude, or insufficient time spent outdoors). Some countries (e.g. Finland) have adopted mandatory vitamin D fortification policies to help reduce this risk.

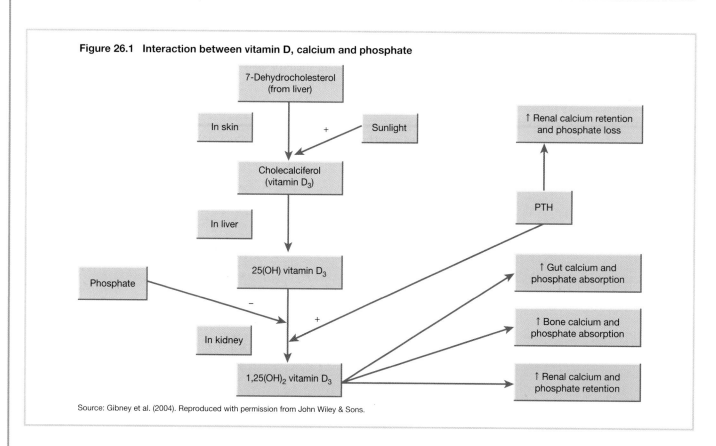

Figure 26.1 Interaction between vitamin D, calcium and phosphate

Source: Gibney et al. (2004). Reproduced with permission from John Wiley & Sons.

Nutrition at a Glance, Second Edition. Edited by Sangita Sharma, Tony Sheehy and Fariba Kolahdooz.
© 2016 John Wiley & Sons, Ltd. Published 2016 by John Wiley & Sons, Ltd.

Even at lower latitudes, ensuring an adequate dietary intake of vitamin D is important for infants and young children, as well as for people with dark skin pigmentation, for those individuals who do not spend time out of doors (e.g. housebound elderly and night shift workers) and for those who, for cultural or religious reasons, cover all their bodies.

As well as inadequate dietary intake or skin synthesis, low vitamin D status may also be brought about by fat malabsorption, by excessive excretion (e.g. due to alcohol or anticonvulsant drugs) or by conditions that interfere with the activation of the vitamin (e.g. liver, kidney or parathyroid gland disease).

Phosphorus

Phosphorus is present as phosphate and is the second major mineral in the bone. In addition, phosphate is widely distributed throughout the tissues in biologically vital compounds such as ATP, creatine phosphate, phospholipids and nucleic acids.

Regulation of plasma phosphate is mainly by renal excretion, which balances with dietary intake and is also influenced by parathyroid hormone and therefore calcium levels. The two minerals are closely associated to maintain a constant ratio.

Depletion of serum phosphate can result in poor mineralisation, but this is most likely to happen in disease states or starvation.

Other minerals and vitamins

Magnesium

Magnesium is involved in the formation of bone crystals and in parathyroid hormone (PTH) function, but there is little evidence that changes within normal limits in magnesium intake have a major effect on bone health.

Potassium

Potassium has been proposed as an important factor in bone health and linked to a higher bone mineral density and thus a lower fracture risk. Fruits and vegetables provide a major source of potassium in the diet, and it has been postulated that the *alkaline residues* from fruits and vegetables minimise the demand for buffering salts to be drawn from the bones, avoiding a potential demineralising effect. This is in contrast to the situation where *acid residues*, for example, from proteins and cereals, require buffering by ions such as citrate and carbonate from bones.

Vitamin A

Large intakes of vitamin A have been associated with changes to the bones, including thickening of the long bones and hypercalcaemia, associated with increased bone resorption. Excessive intakes of vitamin A, taken as supplements, have been reported in some studies to cause bone demineralisation, but this issue requires further clarification.

Vitamin C

Vitamin C is needed for formation of the amino acids *hydroxylysine* and *hydroxyproline*, which are essential for collagen crosslinking. Bone fractures occur in scurvy, and it is possible that even at subclinical levels of vitamin C deficiency, there is an increased risk. This has been reported in smokers, whose vitamin C need is increased.

Vitamin K

This is needed for the γ-carboxylation of glutamate residues on three key proteins found in the bone, including *osteocalcin*, which has high calcium-binding activity. Inverse relationships have been identified in older people between vitamin K status and fracture risk.

Other factors

A number of other minerals have been proposed as being important in bone metabolism. These include zinc, copper, boron, aluminium, manganese and chromium. More research is needed to clarify their exact role.

In addition, other dietary factors are believed to affect bone health. These include:
• Alcohol – generally has a negative effect on bone density, via a toxic effect on the osteoblasts.
• Caffeine – increases calcium loss in the urine; however, additional milk taken with coffee may offset this effect.
• Phytoestrogens – found in soya; have been reported to have a beneficial effect, via a weak oestrogenic action. The amount that needs to be consumed is higher than habitual levels in Western countries.

Lifestyle factors affecting the bone include smoking (which has a negative effect on bone density) and physical activity, which is beneficial and stimulates bone formation and mineralisation at the sites of mechanical strain. Conversely, immobilisation and lack of activity cause a reduction in bone mass.

Diet and phosphates

Phosphates are widely distributed in the diet in both animal and plant foods and are also used as an additive by the food industry. There is some concern about high phosphate intakes from carbonated drinks and their potential to impair calcium absorption from the gut, with a consequent effect on bone mineralisation.

27 Alcohol

Aim

1 To study the measurement and metabolism of alcohol and the consequences of excessive consumption

Although alcohol is not a nutrient, consumption of alcoholic beverages is common in most societies. Alcohol consumption rates vary both within and between countries due to a variety of cultural, religious and socio-economic factors. Some studies suggest that low to moderate intakes of alcohol may be cardioprotective; however, alcohol abuse is widespread, and this issue has important health, social and economic implications.

Measurement of alcohol consumption

Alcohol consumption is expressed in terms of 'units'. In the UK, one unit is defined as 10 mL (8 g) of pure alcohol. This is equivalent to a half-pint (284 mL) of standard strength beer, lager or cider (3–4% alcohol by volume) or a single small shot (25 mL) of 40% spirits. A small glass (125 mL) of ordinary strength wine (12% alcohol by volume) contains one and a half units of alcohol.

The unit of alcohol itself is different depending on the country. For Australia/New Zealand, the USA and Japan, one unit of alcohol is 10, 12 and 14 g of ethanol, respectively.

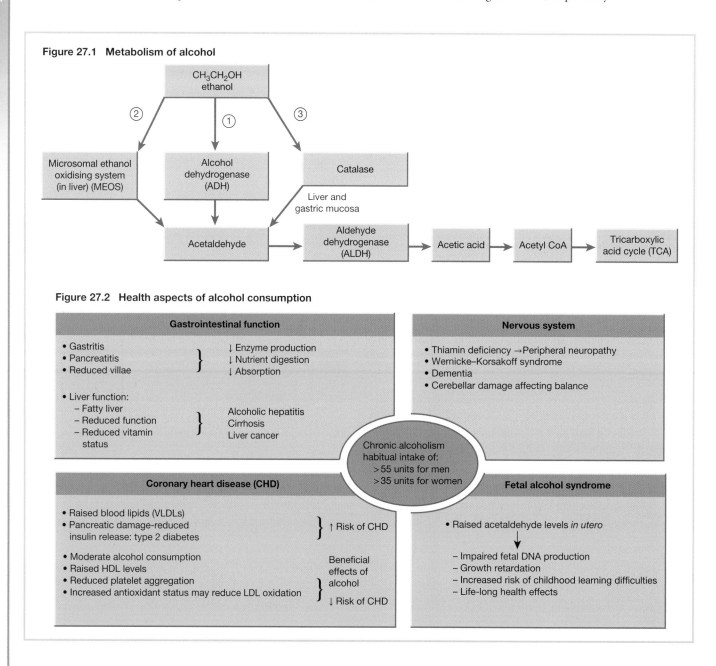

Figure 27.1   Metabolism of alcohol

Figure 27.2   Health aspects of alcohol consumption

Nutrition at a Glance, Second Edition. Edited by Sangita Sharma, Tony Sheehy and Fariba Kolahdooz.
© 2016 John Wiley & Sons, Ltd. Published 2016 by John Wiley & Sons, Ltd.

Recommendations for safe alcohol intake (based on the UK definition) are no more than 3–4 units per day for men and 2–3 units per day for women. Binge drinking is defined as consuming twice this amount in 1 day. In a week, intakes should not exceed 21 units for men and 14 units for women, and there should be alcohol-free days. Weekly alcohol intakes exceeding 55 units for men and 35 units for women are regarded as being 'likely to do harm'. Because of the risk of fetal alcohol syndrome, women who are trying to get pregnant should not drink alcohol, and no alcohol at all should be consumed during pregnancy (see Chapter 28).

Metabolism of alcohol

Within the liver, three main pathways have been demonstrated for the metabolism of alcohol (Figure 27.1), all of which produce **acetaldehyde**:
- The dominant pathway (1) involves the zinc-containing enzyme *alcohol dehydrogenase* (ADH), found in liver cytoplasm. This is the main rate-limiting step. The accumulation of acetaldehyde leads to headaches and cutaneous flushing.
- The *microsomal ethanol-oxidising system* (MEOS) (2) normally metabolises up to 20% of ingested alcohol but becomes more active in chronic alcoholics. Alcohol stimulates the development of microsomal membranes, where *cytochrome P450* (a vitamin C-requiring factor) is induced.
- A third (relatively insignificant) pathway involves the enzyme *catalase*, which is found in many cells of the body (3).

Factors affecting alcohol metabolism

The rate at which alcohol can be metabolised varies considerably from person to person and is related to body size. In a healthy young male, it may be 8–10 g/h. For a given amount of alcohol, women experience a greater increase in blood alcohol concentration than men because they tend to have a greater body fat content, lesser body water and generally lower body weight.

Alcohol metabolism is also affected by:
- Genetic factors
- Lean body mass
- The presence of other foods recently consumed
- Previous history of alcohol intake (rate of metabolism is higher in chronic alcoholics)

Alcohol and energy balance

Alcohol yields 29 kJ (7 kcal)/g. If drunk in addition to a normal food intake, the extra energy is likely to cause weight gain. This is not always the case, however, as alcohol metabolised via the MEOS system produces little ATP. Instead, the process of oxidation leads to heat production, so the energy released via this pathway is dissipated and not stored.

Consequences of alcohol abuse

Alcohol affects *every system* in the body, especially the gastrointestinal, cardiovascular and nervous systems (Figure 27.2). The main clinical risk factor associated with excessive alcohol intake is cirrhosis of the liver.

Alcohol abuse also has important social consequences, including violence, accidents, suicide and family breakdown. In addition, absence from work due to excessive alcohol consumption has economic implications, both for the individuals concerned and for the economy as a whole.

The nutritional consequences of alcohol abuse include the following:
- **Fat metabolism** in the liver becomes abnormal. The large amounts of NADH and NADPH produced by alcohol metabolism stimulate fat synthesis, which leads to high levels of circulating VLDL. In heavy drinkers, the liver increases in size due to the accumulation of excess fat, eventually leading to chronic inflammation.
- **Blood glucose control** is less effective. This reflects reduced insulin production and reduced gluconeogenesis. Hypoglycaemic episodes, resulting in 'blackouts', may occur.
- **Protein synthesis** is reduced, although protein catabolism is unaffected. Tissue repair is compromised and digestive enzyme production is reduced.
- Alcohol induces the breakdown of the active forms of **vitamin D**.
- **Vitamin K** cofactor production in the liver ceases, affecting blood clotting.
- Activation of **B vitamins** is compromised by liver disease.
- Reduced **thiamin** absorption, associated with vomiting and diarrhoea, and increased demand for thiamin result in deficiency, leading to peripheral neuropathy. In its severe form, psychological disturbances, loss of memory and psychosis (Wernicke–Korsakoff syndrome) may develop.
- Low status of **riboflavin**, **niacin** and **pyridoxine** may lead to diarrhoea, dermatitis and psychological problems.
- Reduced **folate** absorption leads to megaloblastic anaemia.
- **Zinc** is a cofactor for ADH. Zinc status may be reduced, which will compromise alcohol metabolism, decrease wound healing, dull the sense of taste and reduce immune function.
- **Iron** status in alcoholics may vary, depending on the type of drink they habitually consume. Spirits provide no iron, but some wines and beers do. Blood loss due to intestinal mucosal irritation may lead to iron depletion.

28 Fetal alcohol spectrum disorder

Aims

1 To define fetal alcohol spectrum disorder (FASD) and consider its origins, development, prevalence and associated costs
2 To understand the vast effects FASD can have on the brain, body and overall development
3 To understand the key role of nutrition professionals in the prevention of FASD and in support of clients with FASD

What is fetal alcohol spectrum disorder?

Consuming alcohol during pregnancy can damage developing cells in the fetus and result in brain dysfunction and disruption of other organ systems such as the heart. Fetal alcohol spectrum disorder (FASD) is the term used to describe the range of impairments that occur; these impairments are lifelong and cause increasing difficulty with age as societal expectations increase for independent functioning.

Alcohol is water-soluble and crosses from the maternal circulation through the placenta to the fetus. The extent of damage depends on many factors including:

- The amount of alcohol consumed
- The timing and frequency of consumption
- Binge drinking, which results in higher blood alcohol levels
- Vulnerable periods in fetal development
- Maternal stress
- Maternal nutritional status
- Maternal and fetal genetic and epigenetic factors

Prevalence and costs of FASD

FASD is a major public health problem. It is rooted in the **biopsychosocial determinants of health**, including poverty, lack of educational opportunities, multigenerational trauma and undiagnosed/unsupported mental health issues. Prevention is complex and requires a multisystem approach.

FASD is common, with current estimates of 1 in 100 in the population. However, prevalence data are lacking because of a lack of capacity for diagnosis and the absence of biological markers. The lifetime cost is estimated to be $1.8 million per case across many systems of care (health, education, children's services, justice, mental health addictions, housing and employment).

Effects of FASD on the brain

Alcohol can damage fetal brain development in a number of ways:
- Through neuronal cell death or *apoptosis*
- Interruptions in cell migration, adhesion and connections
- Alterations in neurotransmitter development

Maternal nutritional status (e.g. *folate, choline*, and *antioxidants*) may play a role in reducing the impact of alcohol on fetal cells, but research in this area is limited and primarily done in animal models.

In clinical settings, routine structural MRI rarely reveals evidence of brain damage except in extreme cases where there may be *absence of the corpus callosum, cerebellar hypoplasia* and *microcephaly*. However, research-level neuroimaging studies are identifying differences in functionality in brain areas, especially in the *frontal cortex* and in the connecting *white matter pathways* between brain regions.

In full fetal alcohol syndrome (FAS) or partial fetal alcohol syndrome (pFAS), there is the visible *facial dysmorphology* of *thin lips* and a *flat philtrum* that results from prenatal alcohol exposure between day 19 and 21 of pregnancy, often when the pregnancy is not yet recognised by the mother. The other facial characteristic is small *palpebral fissures* (measured as the length of the eye slit). This can result from exposure over a longer period in gestation. There are standards for assessment of the facial features, including digital photographs and software analysis.

The characteristic face of FAS or pFAS is found in only about 10% of affected individuals. In the majority of those living with FASD, the disability is invisible, with no physical or biological markers. However, the brain impairment can be severe and result in lifelong problems associated with learning deficits, difficulties in emotional, sensory and behavioural regulation, impairment in memory, difficulties with motor planning, deficits in functional and social communication and impairment in executive functions of the brain (judgement, planning, organising, sequencing, flexible thinking, inhibition, shifting and sustaining attention). A multidisciplinary team is required to assess for evidence of this brain damage.

The brain impairment results in maladaptation and the inability to function independently in life. Without appropriate supports, this puts the individual living with FASD at risk for **social victimisation**, coming into **trouble with the law**, **being homeless** and having **mental health** and **substance abuse** problems. Early diagnosis and access to services have the potential to improve outcomes and quality of life. The ultimate goal is to break the multigenerational cycle in FASD.

Effects of FASD on the body

Alcohol can also have an impact on other developing organ systems in the fetus. Several *cardiac defects* are associated with prenatal alcohol exposure. *Growth deficiency* at birth and throughout life is a hallmark in full FAS but not FASD.

There can be *vision* and *hearing problems* as well, and early detection is imperative.

In infancy, there can be *feeding issues* related to problems in coordinating suck and swallow reflexes. Later on, textural sensitivities can severely hinder dietary intake and result in failure to thrive.

Therefore, in nutrition practice, the history of prenatal alcohol exposure can be important in management. If this is known from birth, anticipatory guidance and developmental and health screening should be provided. This history may not be available, however, as many health providers fail to ask the question of alcohol use in pregnancy to women in a supportive, non-judgemental manner.

Questions about the use of alcohol should be a standard practice for all health-care professionals, especially in caring for women

Nutrition at a Glance, Second Edition. Edited by Sangita Sharma, Tony Sheehy and Fariba Kolahdooz.
© 2016 John Wiley & Sons, Ltd. Published 2016 by John Wiley & Sons, Ltd.

in childbearing years. Incorporating these questions into nutrition counselling is a natural fit and needs to be accompanied by supports for harm reduction, such as brief interventions and referrals to community-based services. Nutrition counselling is an opportunity to have the prevention conversation in a safe and supportive setting.

Screening tools, diagnostic assessment and interventions

Screening tools are being explored at a population and individual level, but at the present time, there is no research-validated tool. Promising areas include using questionnaires to detect the behavioural phenotype patterns in school-age children and individuals in the justice system.

One biological marker is measuring *fatty acid ethyl esters* (*FAEE*) in the *meconium* passed from the gut of all newborns. However, this does not detect exposure in the first 13 weeks of pregnancy, as the gut lumen is not functional until that time for fetal digestion. The first trimester is therefore not sampled. Unfortunately, this is a major time of risk in fetal development and a time that many pregnancies are not recognised by the woman.

The test only determines alcohol exposure as a risk factor and is not a diagnosis of FASD. The exposed infant needs developmental monitoring, and the birth mother needs various supports. There are many legal and ethical issues to be explored too, as child welfare authorities may use this test to remove children from their mother's care.

Currently, the best screen is a child/youth/adult who is struggling in function and a confirmed history of prenatal alcohol exposure. Assessment of brain dysfunction needs to be carried out by a trained multidisciplinary team using current guidelines. The assessment should subsequently lead to interventions that improve quality of life and prevent adverse secondary outcomes. These supports must span many facets of health care and also need to consider transition points in this lifelong disability.

There are many promising interventions, such as early access to educational interventions and stability of the home environment. Medications may be considered for certain targeted behaviours, but there needs to be careful monitoring for side effects and benefit/risk balance. Drugs often have major side effects on nutrition, growth, metabolic state and sleep pattern. The nutritionist can be a key team member in this area.

Role of the nutritionist in FASD

Nutritionists can play an important role in the prevention of FASD by educating all women and their partners about the harmful effects of alcohol use in pregnancy as part of regular nutrition counselling. Nutritionists should ask about past and present alcohol use as part of the history with every client. If risky drinking patterns are identified, hopefully before pregnancy, the nutritionist can provide interventions and referrals to other services.

The nutritionist also needs to be part of the team addressing the feeding issues in children with FASD and in monitoring the side effects of medications on growth.

If a client has FASD, they may not understand or retain information that is provided or be able to follow through because of their brain impairments. The health-care professional needs to take account of these cognitive impairments and change how information is given. Methods can include:
- Breaking down the tasks
- Being more concrete
- Using visual aids in teaching
- Providing repetition

If the client does not adhere to the expectations, blame should not fall on the client. The professional needs to set reasonable expectations and explore with the client how to build in more supports and develop more effective strategies.

Practice points

- Nutrition counselling is an opportunity to educate all women of childbearing age about the harm of drinking alcohol during pregnancy and to provide brief interventions and referrals to community resources.
- Preventing FASD requires a multidisciplinary approach based on addressing the psychosocial determinants of health and access to coordinated interventions and supports in the community.
- FASD is common and costly and impacts the individual living with FASD across their lifespan. Many professional groups will be working with FASD cases, and nutritionists need to know how their clients may be impacted and individualise their practice accordingly. Key areas are awareness that growth deficiency and feeding difficulties can be related to prenatal alcohol exposure, knowledge about the side effects of medications on metabolism and growth and the need to tailor counselling to a client with FASD.

29 Fluids in the diet

Aims

1 To consider the need for water in the body and its role in maintaining health
2 To explore the ways in which water and other fluids can contribute to fluid balance and nutrition

Water makes up 50–60% of the total body weight of an average adult, and even small reductions in levels of hydration can have serious consequences for normal functions. Humans cannot survive beyond about 10 days without water. Water content is higher in males than females because males have a higher percentage of lean mass, which contains more water than does body fat.

Water is required for the following processes:
• Ingestion, digestion and absorption of food, including production of various secretions, movement of the food bolus along the digestive tract and elimination of waste
• Transport of nutrients and metabolites in solution, metabolic processes occurring in fluid environments, establishing osmotic gradients
• Maintenance of moist mucous membranes
• Maintenance of blood volumes and haematocrit, as well as extracellular and intracellular fluid volumes, which affect tissue osmolarity
• Renal function, which is dependent on adequate perfusion pressure
• Body temperature regulation by sweat loss

Fluid balance

Fluid balance represents the relationship between *fluid intake* and *fluid loss* (Table 29.1). Fluid intake is largely under the control of the individual, but people relying on others for fluid (such as young children or dependent elderly people) may be unable to determine their intake. Fluid is lost from the body in a number of ways, which are normally outside the individual's control.

Water gain by the body

Water is gained by the body from foods and drinks.

Metabolism

Small amounts of water are produced during metabolic processes, such as when proteins, fats and carbohydrates are catabolised to produce energy.

Table 29.1 Summary of average values for fluid gain and loss per day for a healthy individual leading a sedentary life (values vary depending on circumstances).

Water gain – route	Water gain – volume (mL)	Water loss – route	Water loss – volume (mL)
Water in food	1000	Urine	1300
Metabolic water	350	Faeces	100
Drinks	1200	Skin	750
		Lungs	400
Total	2550		2550

Water in Food

Water is also ingested with food:
• Some foods are semi-liquid (e.g. yogurts, soups and ice cream).
• Many seemingly solid foods contain a high percentage of water (e.g. fruits and vegetables).
• Even foods that seem quite dry, such as cereals, bread, cheese and meat, contain some water.

Drinks

Consumption of water from drinks is very variable. The choice of drink may make an important contribution to nutrient intake.

Water loss from the body

Water is lost from the body via the urine, faeces, skin and lungs.

Urine

Daily urine production (*diuresis*) closely follows the levels of hydration. Pale, straw-coloured urine indicates good hydration, whereas small volumes of dark-yellow urine indicate significant levels of dehydration.

Faeces

Fluid loss in the faeces is normally small (about 100 mL/day), but in diarrhoeal diseases, faecal losses can increase to 2000 mL/day, representing a major threat to life. Abuse of laxatives can also result in large fluid losses and lead to dehydration.

Skin

Water loss through the skin occurs continuously. Children are particularly at risk because their surface-to-volume ratio is considerably higher than it is in adults. Normal levels of water loss can be doubled in heat, when sweating is taking place for heat regulation. It is estimated that water loss through sweat increases by 500 mL/day for each 1°C rise in body temperature. Even moderate exercise can increase sweat losses to 1000–3000 mL/h.

Lungs

In order for effective gas exchange to occur in the lungs, inhaled air must be moistened. Therefore, exhaled air contains water vapour. Dry climates, air-conditioned offices and high-altitude situations encourage this form of water loss.

Maintenance of normal hydration

Most sedentary adults in a temperate climate need about 1200–1500 mL/day. This assumes that a further 1000 mL of fluid is being obtained from food, resulting in a total fluid gain of about 35 mL/kg body weight per day.

Dehydration

Many population groups are at possible risk of dehydration, including young children, dependent elderly, athletes and people working in hot environments (Table 29.2). Although the prevalence of mild dehydration is not known, significant numbers may be affected.

Nutrition at a Glance, Second Edition. Edited by Sangita Sharma, Tony Sheehy and Fariba Kolahdooz.
© 2016 John Wiley & Sons, Ltd. Published 2016 by John Wiley & Sons, Ltd.

Table 29.2 Population groups at risk of dehydration.

Group at possible risk	Reason(s) for vulnerability
Young children	Poorly developed thirst mechanism/lack of awareness Dependence on others for fluid supply Relatively low body water volume Large surface area for water evaporation
Dependent elderly people	Possible confusion about fluid intake Dependence on others for fluid supply Relatively low body water volume Possible drug therapy (e.g. diuretics) Poor food intake, little metabolic water produced Reluctance to drink because of limited mobility to use lavatory
Subjects with raised body temperature	Increased losses through skin (sweating) and lungs (rapid breathing) Poor appetite, little food intake Possible losses from GI tract in vomiting/diarrhoea Poor thirst mechanism/provision of fluids
Sports people	Large sweat losses to maintain body temperature Increased respiration and lung losses Inability/unwillingness to consume fluid during exercise
People working in heat	Large sweat losses

As the body becomes dehydrated, the thirst mechanism is triggered by a fall in body fluid volume normally associated with a rise in osmolality. However, by the time the signals to consume additional fluid appear, the effects of dehydration will already have begun. Thus, *anticipatory fluid consumption* may be the only way to prevent dehydration, so fluid consumption should become a habit.

The general consequences of dehydration are summarised in Table 29.3. They range from mild effects on physical skills

Table 29.3 Summary of consequences of dehydration.

Degree of dehydration	Amount of fluid deficit	Consequences	Comments
Mild	500–1000 mL; 1–2% body weight	May affect cognitive function	May reduce accuracy in performance
Mild to moderate	1000–3500 mL; 2–5% body weight	Headaches, cognitive impairment, nausea	Substantial detrimental effect on performance in sporting activity; affects temperature regulation
Severe	>6% body weight	Pyrexia, tachycardia, dizziness, weakness	Loss of physical performance skill
Life threatening	10%	Raised blood pressure, renal failure, coma and possibly death	

performance, cognitive function and mood at a 1–2% loss in body weight to tachycardia, weakness and severe reduction in skills performance above 6% body weight loss. When the fluid deficit is greater than 10% of body weight, dehydration becomes life threatening and is generally fatal at 15%.

Dietary factors that influence diuresis

- High-sodium and high-protein diets increase the solute load and therefore obligatory urine loss and require compensatory increases in fluid intake.
- Caffeine is a methylxanthine (found in coffee, tea and colas and some high-energy drinks) and is chemically related to theobromine and theophylline found in tea and chocolate. These compounds have a diuretic action; however, at doses of <300 mg/day, the level of diuresis is offset by the volume of fluid ingested. In practice, this means that caffeine consumption will not lead to a significant level of dehydration.
- Alcohol produces a diuresis. Consuming neat spirit could lead to negative fluid balance, but alcohol in beer will result in a positive balance because of the fluid accompanying the alcohol in the drink.

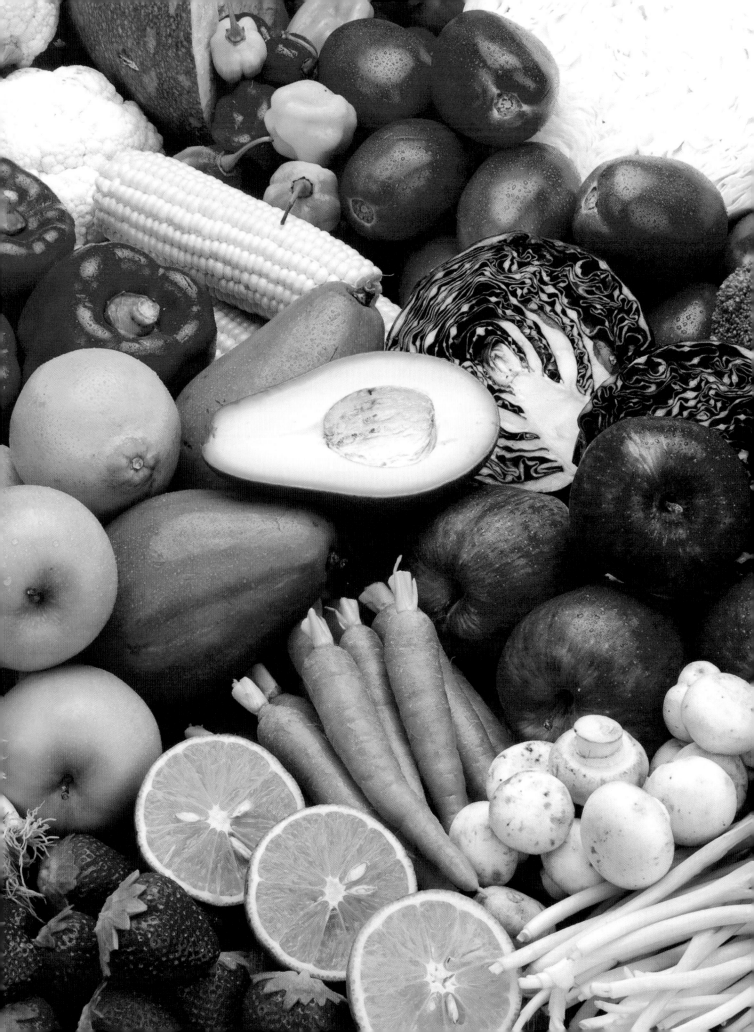

Nutritional epidemiology including assessments, consequences and food choices

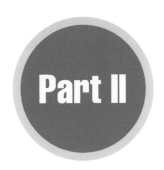

Part II

30 Introduction to nutrition epidemiology: Study designs I

Aim

1 To introduce study design methods (descriptive and experimental studies) and their applications

Understanding the role of nutrition in health or disease is based on information on food intake and health indicators (*exposure* and *outcome*). This is addressed by nutritional epidemiological studies in groups of people, generally over a long period of time.

Study design methods

Descriptive studies

Descriptive studies aim to **determine how common a particular disease (outcome) or exposure** (nutrient intake, e.g. deficiencies or excesses) is within a specific population at a certain time. These studies analyse 'person, place and time' to characterise a given outcome (e.g. prevalence of cardiovascular diseases in men and women in Canada in 2014). The four main types of descriptive studies are presented in Table 30.1.

Prevalence surveys

These surveys try to utilise a representative sample of people to estimate the proportion of (or number of individuals within) a population that are affected by a health outcome. Most data are self-reported. For example, many countries employ regular national surveys (e.g. every 5 years) to determine the prevalence of obesity in a representative sample of the population. Using this approach, changes over time can also be observed.

Case reports

Unusual cases of disease are described in great detail to identify potential causes of that disease. For example, researchers recently described the treatment of sensorimotor neuropathy with intravenous folic acid in a patient suffering from folate deficiency and alcoholism. Data from case reports are very selective and provide limited information about potentially relevant exposures.

Surveillance data

Surveillance data can measure prevalence, distribution and incidence of disease. Surveillance has traditionally been used to monitor infectious disease outbreaks, but it is now used to track many diseases and risk factors. For example, some countries regularly collect data on chronic diseases, such as diabetes, to calculate disease prevalence and incidence. Regular surveillance helps health officials monitor trends, identify potential risk factors and create appropriate plans of action or policies.

Analyses of routinely collected data

Routinely collected data (e.g. death certificates, which use the International Classification of Diseases (ICD) codes), morbidity data (e.g. disease registries) and hospital records are used to calculate incidence and prevalence of a disease. The data include demographics, cause of death and medical history. One drawback is that raw data are often incomplete, or multiple related diseases are mentioned on the death certificate.

Analytical studies

Analytical studies aim to determine **causal associations** between specific factors and an outcome. These studies examine correlations revealed by descriptive studies and attempt to determine the strength of that relationship. For example, analytical studies can examine whether or not obese individuals are more likely to develop coronary heart disease. They can be subdivided into those that are experimental (*intervention*) and those that are non-experimental (*observational*) (see Chapter 31).

Experimental (intervention studies)

Intervention studies, if designed appropriately, utilise current evidence to inform, develop, implement and evaluate programmes to improve health and prevent disease. For example, intervention studies can determine which of several strategies for weight loss is best at decreasing a group's weight. These studies are able to manipulate exposure and observe any changes in outcome.

Uncontrolled trials

Uncontrolled trials provide treatment to all willing participants. For example, investigators may administer a dietary intervention to improve individuals' depressive symptoms. Participants will be assessed on various measures before and after the intervention to detect changes. However, the absence of a control group limits causal interpretation.

Controlled trials

Controlled trials utilise a control group that (ideally) has identical general characteristics to the intervention group. A comparison of these groups allows identification of changes that may occur due solely to the intervention. For example, investigators wishing to assess the effectiveness of a supplement will give half the participants the supplement and the other half (the controls) a **placebo**.

Table 30.1 Examples of descriptive study designs used in epidemiology.

Type of study	Key features
Prevalence survey	Measures rate of health outcome in a representative sample of the population
Case reports	Reports unusual cases of disease in great detail to identify potential causes of that disease
Surveillance data	Regular collection of data to estimate prevalence, distribution and incidence of disease
Analyses of routinely collected data	Analysis of available data to estimate incidence and prevalence of health outcomes

Nutrition at a Glance, Second Edition. Edited by Sangita Sharma, Tony Sheehy and Fariba Kolahdooz.
© 2016 John Wiley & Sons, Ltd. Published 2016 by John Wiley & Sons, Ltd.

Randomised controlled trials

Randomised controlled trials (RCTs) evaluate an intervention by selecting a group of individuals with the same health status and randomly allocating them to either a **control** or an **intervention** group. The control group receives a placebo or standard treatment. The intervention group receives the treatment. Any difference in outcome between the groups can thus be attributed to the intervention. An RCT might examine the effect of a modified diet (intervention group) relative to a standard diet (control group) on serum cholesterol levels. Ethical concerns often prevent human testing, which limits the determination of causality within epidemiology.

Community trials

In this form of RCT, which is often used when individual interventions are impractical, entire communities receive the intervention. These trials evaluate preventative health measures. Communities are randomised to either intervention or control, balancing out characteristics between the groups. For example, the Healthy Foods North (HFN) project was a community-based nutrition and physical activity intervention programme designed for promoting health and reducing risk factors of chronic disease among indigenous peoples in the Canadian Arctic. The impact of the intervention was assessed using pre- and post-intervention changes in prevalence of obesity between case and control communities.

Quasi-randomised controlled trials

Quasi-randomised controlled trials are similar to RCTs, except that a non-random method of group allocation is utilised. Consequently, the risk of selection bias and the potential for confounding between-group differences is high. For example, in a study examining the effect of an educational intervention on fast food consumption, the control and intervention groups are divided based on the participants' dates of birth.

Non-randomised controlled trials

Non-randomised controlled trials are similar to RCTs, except that a completely arbitrary method of group allocation is utilised. For example, studying the effect of an epidural on breastfeeding depends on women choosing to receive an epidural. Investigators cannot assign women to intervention and control groups. This study design confers an additional level of selection bias, as known and unknown variables are not equally distributed between each group.

31 Introduction to nutrition epidemiology: Study designs II

Aims

1 To introduce study design methods (non-experimental studies) and their applications
2 To introduce the concepts of measurement error, the validity of results and the sensitivity of tests

Non-experimental (observational studies)

Observational studies aim to assess the natural course of disease progression, health outcome or exposure in relation to disease occurrence (Table 31.1). These studies do not involve any manipulation of participants. Instead, what happens naturally or what previously occurred is recorded. For example, one might measure the rate of lung cancer and vitamin C intake over a long period of time within a population to determine if there is an association between the exposure, vitamin C, and the outcome, lung cancer.

Cohort studies

A cohort study follows a group of individuals over a time period (*prospectively*) to assess a health outcome of interest. The rate of disease onset among initially healthy individuals is observed. For example, the European Prospective Investigation on Cancer (EPIC) study is following healthy people in 10 European countries over several decades to assess the incidence of cancer and any possible associations to exposures, including dietary intake. Cohort studies provide information on the possible causes of a disease and offer measurement of an individual's risk of that disease. The generalisability of results depends on the participants' characteristics. Changes in participants' diet over time and individuals *lost to follow-up* may influence the results. These studies are expensive, are very long term and may only be suitable for diseases that commonly occur. A wide range of exposures is necessary to assess risks or outcomes, for example, people who consume 0–10 servings of vegetables per day and their risk of developing cancer as both are quantified.

Case–control studies

Case–control studies gather information about a specific disease. Those with the outcome of interest are selected (cases) along with unaffected, matched (usually on age, ethnicity and sex) members of the same population (controls), and detailed descriptions of participants' past exposures of interest are recorded. For example, to determine if fish consumption was associated with a decrease in cardiovascular disease, investigators could compare people with and without cardiovascular disease to determine if their past fish consumption habits differed. Compared to prospective studies, case–control studies are less expensive and quicker. But, again, measuring all relevant past exposures is difficult.

Cross-sectional studies

Cross-sectional studies examine a specific exposure and health outcome within a sample of the population. These studies are simple, easy to conduct, preferred for initial investigations and good for analysing exposures that remain constant over time. They provide a snapshot of the situation on which future investigations can be based. To obtain generalisable findings, the participants must be representative of the population. It is difficult to determine causality in these studies.

Ecological studies

Ecological studies determine disease frequency in relation to frequency of exposure to some factor within an entire population. For example, studies that assess the global prevalence of processed meat consumption and cancer rates follow an ecological study model. Ecological studies are solely intended to consider possible associations at the population level. Ecological studies are often difficult to interpret because unstudied differences between study populations may affect disease prevalence (causality is not clear).

Table 31.1 Examples of analytical study designs used in epidemiology.

Experimental (intervention studies)	
Uncontrolled trials	Intervention applied to all participants; no control group
Controlled trials	
• Randomised (RCTs)	Equal probability for all participants allocated to intervention and control group; completely random
• Quasi-randomised	Unequal probability for participants allocated to intervention and control group; method is not truly random
• Non-randomised	Unequal probability for participants allocated to intervention and control group; method used is completely arbitrary and not random
Non-experimental (observational studies)	
Cohort (retrospective and prospective)	Follow a large group of people over time to assess the incidence of a health outcome of interest. Offer a direct measurement about risk of developing the health outcome
Case–control	Allows for study of rare diseases. Two groups, one with the disease and one without, provide detailed description of past exposures
Cross-sectional	A sample representative of the population is used to provide a snapshot of the situation on which future investigations can be based
Ecological	Examination of disease frequency in relation to frequency of exposure at the population level

Nutrition at a Glance, Second Edition. Edited by Sangita Sharma, Tony Sheehy and Fariba Kolahdooz.
© 2016 John Wiley & Sons, Ltd. Published 2016 by John Wiley & Sons, Ltd.

Measurement error, result validity and test sensitivity

Systematic and random errors

Errors can occur when selecting the study population or when measuring variables. **Systematic errors** occur when a measurement tool is imprecise and affects all participants equally. For example, a scale might repeatedly measure an individual's weight 2 lb lighter than the true weight. **Random errors** occur when measurements are varied and can be reduced by conducting several measurements. For example, due to daily fluctuations in an individual's dietary intake, observations of eating habits over many days will give a more accurate representation of the diet.

The case of validity

Two types of validity require consideration: internal and external. Internal validity requires that the results 'make sense' and that the 'exposure' caused the 'outcome' (i.e. that the results are free from bias, confounders (other independent variables) and random chance). External validity relates to how readily the results can be applied to a general population. External validity depends on the study population; results from an extremely specific sample population may not apply to a broader population. For example, the impact of a diet and physical activity intervention among individuals with depression could not be generalised to a healthy population. If a study has external validity, the results are applicable to another setting.

Testing the test

The quality of a clinical test can be evaluated by testing its **sensitivity** and **specificity**. If a test is sensitive, individuals with a disease will test positive for that disease. If a test is specific, those without the disease will test negative. A test that is both specific and sensitive is desired.

Summary

Almost all aspects of the study of nutrition have potential drawbacks. Some can be eliminated with careful study planning and design and, where possible, with repeated measures. In attempting to link *exposure* to a causative (or preventive) factor and a health (or disease) *outcome*, the multifactorial nature of relationships needs to be considered to prevent inappropriate conclusions being drawn.

32 Research ethics

Aims

1 To identify the three core ethical principles
2 To recognise ethical considerations and standards for dietetic, health and research professionals

Core ethical principles

Ethics refers to moral principles that govern a person's behaviour or those pertaining to an activity, such as research. There are three basic ethical principles (Figure 32.1):
- Respect for persons
- Beneficence
- Justice

The welfare and integrity of individuals must take priority over all else when practising in the field of nutrition, whether in research or dietetics.

The principle of **respect for persons** includes respect for an individual's autonomy as well as the protection of vulnerable persons. Autonomy refers to the ability to determine what is best for oneself. Therefore, respect for autonomy simply means that the self-determination of people, who are capable of making informed decisions about their personal choices, should be treated with respect.

'Vulnerable persons' refers to individuals who lack the capacity to protect their own interests. These individuals are considered to have impaired or diminished autonomy and include such groups as children and people with cognitive impairment or mental health issues. Protection of vulnerable persons is critical, and special considerations should be made when working with these individuals to ensure that they are safeguarded against harm or abuse.

Beneficence refers to the ethical obligation to maximise benefit and minimise harm. Before undertaking any research, all potential benefits and predictable risks and burdens to individuals and groups involved should be carefully assessed. Research may only be conducted if the importance of the objective outweighs the risks and burdens to the research subjects. As well, measures to minimise the risks must be employed and risks must be continuously monitored, assessed and documented. Nonmaleficence, the obligation to do no harm, is vital when conducting research.

Justice refers to the ethical obligation to treat each person in a manner that is morally right. Distributive justice requires that both the risks and benefits of participation in research or care are distributed equally.

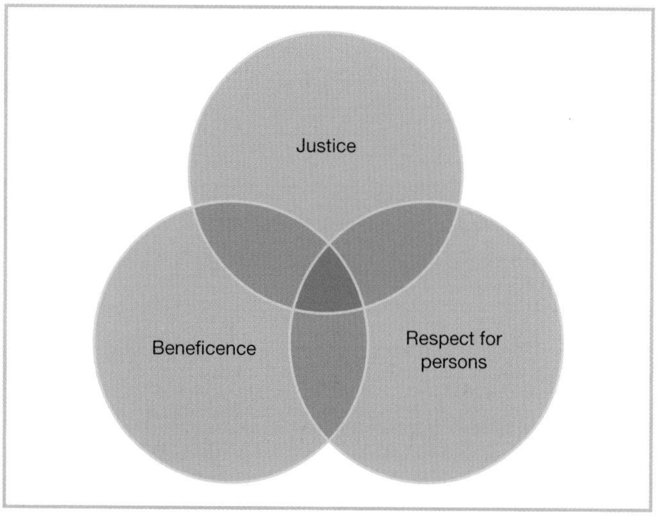

Dietetics

The International Confederation of Dietetic Associations published the International Code of Ethics and Code of Good Practice in 2008. The document was prepared with the input of dietetic associations around the world, and although it is not meant to replace any national standards, it serves to establish the common ethical considerations of dietetics professionals globally.

International Code of Ethics

Dietitians practice in a just and equitable manner to improve the nutrition of the world by:
- Being competent, objective and honest
- Respecting all people and their needs
- Collaborating with others
- Striving for positive nutrition outcomes for people
- Doing no harm
- Adhering to the standards of good practice in nutrition and dietetics

In addition to the International Code of Ethics, there is an International Code of Good Practice to which dietitians should adhere. This can be found on the International Confederation of Dietetic Associations' website.

Nutrition research

Research is fundamental in expanding general knowledge on nutrition and in improving quality of life in many areas of nutrition, whether in the community or clinical practice.

Although research has the potential to improve the quality of life of people across the many borders, respect for research participants and their well-being is absolutely imperative; the well-being of some must not be knowingly compromised for the potential benefit of many.

Events during the Second World War, specifically widespread atrocities committed by Nazi physicians and scientists conducting 'medical experiments', prompted public outrage and spurred the establishment of a code of conduct for human research. The result was the Nuremberg Code, 1947, a set of 10 guiding principles for conducting research with human subjects. Since then, several versions of ethical guidelines for the conduct of research – national and international – have been developed, the most recent internationally recognised guidelines being the Declaration of Helsinki, last updated in 2013.

Figure 32.1 Three core ethical principles

Nutrition at a Glance, Second Edition. Edited by Sangita Sharma, Tony Sheehy and Fariba Kolahdooz.
© 2016 John Wiley & Sons, Ltd. Published 2016 by John Wiley & Sons, Ltd.

A critical component of ensuring that research is conducted in an ethical manner is the review and approval of the study protocol by a Research Ethics Committee (REC) prior to initiating the study. A researcher must not conduct research, including contacting or recruiting participants, without receiving ethics approval from the appropriate institution.

The primary task of an REC is the ethical review of research protocols and their supporting documents. The REC decides whether to approve a research proposal based on its adherence to ethical principles and its scientific validity. The review takes into account any prior scientific reviews and applicable laws. In certain cases, approval may be required from more than one REC; this is especially true when working with vulnerable populations. For instance, when conducting research with indigenous populations in Canada, the ownership, control, access and possession (OCAP) principles, sanctioned by the First Nations Information Governance Centre (FNIGC) and First Nations Regional Longitudinal Health Survey (RHS), provide a framework for conducting research that enables self-determination of all aspects of research conducted with First Nations peoples.

In addition to approval by a Research Ethics Committee, some research activities may also require a research licence. For example, prior to conducting any research in Arctic Canada, the territories of Northwest Territories, Nunavut and the Yukon specifically, the researcher must have a research licence approved.

33 Nutritional assessment methods: Anthropometric assessment

Aims

1 To describe different methods of anthropometric assessment
2 To consider the advantages and disadvantages of each method

Anthropometry

Anthropometric measurements include the following:

Height and weight – The equipment required for measuring height and weight is simple and widely available, so these measures are frequently used in anthropometric assessments.

Height can be measured using direct or indirect methods. Direct measurement is carried out using a measuring rod or *stadiometer*. This requires the individual to be able to stand straight or lie flat. Indirect (surrogate) measures such as knee height/lower leg length may be used (with application of appropriate equations) for those individuals who are bedridden or chair-bound or who cannot stand straight or lie flat.

Although results for height may vary between these measures, they are adequate for body mass index (BMI) assessment.

Weight is measured in young children and adults often using a digital scale.

For monitoring growth and development in children, **growth charts** can be used to plot serial measurement of the child's height/length, weight and head circumference. Growth should follow a *percentile* line; substantial drift from this line needs to be investigated.

Calibration of stadiometers, measuring tapes and weighing scales should be carried out regularly.

Specific measurements of body size and changes in body proportions may be important indicators of nutritional status (Table 33.1). Anthropometric measurements can be compared with validated standards based on age and gender, allowing health professionals to track the growth and development of an individual, as well as evaluate potential over- or undernutrition. Z-score is a statistical measurement indicating the association between a particular score and the mean in a group of scores. When the Z-score is 0, the score is equal to the mean. Positive or negative Z-scores demonstrate a score being above or below the mean, respectively, and the value indicates how many standard deviations from the mean it lies. A Z-score can be used to evaluate underweight (weight for age, <2 Z-scores below reference), stunting (height for age, <2 Z-scores below reference) and wasting (weight for height, <2 Z-scores below reference).

BMI – Determination of height and weight allows the calculation of BMI. This is obtained by dividing weight, in kilograms, by height^2, in metres.

The use of BMI to evaluate nutritional status has been validated by many epidemiological studies and is used internationally to assess the risk of disease. The WHO has developed BMI ranges that classify individuals according to their degree of underweight or overweight, and these ranges represent risk of associated diseases (Table 33.2). In some populations, health risks may increase at lower levels of BMI, so different BMI thresholds are used. For example, in South Asians, the desirable BMI range is from 18.5 to 23, and the cut-off for obesity is >27.5, which is lower compared to the BMI for other ethnic groups.

The use of BMI as an anthropometric measurement is limited by the fact that it does not differentiate between the contribution of muscle, fat or oedema to body weight. Thus, in heavily trained, muscular individuals, a high BMI may be misinterpreted as signifying overweight or obesity. Individuals with significant oedema (e.g. due to kwashiorkor or chronic renal failure) may be misclassified also as being normal weight. BMI is not appropriate for infants or pregnant women, and when used for children and adolescents aged 2–18, its interpretation is different from that among adults. As BMI increases with age, individuals aged 65 years and over may require a separate set of BMI ranges to account for changes in body composition. In addition, it may not be suitable for very tall or very small people.

Circumferences

Circumference measurements can be used to characterise body fat distribution. Body fat can be distributed in varying proportions between the intra-abdominal areas, subcutaneous tissue and within the muscle, and specific fat distribution patterns have been recognised as indicators of disease risk. For example, individuals

Table 33.1 Internationally used standards for assessment of undernutrition.

Measurement	Implication
Children	
Weight for age, <2 standard deviations (SD) (or 2 Z-scores) below reference	Underweight: current insufficient food intake
Height for age, <2 SD (or 2 Z-scores) below reference	Stunting: chronic undernutrition, affecting linear growth
Weight for height, <2 SD (or 2 Z-scores) below reference	Wasting: acute growth disturbance, change in body proportions
Adults	
BMI <18.5 kg/m²	Chronic energy deficiency due to poor food intake or chronic disease
BMI <17.0 kg/m²	Reduced physical capacity likely to increase susceptibility to illness

Table 33.2 Classification of body fatness based on BMI (WHO).

Category	BMI range (kg/m²)
Normal weight	18.5–24.9
Overweight	25–29.9
Obesity – class 1	30–34.9
Obesity – class 2	35–39.9
Obesity – class 3 (morbid obesity)	>40.0

Nutrition at a Glance, Second Edition. Edited by Sangita Sharma, Tony Sheehy and Fariba Kolahdooz.
© 2016 John Wiley & Sons, Ltd. Published 2016 by John Wiley & Sons, Ltd.

with a large proportion of abdominal fat have an increased risk for metabolic syndrome.

Waist circumference, midway between the lower rib margin and the iliac crest, taken at the end of exhalation, reflects visceral adiposity and is sensitive to weight changes.

If **hip circumference** is also measured at the largest part of the buttocks, the waist-to-hip ratio (WHR) can indicate the distribution of body fat between central and peripheral regions. A ratio above 0.8 in women and 0.9 in men is interpreted as abdominal obesity. Increasing values for WHR indicate higher levels of risk for cardiovascular diseases.

Mid-arm circumference (MAC) is the circumference at the midpoint of the upper arm. If the amount of subcutaneous fat in the upper arm is also measured (by measuring skinfold thickness at the mid-triceps), this allows mid-arm muscle circumference (MAMC) to be calculated. This is a useful screen for muscle wasting. However, this measurement is very limited if the arms are muscular.

Head circumference is often used to monitor growth in infants.

Body composition

Humans are made up of:

- Fat mass
- Fat-free mass (protein and minerals)
- Water

Skinfold thickness – This is a measure of subcutaneous adipose tissue. By measuring skinfold thickness at various sites (e.g. mid-biceps, mid-triceps, subscapular and suprailiac) by means of callipers, the percentage body fat can be estimated using appropriate prediction equations.

Other methods for measuring body composition include:

Densitometry – Subjects are weighed in air and immersed in water, and appropriate equations are used to calculate percentage body fat from the difference in weights.

Air displacement plethysmography (BOD POD) – This technique for measuring total body density is based on the same principles as densitometry, except that the individual displaces air rather than water. This makes it much easier for individuals to undergo the procedure. Air displacement plethysmography has been proven to be an accurate method of assessing body composition.

Imaging techniques – *Computed tomography* (CT) or *magnetic resonance imaging* (MRI) can visualise discrete deposits of body fat, especially in the visceral region. *Dual-energy X-ray absorptiometry* (DEXA) can also be used to predict visceral fat deposits.

Bioelectrical impedance analysis (BIA) – This technique measures resistance (impedance) when a small electric current is passed between electrodes attached to the hands and feet. Impedance is related to the volume of total body water and fat-free mass, which is inversely related to fat mass. Although widely used, the technique is subject to errors related to level of hydration and environmental temperature.

Dilution techniques – Body water can be estimated from the concentration of radioactive isotopes injected into the body (see Chapter 5).

Summary

Anthropometric assessment of individuals includes a number of approaches. Describing and assessing anthropometric status can indicate where potential problems may exist and suggest beneficial interventions.

34 Nutritional assessment methods: Dietary assessment I

Aims

1 To describe methods of assessing dietary intake
2 To consider the advantages and disadvantages of each method

The focus of this section is on dietary assessment methods at the national, household and individual level. Nutrient intakes can be calculated and compared to nutrient recommendations to assess dietary quality and dietary inadequacies or excesses.

Assessing food availability (supply) at the national level: Food balance sheets

Food balance sheets are the most common method used to assess the quantity of **food available for consumption** within a country during a specified time period. **Domestic food supply** is calculated using data that describe national food production (in terms of commodities), as well as food imports and existing food reserves. **Domestic food utilisation** is then calculated using data that describe food exports, food added to reserves, food lost to pests and other forms of spoilage and manufacturing, and food used for purposes other than human consumption. By subtracting food utilisation from food supply, the amount of food available for consumption by the population can be calculated, and this can then be converted into a **daily per capita amount** using population data.

The Food and Agriculture Organization of the United Nations (FAO) publishes annual food balance sheets for most countries, dating back to 1961 in most cases. These data can help in the development of agricultural policies that aim to improve production, distribution and consumption of food. They also allow the identification of changes in nutrient intake by tracking trends in the food supply over time, and this information can be used to pinpoint countries that are at an increased risk of dietary inadequacy.

Determining food supply at the national level has a number of inherent limitations. Many calculations are required to determine per capita food supply, and each step can introduce errors. Under-reporting is common for developing countries as food balance sheets do not take into consideration food grown, hunted or gathered for personal use. In addition, food balance sheets cannot describe the disparities in food supply that exist within countries due to economic, seasonal, regional, demographic or socioeconomic differences.

Assessing food consumption at the household level

Household food consumption determines the average food consumption per person based on demographic data available for the household. Per capita nutrient intake is then calculated using food composition data.

Household food consumption record

A household food consumption record provides information on the food consumed within a household. For at least 1 week, the head of the household or a staff member records a description of all foods consumed, including brand, method of preparation and weight. Adjustments are made to incorporate non-household members at meals, as well as meals eaten outside the home. This method requires more effort by respondents, has a low response rate and does not usually determine the amount and types of foods consumed by each individual.

Household 24-h recall method

This method provides information on food consumption for the previous 24 h. The individual who prepares all food within the household is interviewed to obtain detailed descriptions of the quantity of food consumed. This information is converted into a 'per person' food intake by dividing the total amount of food consumed by the number of individuals residing in the household without considering the age and sex distribution of the family members. The household 24-h recall can be used to assess the variety of foods and food groups consumed and the number of households that meet the daily minimum requirements for energy and other nutrients. This method requires the respondent to have a good memory (subjects may not accurately recall their dietary intake).

Assessing food consumption at the individual level

Individual food intake measurement is the most common tool used in nutritional epidemiology. Under-reporting of food intake can occur in all methods as subjects may either fail to record foods eaten or may alter their eating habits. These include 24-h recalls, food records (also called diaries) and weighed food records. These methods assess diet over a 24-h period or longer. If the number of assessment days is increased, an individual's usual food intake can be determined more accurately.

Other dietary assessment methods include dietary histories and food frequency questionnaires. These methods provide information on food patterns and can provide insights into overall usual intake.

The common methods include:

24-h recall method

A 24-h recall provides information on all foods and beverages consumed by an individual during the previous day. Initially, respondents provide a list of all beverages and foods consumed; next, each item is described in detail, including brand name, cooking method and estimated portion size. Food models or common household utensils (such as spoons, cups, etc.) are often provided to assist individuals in estimating portion sizes. Finally, the interviewer checks with the respondent to ensure that no items have been missed, including nutritional supplements or hidden foods like sugar in tea. To prevent biases during recording, interviewers must avoid judgemental comments or leading questions. A series of 24-h recalls performed over weekdays and weekends can be used to assess an individual's usual intake. Respondent burden is minimal, compliance is high, cost is relatively low, and individuals with low literacy levels can participate. Limitations include errors made by respondents with poor memory, difficulty determining whether a single 24-h recall represents typical daily consumption and under-reporting.

Nutrition at a Glance, Second Edition. Edited by Sangita Sharma, Tony Sheehy and Fariba Kolahdooz.
© 2016 John Wiley & Sons, Ltd. Published 2016 by John Wiley & Sons, Ltd.

Food record

A food record is an individual dietary assessment method that requires the respondent to record all beverages and foods consumed at the time of consumption. The record should include detailed descriptions of each food item, including brand name, cooking method and weight or volume. Although this method is quite useful, low response rates are common. Also, individuals often alter their eating habits to decrease the effort required to complete the food record. This method is inaccurate when eating away from the home.

Weighed food records

Individuals are required to weigh all beverages and foods and provide a description of the food, brand name and preparation method. To ensure that the record is indicative of usual intake, weekend days must be included in the record. This method can be accurate and can decrease the likelihood of under-reporting. However, individuals often change their eating habits to make participation more convenient or to impress the investigator. Additionally, respondents must be literate and the high response burden often results in low compliance.

35 Nutritional assessment methods: Dietary assessment II

Aims

1 To describe the purpose, development and use of food frequency questionnaires

2 To consider the strengths and weaknesses of food frequency questionnaires as a tool for dietary assessment

Food Frequency Questionnaires (FFQs) are designed to measure the **frequency** with which foods or food groups are consumed over a specific period of time. They are one of the most widely used methods of dietary assessment in nutritional epidemiology and are particularly suitable for large-scale studies that attempt to evaluate associations between dietary habits and risk of disease.

Like 24-h recalls and diet histories, FFQs are a *retrospective* method of dietary assessment, in that their aim is to measure past consumption of foods.

The underlying principle of the FFQ is to sacrifice precise measurement of food intake (and therefore of nutrient intake) for more crude information relating to an extended period of time. Thus, the FFQ approach is aimed at measuring the *usual* diet rather than *actual* intake.

Format

An FFQ consists of a list of foods or food groups and a number of frequency response categories or options that subjects may choose from (e.g. twice a day, once a week, once a month, etc.)

Generally, FFQs measure food consumption over a 1-week or 1-month period, but sometimes they cover an entire year. The frequency options shown on the FFQ must cover all relevant time periods so that there are no gaps.

The length of the food list depends on the focus of the questionnaire. If the intention is to measure intakes of single nutrients such as calcium or vitamin D, or particular food groups such as fruit and vegetables, the questionnaire may contain relatively few items. However, if the focus is on measuring energy intake or dietary diversity, it could contain 100–200 items or sometimes even more.

> There are three types of FFQ:
> 1 **Qualitative** – These do not measure portion size.
> 2 **Semi-quantitative** – These use standard or reference portion sizes.
> 3 **Quantitative** – These attempt to measure actual portion sizes consumed, with various tools being used to aid estimation.

Development and use of FFQs

FFQs are generally designed so as to rank individuals into broad categories (e.g. *quantiles*) of intake rather than to calculate exact mean intakes. They can either be developed from scratch or adapted from existing, previously validated FFQs.

The choice of foods to include on the FFQ depends on the objectives of the study and on the population being studied, but the foods listed must be *informative*. In other words:

• Each item should be *widely consumed* by the population of interest and/or contain a *large amount* of a particular nutrient of interest.

• To be discriminatory, use of that item should *vary* between individuals.

This requires previous dietary information regarding the target population.

Once the list of foods or food groups has been developed, frequency categories must be assigned that are appropriate to the time frame of interest.

Then, the *reproducibility* and *relative validity* of the FFQ must be evaluated:

• **Reproducibility** refers to the consistency of questionnaire measurements when administered on more than one occasion to the same person at a different time.

• **Relative validity** is the degree to which the questionnaire actually measures what it was designed to measure.

Advantages and disadvantages of FFQs

Advantages

FFQs have a number of advantages over other dietary assessment methods:

• They provide a relatively simple, inexpensive and standardised way of collecting data from a large number of individuals.

• They can easily be interviewer administered, self-administered (if respondents are literate) or even computer administered.

• The time taken to complete an FFQ depends on the length of the food list and on the respondent, but most questionnaires can be completed in 15–30 min. This is a low burden for respondents and so leads to better compliance.

• Data can be processed and computerised easily, and data entry does not require nutritional expertise.

Disadvantages

FFQs also have several limitations:

• Before they can be used in dietary intake studies, FFQs must be validated. This involves comparison with results obtained from a superior standard method (such as a weighed food intake record or multiple 24-h recalls) and calibration studies. This process is time consuming and burdensome.

• When the time frame of an FFQ is short (e.g. 1 week or 1 month), seasonal effects cannot be captured.

• FFQs have a low capacity to obtain information about actual foods consumed because this type of questionnaire provides little information about how foods are consumed (such as cooking methods) and no information about food combinations within a meal.

Nutrition at a Glance, Second Edition. Edited by Sangita Sharma, Tony Sheehy and Fariba Kolahdooz.

- Intake is dependent on the number of items on the food list; the longer the food list, the more likely it is that intake will be overestimated, and conversely, the shorter the list, the more likely it is that intake will be underestimated.
- The complexity of the task that respondents are asked to perform leads to large random errors, which implies an increased variance and so a decrease in precision of the dietary estimates. The effects of random errors can be reduced by increasing the number of observations.
- Use of FFQs is very dependent on having reliable food composition tables for the analysis. The list of foods and portion sizes must be relevant to the population being studied. For a little studied population, this can be a lot of work.

36 Inadequate nutritional intakes: Causes

Aim

1 To consider environmental factors that may contribute to inadequate nutritional intakes

Inadequate intakes of specific nutrients and *excessive or unbalanced* intakes can both result in *malnutrition*, which may cause illness (morbidity) and possibly death (mortality).

Nutritional adequacy is best viewed as a spectrum, rather than having fixed boundaries (Figure 36.1).

Causes of inadequate nutrition and associated diseases

Who is at risk?

Individuals who live in countries with poor food security, or who themselves are food insecure, are at risk of undernutrition, which can manifest as specific nutrient deficiencies, hunger (chronic or seasonal) or prolonged periods of starvation/famine.

Contributory factors

Disease prevalence is affected only in part by medical practice and treatment. Many *environmental* factors have a much greater impact on health outcomes, as they affect all aspects of people's lives (Table 36.1). Examples include globalisation (which affects food availability, pricing and dietary patterns), the political and legislative framework within a country, the extent to which people have access to clean water, sanitation, nutrition and health knowledge and appropriate health care, and their socio-economic status (including the overall status of women in society).

The actual impact these factors may have on the health of any given individual depends on the *personal choices* they make (or are able to make) and their individual *genetic susceptibility*. Owing to this *individual level of response*, the effects of undernutrition may not be seen equally within a household, community or region.

Food supplies may be inadequate in quantity as well as quality. Therefore, inadequate energy intakes may be present in addition to insufficient nutrient intake.

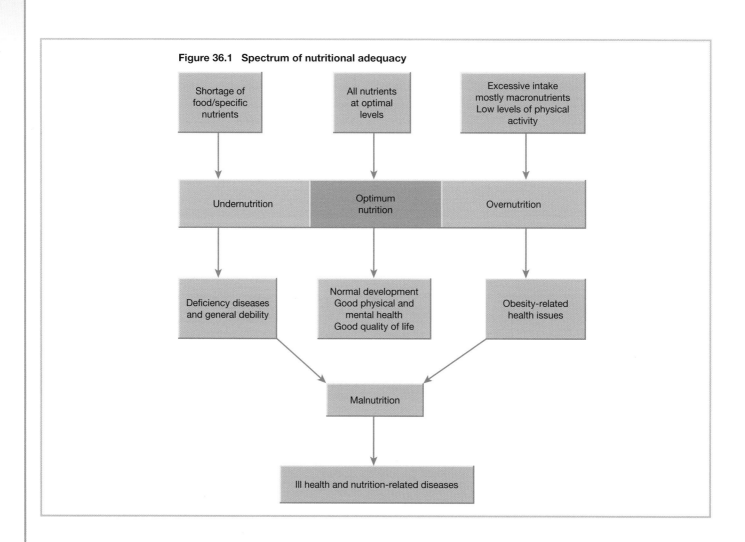

Figure 36.1 Spectrum of nutritional adequacy

Nutrition at a Glance, Second Edition. Edited by Sangita Sharma, Tony Sheehy and Fariba Kolahdooz.
© 2016 John Wiley & Sons, Ltd. Published 2016 by John Wiley & Sons, Ltd.

Table 36.1 Potential impact of environmental factors on health outcomes.

Environmental factor	Consequence with potential impact on nutrition and health
Globalisation of crop production, trade and food supplies	Changes to food availability, access, pricing and dietary patterns
Political and legislative measures	Policies on health, education, agriculture and land ownership, import/export policies, employment, social/welfare policies, and transport (food supplies, access to markets)
Socio-economic status of groups within population	Access (physical and financial) to safe food of adequate nutritional quality
Health-care provision	Access to appropriate health care at all life stages (e.g. immunisation, antenatal care, information on infant/child feeding practices, and early recognition of disease)
Clean water and sanitation	Less infectious diseases and environmental contamination; reduced nutritional needs to fight infections
Education/health and nutrition knowledge	Awareness of the importance of diet and health care, lifestyle habits Better food production techniques by farmers
Status of women	Generally, women may be more likely to integrate health measures within a family; higher status allows women to be involved in decision-making

In some diets, nutrients may appear to be present in sufficient amounts but may be unavailable as a result of:
- **Binding** to other components of the food (e.g. phytate, dietary fibre, proteins)
- **Inactivation** by food preparation methods
- **Inhibition of absorption** by other dietary factors eaten concurrently (e.g. factors that affect intestinal pH)
- **Competition** by parasitic infestation within the gut
- **Poor utilisation** (e.g. lack of carriers for absorption or transport in the blood, due to malnutrition or a genetic defect)
- **Treatment with drugs** that prevent utilisation

Magnitude of the problem

It is difficult to obtain accurate information regarding the extent of undernutrition in the world today because data are either not collected routinely or are affected by sudden crises such as the outbreak of war or the occurrence of environmental disasters. The growing burden of HIV/AIDS and tuberculosis makes an important contribution to undernutrition as well; however, these effects are difficult to quantify.

Despite a theoretically adequate global food supply, the Food and Agriculture Organization (FAO) of the United Nations estimates that there are approximately 868 million undernourished people in the world. The majority live in developing countries, but about 16 million live in developed countries.

Groups at risk for inadequate intakes in developed countries include:
- Large families on low income
- Marginalised groups in society (e.g. minority ethnic groups, refugees)
- The homeless
- Individuals with addictions (e.g. to drugs, alcohol, etc.)
- Those in need of care, but who are not receiving a sufficient amount (e.g. people with disabilities)

Progress is being made internationally in reducing the number of people affected by undernutrition, but results vary from one region to another. The consequences of inadequate nutrition are discussed in Chapter 37.

37 Inadequate nutritional intakes: Consequences

Aim

1 To consider the consequences of inadequate intakes of macronutrients and micronutrients

Assessment

Inadequate macronutrient intake will most obviously be reflected in disturbed growth among children and body weight changes among adults. These effects can be monitored using anthropometric tools (see Chapter 33). Assessment of adolescents is often neglected due to the difficulty of relating measurements to reference standards during puberty. While undernutrition in the elderly is poorly reported, it is believed to be widespread, as this age group may become increasingly dependent for food on other members of their family or communities, and develops a greater risk of disease, which can compromise nutritional status.

Consequences of undernutrition

Undernutrition can have both short- and long-term consequences, including impaired growth rate and cognitive development, reduced work capacity, compromised ability to recover from injury or trauma, increased risk of infection and developing chronic diseases (Figure 37.1). There may also be intergenerational effects through poor pregnancy outcomes and low birth weight.

Macronutrient inadequacies

Protein–energy malnutrition, which reflects serious undernutrition, may present as **marasmus**, **kwashiorkor** or a mixed picture of the two, known as **marasmic kwashiorkor** (Table 37.1). The exact form of the condition depends on feeding patterns.

Micronutrient inadequacies

Deficiencies of **iron**, **zinc**, **vitamin A** and **iodine** affect the greatest numbers of people worldwide (Table 37.2). **Vitamin D** and several other micronutrients may also be widely deficient in populations and contribute to morbidity.

Some micronutrients may become deficient when diets lack specific food groups. These include:
- Vitamin B$_{12}$, when vegan diets are consumed
- Calcium, when dairy products are excluded from the diet
- Riboflavin, when diets are low in green vegetables and dairy products

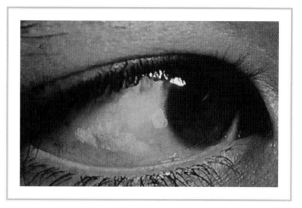

Figure 37.1 Physiological and functional consequences of undernutrition: Bitot's spots, a clinical sign of vitamin A deficiency.

Table 37.1 Conditions associated with a lack of macronutrients.

Condition	Diagnostic signs
Marasmus	Extreme wasting of fat stores and atrophy of visceral tissues; attributed to a severe lack of dietary energy
	Alert but minimal physical activity undertaken
	Normal but shrivelled skin
	Very susceptible to infection
Kwashiorkor	Oedema affecting face, limbs and abdomen, also enlarged liver
	Irritable, lethargic and anorexic
	Skin often cracked and ulcerated, hair colour changes
	Attributed to low protein intake, associated with excessive free radical damage to liver, with insufficient antioxidants
Marasmic kwashiorkor	Severe muscle wasting together with oedema
	Prognosis poor

Consumption of a balanced diet that contains appropriate amounts of foods from all major food groups (see Chapter 39) increases the chance of achieving adequate nutrition. Dietary variety helps to ensure an adequate diet, but may not always be possible if food supplies are limited.

Nutrition at a Glance, Second Edition. Edited by Sangita Sharma, Tony Sheehy and Fariba Kolahdooz.
© 2016 John Wiley & Sons, Ltd. Published 2016 by John Wiley & Sons, Ltd.

Table 37.2 Conditions associated with micronutrient deficiencies.

Nutrient	Numbers affected	Causes	Consequences for health
Iron	About 2 billion people worldwide; mainly women and children	Low iron intake or blood loss due to parasitic and malarial infections	Anaemia; affects cognitive development and behaviour in children, immune function, pregnancy outcome, work capacity
Vitamin A	Up to 250 million children with subclinical vitamin A deficiency; up to 500 000 become blind each year. Pregnant women also affected, transmits to next generation	Low intake of preformed sources of vitamin A and low absorption rates of precursor carotenoids	In the eye: loss of night vision; Bitot's spots, damage to cornea, leading to ulceration and blindness Impaired resistance to infection, increased mortality Affects fetal development, physical growth, haemopoiesis, spermatogenesis Maternal mortality
Iodine	Over 16 million children born with cretinism; up to 50 million affected with poor cognitive development	Low levels in soils; goitrogens interfering with utilisation from the diet Low selenium levels may exacerbate low iodine intakes	Poor mental development in infants born to deficient mothers Stillbirths
Zinc	Up to 2 billion people	Low dietary intake, high levels of absorption inhibitors	Increased risk of infection, reduced resistance Prematurity in infants, growth failure throughout childhood, delayed sexual maturity
Vitamin D	Up to 1 billion people and especially those living in northern climates or who usually cover up	Lack of skin synthesis from sunlight (due to season/latitude, pigmentation, cultural factors or lifestyle), poor dietary intake, high levels of binding factors (e.g. phytate) in diet	Poor bone development in childhood and loss of bone minerals from mature bones

38 Definitions of an adequate diet

Aims

1 To define nutritional requirements
2 To explain the basis of dietary recommendations for energy and nutrients and the use of Dietary Reference Intakes (DRIs)

In defining an adequate diet, it is important to distinguish between the *physiological need* for essential nutrients and the *balance of foods that must be eaten* to provide these nutrients:

- Studies of nutritional requirements provide information about appropriate quantities of nutrients, which can lead to the development of **dietary intake reference values** and **nutrient-based dietary goals** aimed at groups or populations.
- However, people generally do not eat food with the conscious awareness that they are consuming nutrients. Therefore, for practical purposes any definitions of an adequate diet must be expressed in terms of **food-based dietary guidelines**. To do this, knowledge of the major nutrient groups provided by different foods is required (this is considered in Chapter 39).

Nutritional requirements

A certain amount of every nutrient is used up by the body every day, and this amount must be replaced through the diet or derived from body stores.

For some nutrients, a daily intake is not critical as only a small proportion of available stores is used each day. However, if the daily needs are provided from body stores over an extended period of time, these stores gradually become depleted, the functional form of the nutrient becomes unavailable, and eventually a clinical deficiency develops. For some nutrients, there is only minimal storage capacity, and therefore, a regular intake is necessary. Given the uncertainties, it is preferable to aim for an adequate intake of all nutrients every day.

A *requirement* is defined as the amount of a specific nutrient required by an individual to prevent clinical signs of deficiency. Two problems arise from this definition:

- The possibility that depletion of reserves to a level just short of clinical deficiency may still be harmful to health or that amounts greater than the minimum may have a positively beneficial effect.
- It is difficult to quantify requirements for nutrients that have no definable deficiency state.

Nevertheless, ascertaining nutrient requirements is necessary for guidance on adequate diets.

Dietary Reference Intakes

Requirements within a population are generally assumed to be normally distributed (Figure 38.1). Dietary Reference Intakes (DRIs) are reference values for normal and healthy individuals and include the Estimated Average Requirement (EAR), Recommended Dietary Allowance (RDA), Adequate Intake (AI) and Tolerable Upper Intake Level (UL).

EAR – The EAR is the median daily nutrient intake that satisfies the needs of approximately half of the healthy individuals in a specific age or gender group. Some individuals will have needs greater than or less than the EAR. This value is not ideal for advising individuals' nutrient requirements, but can be used to determine the percentage of a group that has inadequate nutrient intake. For energy, the Estimated Energy Requirement (EER) is used. For certain nutrients, the EAR has not been determined (e.g. vitamin K, pantothenic acid, biotin, Manganese, and choline).

RDA – The RDA is the daily average minimum nutrient intake that is sufficient for approximately 97.5% of the healthy individuals in a specific age or gender group. An RDA is considered to be two standard deviations above an EAR.

AI – For nutrients where there is insufficient information to set an RDA, an AI may be set to give a general target figure. The AI is a daily median nutrient intake value based on approximations from studies of healthy individuals. Similar to RDAs, an individual whose usual intake meets or exceeds the AI is at low risk of inadequate intake. AIs are much less reliable than RDAs and must be used with caution. Unlike RDAs, AIs can be used for a group; however, RDAs and AIs are more suitable for individuals. AIs are used in cases where RDA is unavailable (e.g. fibre and vitamin K).

UL – The UL indicates the largest daily nutrient intake shown to harbour no adverse side effects to a large majority of the individuals in a particular age or gender group. Any intake beyond the UL increases an individual's risk of experiencing adverse effects. ULs can be used to estimate the number of individuals within a group that are at risk for adverse effects due to excessive consumption of a particular nutrient. ULs are unavailable for biotin, pantothenic acid, riboflavin, thiamin, vitamin K and vitamin B_{12}; however, caution must still be used when consuming these nutrients.

Macronutrient recommendations

Carbohydrates, fat and protein are energy sources that can compensate for one another to some extent to meet an individual's energy requirements. In some countries (e.g. the USA and Canada), recommendations for adequate macronutrient intake are given in percentage ranges called **Acceptable Macronutrient Distribution Ranges** (AMDRs). These values are expressed as a percentage of the total energy consumed (Table 38.1).

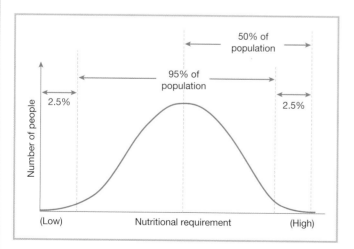

Figure 38.1 Basis of dietary reference values

Nutrition at a Glance, Second Edition. Edited by Sangita Sharma, Tony Sheehy and Fariba Kolahdooz.
© 2016 John Wiley & Sons, Ltd. Published 2016 by John Wiley & Sons, Ltd.

Table 38.1 Acceptable macronutrient distribution ranges for men and women.

Age (years)	Total carbohydrate (%/total energy)	Total protein (%/total energy)	Total fat (%/total energy)	n-6 Polyunsaturated fatty acids* (%/total energy)	n-3 Polyunsaturated fatty acids† (%/total energy)	Added sugars (%/total energy)
1–3	45–65	5–20	30–40	5–10	0.6–1.2	≤25
4–18	45–65	10–30	25–35	5–10	0.6–1.2	≤25
≥19	45–65	10–35	20–35	5–10	0.6–1.2	≤25

*Linoleic acid.
†α-Linolenic acid.

AMDRs are based on evidence relating to the risk of reducing chronic diseases, such as diabetes and obesity. Additional recommendations have been made for added sugars, *trans-* and saturated fatty acids and cholesterol. There is no calculated range for *trans-* and saturated fatty acids and cholesterol, but individuals are recommended to keep their intake as low as possible to avoid increasing their risk of developing coronary heart disease.

Summary

DRIs are sets of nutrient reference values that can be used to assess diets, help prevent disease and avoid overconsumption of specific nutrients. DRIs are based on the dietary requirements of healthy populations and are to be used by healthy individuals and groups. They can be used to assess the usual intakes of both individuals and populations, but they are not recommended for use as indicators of dietary adequacy because DRIs are mean values. EAR can be used to determine the percentage of a group that has inadequate nutrient intake.

While DRIs can provide the basis for dietary advice, to be useful to the general public, these values need to be expressed in terms of foods. This is considered in Chapter 39.

Information about requirements

Information about nutrient requirements is obtained in a variety of ways, depending on the nutrient:
- Actual intakes in apparently healthy populations
- Amounts needed to achieve balance in the body (amount taken in = amount utilised or lost)
- Amounts needed to reverse clinical signs of deficiency
- Amounts needed to achieve tissue saturation or normalise a biochemical or biological marker

39 Creating an adequate diet

Aims

1 To describe 'healthy eating'
2 To show how dietary recommendations can be used in variety of ways to produce guidelines for an adequate diet

An **adequate diet** is one that:
- Contains all the nutrients listed in the Dietary Reference Intakes (DRIs) tables, in amounts that meet the requirement for an individual's age and sex
- Supports health and allows the individual to fulfil all their work and leisure activities
- Provides sufficient reserves to protect against nutritional deficiencies during periods of poor food intake (e.g. short periods of illness)
- Offers some protection against diseases

These points encompass the principles of *healthy eating*. However, it can be difficult for most people to evaluate their diet by these standards without information about nutrient content of foods, which has to be obtained from food composition tables. Practical suggestions for healthy eating can be provided to consumers in the form of **food-based dietary guidelines** (Appendix B1).

A balanced diet

The concept of a *balanced diet* is based on the nutritional composition of related foods, which can be classified into food groups. Diets containing appropriate amounts of these food groups, relative to one another, are nutritionally 'balanced'.

This concept is utilised in a variety of *food planning guides*, such as the 'pyramid' (as used in some countries in Asia, the USA and the Mediterranean) or 'plate' (as used in the UK) models. In general, these models recommend a diet that is mainly composed of plant foods (grains, pulses, fruits and vegetables), dairy products, meat and fish.

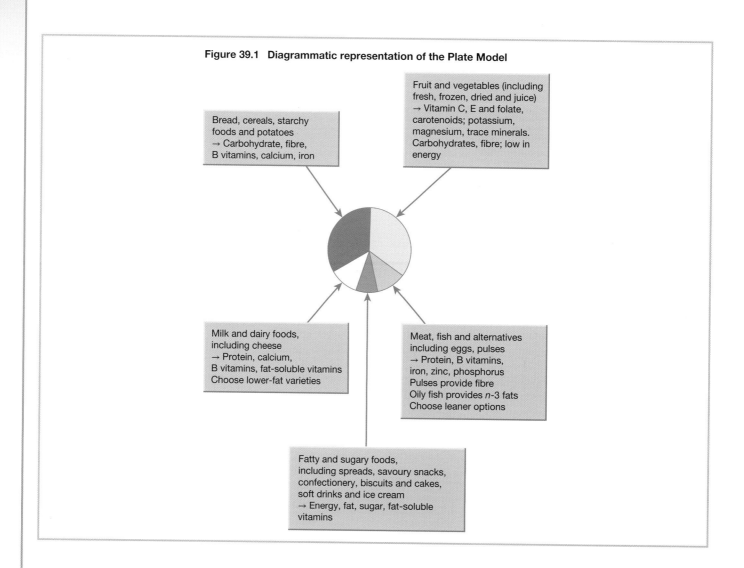

Figure 39.1 Diagrammatic representation of the Plate Model

Bread, cereals, starchy foods and potatoes
→ Carbohydrate, fibre, B vitamins, calcium, iron

Fruit and vegetables (including fresh, frozen, dried and juice) → Vitamin C, E and folate, carotenoids; potassium, magnesium, trace minerals. Carbohydrates, fibre; low in energy

Milk and dairy foods, including cheese
→ Protein, calcium, B vitamins, fat-soluble vitamins
Choose lower-fat varieties

Meat, fish and alternatives including eggs, pulses
→ Protein, B vitamins, iron, zinc, phosphorus
Pulses provide fibre
Oily fish provides *n*-3 fats
Choose leaner options

Fatty and sugary foods, including spreads, savoury snacks, confectionery, biscuits and cakes, soft drinks and ice cream
→ Energy, fat, sugar, fat-soluble vitamins

Nutrition at a Glance, Second Edition. Edited by Sangita Sharma, Tony Sheehy and Fariba Kolahdooz.
© 2016 John Wiley & Sons, Ltd. Published 2016 by John Wiley & Sons, Ltd.

The Plate Model (Balance of Good Health)

According to the Plate Model, the cereals and starchy foods group and the fruits and vegetables group should each comprise one-third of the diet. The remaining third should be composed of meat, fish and alternatives (12%) and dairy products (15%), with only a small proportion of the diet coming from foods that are rich in fat and sugar (8%) (Figure 39.1).

This balanced diet should be achieved over the course of the day, but not necessarily at every meal. Additional advice has evolved from the Plate Model, such as the promotion of *five a day* for fruits and vegetables or *three a day* for dairy products. It should be remembered that the Plate Model, like other pictorial representations used in various countries, is simply a guide and provides an overview of the relative proportions of the diet. The *key objective is to consume a mixture of foods* and include as much variety as possible. No foods are specifically excluded, and none are essential – there is no implicit labelling of 'good' and 'bad' foods. Nevertheless, some foods should be eaten in greater amounts such as fruits and vegetables and others only occasionally.

'Traffic light' labelling

Advances in the way foods are labelled are being developed in many countries, to make it easier for people to choose foods that contribute to a balanced diet. For example, in the UK, foods may be labelled with series of traffic light symbols – green, amber and red, based on target levels of intake for particular nutrients – to provide a guide to foods that can be eaten freely without compromising dietary quality and those whose intake should be limited. This is an area of considerable debate, however, as some foods may be 'green' for one nutrient but 'red' for another.

Summary

Food-based dietary guidelines, pictorial representations of a balanced diet and additional information on food labels can help consumers achieve an adequate and healthy diet even though they may be unaware of nutritional requirement figures.

Healthy eating

Healthy eating advice can be formulated in fairly general terms, for example:
- Eat lots of fruits and vegetables.
- Eat more fish – including a portion of oily fish each week.
- Cut down on saturated fat and sugar.
- Try to eat less sodium – no more than 2 g a day (equivalent to 5 g of salt daily) for adults.
- Get active and try to maintain a healthy weight (exercise 30 min a day).
- Drink plenty of water.
- Don't skip breakfast.

Applying food-based dietary guidelines

Although the principle of food-based dietary guidelines is straightforward, their application may sometimes be confusing. Common questions include:
- Which food groups do composite dishes count towards (e.g. meat and vegetable mixtures, pizza)?
- How big is a portion?
- What about alcohol?
- Do the guidelines apply to young or old people, to people with small appetites or to those on special diets?
- Do they apply to people from different cultures?

40 Optimising nutrition

Aims

1 To consider the concept of 'optimal nutrition'
2 To discuss different ways in which optimal nutrition might be achieved

Advances in nutritional knowledge have led to awareness that:
- For each nutrient, a certain *minimum quantity* must be provided so that its *basic physiological role* is carried out.
- *Amounts greater than this* can maintain normal function in health and, in addition, provide a *reserve* against inadequate intakes or greater needs.
- *Intakes above these levels* may operate in *non-nutritional* or protective ways, but for some nutrients, there is an upper level of acceptance.
- *Other factors in foods*, which *do not have a clear nutritional role*, may also be beneficial to health.

Thus, the concept of nutritional adequacy can cover a very wide spectrum ranging from 'preventing deficiency' to 'optimal nutrition' to excessive.

Some populations in the world have inadequate access to food because of limited resources or poor availability and may not be able to reach even the very minimum level of nutritional adequacy, while at the other end of the spectrum, in the richer countries, food companies produce an ever-expanding range of special products that aim to optimise health through nutrition and can even cause excessive intake.

Balanced diet

In essence, a balanced diet is constructed using *major food groups*, which are broadly classified according to the main nutrients they provide. These are quantified into numbers of servings so that the individual will consume a mixture of foods, and therefore nutrients, that should be sufficient to meet their requirements.

Optimal nutrition

The recognition that there are dietary links in the aetiology of many diseases has led to the concept of optimal nutritional status.

For a dietary constituent, this is the level of intake that is required for:
- Maintenance of good health and prevention of overt nutritional deficiency and its associated health risks
- Reduction of chronic disease risk

Achieving optimal nutrition

Nutritional status can be improved in a number of ways for those at risk of deficiency, including:
- Supplementary feeding
- Fortification of specific food commodities
- Use of dietary supplements
- Introduction of functional foods into the diet

Changes in nutritional behaviour can also be brought about through approaches that change knowledge, skills and attitudes.

Supplementary feeding

Vulnerable groups in the population may be targeted with a specific supplementary feeding programme based on an assessed need.

This may be achieved by providing:
- A balanced supplement containing macro- and micronutrients
- One that contains a particular micronutrient that had been found to be lacking (e.g. iron)

This type of programme is most commonly used with vulnerable groups (e.g. pregnant women and children) in situations of under-nutrition or disrupted food supplies.

Fortification of foods

The addition of a nutrient or nutrients to a widely consumed food can target an entire population group. Issues to consider include the chemical form of the nutrient, the vehicle used for fortification, its acceptability, its stability and its cost.

Some food products (e.g. white flour, bread, other grain products, margarine, salt and milk) are fortified by law in different countries (i.e. mandatory fortification):
- There can also be voluntary fortification of certain products by food companies, including breakfast cereals, dairy products (e.g. yogurts, milk and spreads), infant foods, fruit juices and other beverages.

There is a growing trend towards the production of fortified foods that promise protection against disease, such as osteoporosis, heart disease and cancer, and containing a range of vitamins or minerals.

The impact of fortification on nutritional status depends on the degree of 'market saturation' with the fortified product. If alternatives are available, then its effectiveness will be reduced.

Points to consider include:
- Mandatory addition of folic acid to flour in the USA, Canada and other countries has resulted in a measurable reduction in the incidence of pregnancies affected by neural tube defects.
- Iodisation of salt is an extremely effective public health measure for reducing the incidence of goitre and cretinism.
- Even with a choice of products available, fortification of a relatively common product (e.g. breakfast cereal) can raise the nutritional status of vulnerable groups, such as older adults, across a range of nutrients.

Functional foods

This term covers a wide variety of products that carry the common claim of possessing some health-promoting properties. This could be applied to many normal foods but is more specifically used to describe foods that are rich in non-nutritional factors that are either naturally present or have been added to achieve a possible health benefit (see Chapter 74).

Nutrition at a Glance, Second Edition. Edited by Sangita Sharma, Tony Sheehy and Fariba Kolahdooz.
© 2016 John Wiley & Sons, Ltd. Published 2016 by John Wiley & Sons, Ltd.

Other dietary supplements

There is a wide diversity of dietary supplements on the market, some of which are derived from common foods and others from plants that are not normally consumed as part of the diet. Although they may be perceived as enhancing *nutritional status*, this can only be the case when the supplement taken is a nutrient. In all other cases, the effect is non-nutritional.

Non-nutritional supplements may be taken to:
• Prevent or treat diseases that are not the result of deficiency (e.g. reducing menstrual symptoms, trying to prevent a cold, stimulating the immune system, increasing mental alertness, relieving arthritic pain)
• Enhance sporting performance (e.g. ergogenic aids, muscle-building products, body-shaping products)

In both cases, the evidence is generally weak and not supported by clinical trials.

Preventing deficiency

Figures published in Dietary Reference Intake (DRI) tables provide the scientific basis on which nutrient-based guidelines and dietary goals are formulated.

In practical terms, it is easier for consumers to relate to *food-based guidelines*, which therefore form the basis of advice about balanced diets.

Quantifying optimal nutrition

At present, information about optimal levels of nutrients is incomplete. More research is needed about both individual influences and nutrient functions, including:
• What is the functional bioavailability of a nutrient?
• What is the key marker of nutrient *status* that is sensitive to changes in intake?

• What is the key marker of nutrient *function* that is sensitive to changes in status?

There are many factors that may influence the above, related to:
• Individual variability (genetic, ethnicity, environment, social factors, age, and sex)
• Different responses at certain life stages and how these can lead to disease
• Interaction between dietary constituents, affecting their bioavailability

Reduced-nutrient foods

Some foods may have a reduced content of a nutrient:
• Lower fat or lower sugar products are designed to achieve a reduction in calories.
• Low-salt foods may be formulated to reduce the sodium content.
• There are also special products that cater for consumers requiring products low in lactose, milk-free, gluten-free, etc.

Organic foods

Consumers generally believe that foods produced organically, often by more traditional agricultural methods, have superior nutritional quality. This is not currently supported by the scientific literature, in which studies find no difference in nutrient content between organic and non-organic produce; there is also no information about impact on human health. It is, however, probable that organic foods contain little or no residual levels of pesticides and herbicides.

At the present time, organic food is more expensive, and this may mitigate against consumption of an adequately diverse diet. It is preferable therefore to ensure adequate intake of a balanced diet, even if this is not organically produced. There is more evidence supporting the need for a good healthful range of foods than for the benefits of organic food.

41 Excessive or unbalanced nutritional intakes

Aims

1 To discuss malnutrition resulting from overnutrition and unbalanced diets

2 To identify dietary factors commonly associated with overnutrition and unbalanced diets

Overnutrition and unbalanced diets can lead to increased morbidity and mortality from *nutrition-related non-communicable diseases* (NR-NCDs) such as cardiovascular disease, diabetes and cancer. NR-NCDs may coexist with undernutrition within some populations (Table 41.1). Both overnutrition and unbalanced diets result in various forms of malnutrition with consequent ill health. These are summarised in Figure 41.1.

NR-NCDs may occur in societies that have undergone a number of transitions or are currently undergoing transitions (see Chapter 68) including:

• Improvements in health care and infection control, resulting in increased lifespan

• Opportunities to improve living standards and acquire more food

• Increased industrialisation and urbanisation, resulting in reduced workloads and energy expenditure

• Globalisation, which leads to the introduction of foods with higher energy density resulting in increased energy consumption

Dietary components and nutrients responsible for overnutrition and unbalanced diets

A number of dietary factors play key roles in the development of nutrition-related diseases.

Fat

Many 'fast foods' and 'convenience food products' contain large amounts of fat. A diet rich in fat is likely to confer a positive energy balance because fat is energy-dense. Reducing the percentage of fat in the diet is generally associated with weight loss.

Specific components of fat intake that are potentially associated with diseases are listed below:
• Saturated fats are positively related to plasma cholesterol levels and risk of coronary heart disease.
• An appropriate ratio of saturated, monounsaturated and polyunsaturated fats is important for protection against coronary heart disease.
• An appropriate ratio of *n*-6 to *n*-3 fatty acid consumption (between 2:1 and 3:1) is desirable for brain development and

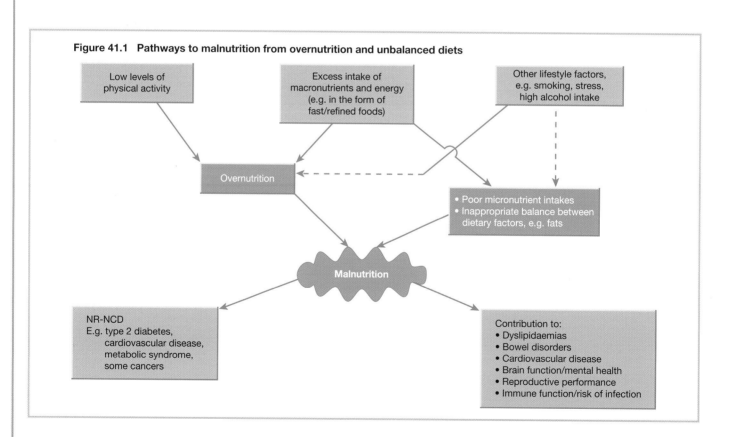

Figure 41.1 Pathways to malnutrition from overnutrition and unbalanced diets

Nutrition at a Glance, Second Edition. Edited by Sangita Sharma, Tony Sheehy and Fariba Kolahdooz.
© 2016 John Wiley & Sons, Ltd. Published 2016 by John Wiley & Sons, Ltd.

mental health and may influence coronary heart disease risk and inflammatory responses.

Consumption of *trans*-fatty acids has been associated with many NR-NCDs, including cancer, coronary heart disease and type 2 diabetes.

Sugar

Foods and drinks containing large amounts of sugar have spread around the world due to globalisation of the food supply:

• Excessive sugar intake is associated with dental caries. Infants and young children are particularly prone to dental caries due to frequent consumption of sugar-rich liquids and/or foods.

• Consumption of soft drinks, which contain 'hidden' sugar, results in excessive energy consumption and may contribute to overweight, especially in young people.

Complex carbohydrates

Generally, digestion and absorption of complex carbohydrates take longer than simple sugars, resulting in slower release of glucose into the bloodstream. Consequently, these carbohydrates have a lower glycaemic effect and fewer metabolic consequences:

• Many foods rich in complex carbohydrates are also rich in dietary fibre. Fibre is beneficial for weight control, bowel function and serum cholesterol.

Alcohol

Alcohol can contribute to excessive energy intake. However, not all studies show an association between large intakes of alcohol and weight gain.

Alcohol consumption can lead to decreased breakdown of fatty acids for fuel and may increase fatty acid biosynthesis.

Alcohol consumption may disrupt normal food intake in heavy drinkers, leading to undernutrition or potentially malnutrition. The most common nutrient deficiency in heavy drinkers is thiamin deficiency.

Antioxidant nutrients

Antioxidants, including vitamins C and E, the carotenoids and certain other phytochemicals, may be inadequate in low-quality diets that are high in macronutrients. Such diets are likely to be lacking in fruit and vegetables. A large body of research implicates low antioxidant status in the development of NR-NCDs, although supplementation trials with individual antioxidants have not always yielded positive results.

Table 41.1 Key dietary factors linked to overnutrition or unbalanced diets.

Overconsumption	Underconsumption
Total fat; also saturated and possibly *n*-6 fatty acids	*n*-3 fatty acids, especially in relation to high intakes of *n*-6 fatty acids
Sources of refined carbohydrate, for example, sugars	Complex carbohydrates, with low glycaemic index, for example, whole plant foods
Alcoholic beverages	Antioxidant nutrients, present in foods of plant origin, such as fruit and vegetables
Salt (as sodium), particularly from processed foods	Potassium (e.g. from fruit and vegetables), which may counterbalance high sodium intakes

Nutritional supplements

Excessive intakes of nutrients, usually in the form of supplements, can be harmful:

• There are physiological mechanisms regulating nutrient absorption, transport and excretion that protect against potentially toxic levels of nutrients. These mechanisms may fail under certain circumstances (examples include excessive alcohol intake, some genetic disorders and renal insufficiency).

• Excessive absorption of various nutrients can be harmful. These nutrients include some fat-soluble vitamins (e.g. vitamins A and D) and many minerals (e.g. copper, iron, magnesium and selenium).

• To protect the public against excessive intakes, many countries and the FAO/WHO have established upper limits for safe nutritional supplement intakes.

Summary

The lifestyle and diet changes during the last decades influence diet quality, which affects the prevalence of nutrition-related chronic diseases including high prevalence of overweight and obesity. However, undernutrition remains a serious problem in many populations. This poses a major challenge for health-care systems, which may be faced with the two extremes of the food consumption spectrum and thus have to deal with a *double burden of malnutrition*.

Food choice: Individual, social and cultural factors

Aim

1 To describe the factors that can influence an individual's choice of foods

To achieve an intake of nutrients that will meet the physiological requirements and provide optimal health, it is necessary to make an *appropriate choice of foods*. Food choice is affected by many factors, including those that relate to:

- The individual (internal factors)
- The cultural and social context within which the food is consumed (external factors)
- The food itself (discussed in Chapter 43)

Understanding these factors is critical when undertaking any initiative that tries to change peoples' food intakes.

Food habits

Food choices are a component of *food habits*, the typical behaviours surrounding food as practised by a group of people. Food habits determine not only the type of foods chosen but also mealtimes, number of meals consumed, food preparation methods, meal participants, portion sizes and ways of eating (Figure 42.1).

Internal (individual) factors determining food choices

The drive to eat is underpinned by **physiological** and **psychological** factors (Table 42.1). Psychological influences may modify or override the physiological need for food; examples of this include binge eating and refusal to eat as a result of depression. Internal factors cannot be separated from the external environment in which these responses have developed.

Table 42.1 Summary of the main physiological and psychological factors believed to have a role in the internal control of food choice.

Factor	Expression	Comments
Physiological factors		
Hunger	Need to eat	Often determined by habit
Satiation/ satiety	Stops food intake/ prevents subsequent eating	May be overridden if presented with a variety of foods
Psychological factors		
Appetite	Desire for specific foods, based on experience	Not thought to be linked to nutritional need
Aversion	Avoidance of specific foods, from (perceived) experience	May severely restrict food choices
Preference	Established by frequency of exposure and early learning. May also be linked to genetic differences in taste sensitivities	Sets specific taste thresholds, for example, to sugar and salt; also resistance to new tastes (neophobia)
Emotions (mood, stress)	Specific foods associated with positive or negative emotions	May lead to comfort eating or food refusal

External factors

These are determined by the social and cultural context and inevitably affect both development and persistence of internal factors, as well as food availability and accessibility.

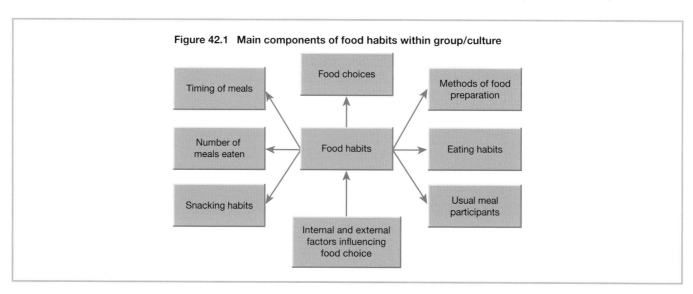

Figure 42.1 Main components of food habits within group/culture

Timing of meals

Food choices

Methods of food preparation

Number of meals eaten

Food habits

Eating habits

Snacking habits

Usual meal participants

Internal and external factors influencing food choice

Culture

Culture is a major determinant of food choice because it confers and reinforces identity and belonging, and underlines differences from other cultures. Cultural influences may be overt (staple food or most popular dish) or subtle (seasonings used or method of cooking). The finding that migrants maintain their cultural identity by retaining food choices has been reported in many studies.

Culture defines what is acceptable as food and may identify subgroups for which certain foods are unacceptable. For example, not all food is considered appropriate for children or during pregnancy (e.g. alcoholic drinks).

Religion

Religion frequently determines the broad context of food choice. Many religions lay down rules about which foods are permitted and when these foods may or may not be eaten. Common examples include prohibitions on specific types of meat and methods of slaughter. Restrictions may also be placed on cooking methods and food combinations, and rules may also include periods of fasting, rituals and festivals. Followers of different faiths may experience constraints in food choice but may gain a sense of identity through adherence to their religion's dietary guidelines.

Ethical decisions

The way food is produced may affect people's food choices. Many people have concerns about the way in which animals are reared and slaughtered, as well as the potential for some agricultural methods to be environmentally damaging. People who have these concerns may alter their food choices to match their ethical principles, such as by choosing organically produced food or by becoming vegetarian.

Economic factors

Within any cultural or religious grouping, the ability to access food in exchange for money, goods or services is a critical factor determining food choice. Better economic status can enable individuals to obtain larger amounts and increased variety of food choices, whereas people living in poverty or on low incomes may have fewer food choices. This may be the result of limited food availability or food accessibility or a combination of both.

Social norms

The accepted behaviour within an individual's social circle in relation to food plays a strong influence on food choice. This is exerted through peer pressure and reinforces expectations about food. It may perpetuate food choices along gender lines, where some foods are perceived as being more 'masculine' (red meat and beer), whereas others are more 'feminine' (salads and white wine). Social norms may also determine the status of foods, with some foods being perceived as more prestigious (often expensive), for example, caviar and champagne, and therefore used to impress others or used on special occasions only.

Media and advertising

Media and advertising often focus on foods that have been processed or manufactured and are less nutritionally dense. Exposure to advertising increases awareness of and demand for the promoted foods. Children who watch television regularly have the highest intake of advertised foods.

Summary

Social and cultural factors have a significant influence on food choices, even among consumers who are not conscious of this. These modify or override physiological and psychological factors and can have either positive or negative consequences on total food intake.

43 Food choice: The food environment

Aims

1 To consider the way in which foods are classified within diets
2 To show how the nature of food influences people's food choices

Over recent decades, the rapid globalisation of the food industry (including the ways in which food is produced, processed, transported, stored and marketed) has had a major effect on the nature of the dietary patterns around the world. This changing food environment inevitably affects people's food choices, as traditional foods lose their predominance in the diet and are replaced by store-bought foods. People's expectations of food availability and food choices also change as foods that were only seasonally available may now be obtained all year-round.

Classification of foods

Traditionally, diets have been described as being composed of **core**, **secondary** and **peripheral** foods (Table 43.1). Core foods would consist of staple foods (e.g. bread, potato or rice), or foods that tend to be consumed several times a day. Secondary foods would be foods that enhance a meal, but would not necessarily be consumed at every meal. Peripheral foods would not be considered an essential part of the diet, but might be consumed as a treat.

The knowledge of what constitutes a 'meal' has been transmitted through generations, and new foods have been subsumed into this structure accordingly as they have become available. Food choice, therefore, has been made on the basis of foods that when eaten together would constitute a meal or were suitable as a snack. The concept of a meal is also changing with some people consuming a pattern of smaller snacks throughout the day rather than following the traditional pattern of larger meals. Some snacks continue to fit into the patterns shown in Table 43.1. For example, a sandwich consists of bread (a core food) plus filling (secondary food), while a packet of chips is essentially a starchy food (potato), albeit with added fat and salt. Other snacks comprise just a secondary food, such as a piece of fruit, or a milk-based drink. Confectionery or soft drinks, which are often consumed as snacks, are peripheral foods, often with low nutritional value.

Recent developments in food technology have led to the creation of new foods that do not fit very easily into the traditional pattern of meals. For example, breakfast cereal bars, which are designed to be eaten on the way to work, and meal replacement drinks, which are sold to encourage weight loss, do not really fit into any of the above categories. Likewise, the addition of nutrients to certain products to enrich them (e.g. orange juice fortified with calcium) alters the nutritional identity of such items and creates difficulties for health educators when it comes to advising the public on how to make dietary changes.

The nature of the food available

In order for an individual to make a particular food choice, the food itself must be available and palatable, and the person must know about it. Food availability depends on a person's ability to access shops and markets and to afford the food available within them, which is variable. Indeed, some urban areas referred to as 'food deserts' have been described as having few or no food stores at all.

Environmental concerns may also influence food choices for some people, since there is a growing awareness about how far food is transported and the environmental costs of *food miles*.

Palatability is the ultimate determinant of food choice, as foods that people perceive as unpalatable will not be purchased in the first place and foods that people discover to be unpalatable will not be repurchased. This creates a challenge for food producers, technologists and quality controllers to minimise spoilage and maintain safety of the product. Aspects involved in availability and palatability are summarised in Table 43.2.

Table 43.1 Traditional classification of foods within diets.

Core foods	Secondary foods	Peripheral foods
Foods that tend to occur in the diet several times in the day – usually include the 'staple' food of the population group, for example, cereal and starchy foods *Nutritionally*: generally a source of energy, carbohydrate, some protein, some minerals and vitamins	Foods that enhance the meal by adding variety and extra colour/texture/flavour; not considered vital to have at every meal Often include sources of protein, for example, meat, fish, dairy products and pulses, vegetables and fruit *Nutritionally*: often a source of protein, additional minerals and vitamins	Foods that are not considered an essential part of the diet, but are pleasant to eat May be seen as a treat or extra item May also include foods only eaten at special occasions Includes drinks, for example, tea and coffee *Nutritionally*: may be rich in fats, salt and sugars

Nutrition at a Glance, Second Edition. Edited by Sangita Sharma, Tony Sheehy and Fariba Kolahdooz.
© 2016 John Wiley & Sons, Ltd. Published 2016 by John Wiley & Sons, Ltd.

Table 43.2 Summary of the major factors associated with availability and palatability of foods.

	Factors involved	Comments
Availability of food	Physical/geographical factors in production	Large out-of-town shops may limit access for some consumers
	Transport and marketing arrangements (for both the food and the consumer)	24-h shopping can increase availability
	Storage facilities	Small convenience stores may not sell healthy items
	Seasonality	Some food and drink items may only be available during particular seasons
Palatability	Appeal to the visual and olfactory senses is the key to initial selection	Criteria of palatability vary with different foods
	Taste, flavour and texture (hedonic appeal) also determine palatability	Fat and sugar combinations often associated with high levels of hedonic appeal
		Advertisers have to overcome resistance to new, unknown flavours and textures

Changing food choices

Research on moving consumers towards healthier food choices has not been very systematic to date. It is very difficult to make a large change in food choice, monitor and measure this and study any health outcome. Thus, tailored approaches are needed that address different groups in the population and particular aspects of food choice.

Specific strategies that are appropriate for the target group might include computer or social media-based interventions, supermarket-based interventions, sports club-based interventions and peer-led interventions for children, adolescents and ethnic minority groups.

The environment in which change is expected must be supportive and not conflict with the aims of the change process.

Only by integrating what is known about factors that influence food choice with proposed intervention methods can change be achieved.

Table 43.3 Summary of influences on food choice.

Internal (individual) factors	External (social/cultural) factors	Nature of the food
Appetite	Culture	Availability
Aversion	Religion	Palatability
Preference	Ethical decisions	
Emotions	Economic factors	
Personality traits	Social norms	
Mood and stress	Education/health awareness	
Health/illness	Media and advertising	
	Availability and accessibility of food	

Summary

Food choice is an immensely complicated issue. Individual, social and cultural factors interact with the food environment to influence individual behaviour. The food environment itself is the product of many commercial decisions, reflected in marketing strategies, pricing policies and advertising. The influences discussed in Chapters 42 and 43 are summarised in Table 43.3.

44 Nutrition in ethnic minority groups and potential impact of religion on diet

Aims

1 To consider the dietary implications of migration
2 To consider the dietary practices associated with certain religions and their potential nutritional implications

Global migration

Global migration is accelerating as the world's population increases and as many countries face labour shortages and ageing populations. In 2010, the WHO estimated the total number of international immigrants to be 214 million.

The extensive movement of people around the world means that immigrants often represent a sizeable minority of a country's population, which has important implications for its health policies and programmes.

In 2011, 1.7 million people emigrated to the European Union (EU), with an additional 1.3 million people moving between member countries within the EU. The UK received the largest number of immigrants, with more than 566 000 people calling the UK their new home. Germany with 489 000 new immigrants, Spain with 458 000 new immigrants and Italy with 386 000 new immigrants rounded out the top four host countries with the most new settlers. As of 1 January 2012, there were 20.7 million foreign-born individuals residing in an EU country, representing 4.1% of the total EU population.

The USA reported having approximately 13.3 million legal permanent resident immigrants at the beginning of 2012. In addition to the immigrant population, more than 58 000 people entered the USA during 2012 as refugees, and almost 30 000 people were granted asylum.

Within Canada, 20.6% of the population in 2011 was foreign born, representing some 6 775 800 individuals, and 6 264 800 individuals self-identified as a visible minority, an almost 3% increase over 2006 census data. This increase in visible minorities is due to a larger proportion of immigrants coming to Canada from non-European countries, with visible minorities representing 78.0% of immigrants between 2006 and 2011 compared to 12.4% prior to 1974.

The nutritional relevance of migration

There is a long tradition of migration around the world, and the offspring of the original migrants may either come to see the host country as their own or retain a feeling of *otherness*. Retention of dietary practices that reflect the 'home' country serves to maintain a cultural connection. Although these traditional dietary practices may be healthy and balanced, they may become less so when practised in the host country and consequently lead to nutritional vulnerability.

Compared with the general population, immigrants face the same economic and social forces that guide food access and availability, such as income, religion, health, gender and time availability. However, they often experience these forces more acutely due to having lower incomes, traditional foods not being readily available and the cost of traditional foods being much greater than other foods within the host country.

Adoption of a Western-type diet is common when individuals move to a Western country. These dietary changes most often result in an increased intake of **simple carbohydrates**, **total fat**, **sodium**, **processed foods**, **animal proteins** and **overall calories**. This is usually the result of a *decreased consumption of plant-based foods* and an *increased consumption of animal-based foods*. However, the flow of dietary practices goes both ways, and increased familiarity with ethnic foods can enrich the diet of a country's original population.

Dietary acculturation

Dietary acculturation is often experienced by immigrants once they begin to settle, including the adoption of mainstream eating habits and food choices. The process of dietary acculturation is experienced differently by individuals, depending on gender and generation, with children more likely to adopt the eating habits of their peers. New members of a country often try to incorporate their traditional foods into the mainstream food culture, adopting new methods of cooking and use for familiar foods.

Not all traditional foods are abandoned at the same rate, and not all new foods are adopted at the same rate. Foods that comprise a cultural dietary pattern fall into three categories:

- **Staple foods** – carbohydrate-rich foods
- **Complementary foods** – often sources of protein and vegetables
- **Accessory foods** – sweets, fats, drinks and spices

Staple foods are most closely tied to *cultural identity* and, as such, are the most resistant to change when individuals migrate. The first foods to change are accessory foods because they are the least associated with cultural identity and are chosen based on personal taste preference. Many traditional diets contain few energy-dense, high-fat foods or sugar-sweetened drinks as accessory foods, but these are the foods that are most easily adopted by new immigrants upon relocation to their host country, and this has significant implications for future health.

Several studies have shown that some members of minority groups consume more vegetables and fruits than their native counterparts, in particular immigrants to North America and the UK.

Nutrition-related health effects of migration

When immigrants start to settle, their overall health is often superior to that of the general population. This phenomenon is known as the *healthy immigrant effect* and can be found globally, regardless of the host country.

However, as immigrants begin to immerse themselves in the new culture, they experience a rapid decline in health, taking on the health profile of their host country. A significant driving force for this decline is the adoption of mainstream dietary habits and dietary acculturation:

- Immigration and adoption of the host country's norms, including diet and physical activity, have a large impact on health and often result in the development of chronic diseases.

Nutrition at a Glance, Second Edition. Edited by Sangita Sharma, Tony Sheehy and Fariba Kolahdooz.
© 2016 John Wiley & Sons, Ltd. Published 2016 by John Wiley & Sons, Ltd.

- The longer the term of residence in the host country, the greater the risk of disease development, with many immigrants experiencing worse health outcomes than the general population.
- The very act of immigrating has been identified as an independent risk factor for cardiovascular disease.

Increased rates of cardiovascular disease, type 2 diabetes and obesity have been observed in immigrant populations in the UK, the USA, the Netherlands, Israel, Luxembourg, Japan and Canada. These chronic diseases have direct links to dietary intakes, suggesting that dietary changes made by immigrants in their host countries significantly impact their overall health and well-being.

Religion and diet

Religious adherence may have an important influence on dietary practices for many people in these groups.

Dietary restriction is reported to be practised by 80–95% of the groups of Asian origin. The main religious groups are **Muslim**, **Hindu** and **Sikh**. Other religious groups among whom diets are likely to be altered include **Buddhists**, **Rastafarians**, **Seventh-Day Adventists** and **Jewish people**. Adherence to religious practice is important as part of a sense of faith and belonging but will nevertheless *vary in its rigidity* between individuals. For example, strict Hindus, Sikhs, Jains and Buddhists follow the dietary principle of no killing for food and comply with vegan/vegetarian diets; if less strict, individuals may eat some animal food such as pork, lamb, chicken, eggs, fish and dairy products. Islamic and Orthodox Jewish doctrines advise their adherents to consume food prepared with halal and kosher rules, respectively. Rigid Muslims and Jewish people may only eat halal or kosher animal food and fish with fins and scales, and avoid pork. Rastafarians and Seventh-Day Adventists may prefer fresh plant-based food and avoid additives, seasonings and condiments. Fasting is common among these religious groups and often related to festivals. Many strict adherents to these religious dietary practices may avoid alcohol, although strict Jewish people would use kosher wine for rituals.

Influences that may contribute to nutritional risk include:
- Discrimination, which affects many aspects of life, including housing, education, access to shops, access to benefits and ability to save and invest for the future.
- Communication difficulties, affecting access to health care and social integration.
- Low income, often linked to poorly paid employment/unemployment, resulting in food poverty.
- Adaptation of the culturally traditional diet to include some items from the host country's diet may result in an unbalancing of nutritional intakes, as nutritionally poor snack and convenience items are included.
- Dietary advice on healthy eating may not be seen as relevant or appropriate for the dietary customs.
- The balance between 'continuity' and 'change' results in considerable diversity for individuals, families and communities, leading to very variable experience and level of risk.

Risk factors for nutrition-related non-communicable diseases

Studies of the causes and risk factors for nutrition-related non-communicable diseases (NR-NCDs) in these groups have identified a number of possible indicators, including:
- High incidence of smoking and poverty-affected lifestyle
- Higher risk of raised blood pressure (especially in African origin groups)
- Short stature, which increases risk
- Higher levels of lipoprotein(a)
- Small babies and rapid weight gain in early life
- Low folate status, which raises homocysteine levels
- Low levels of physical activity

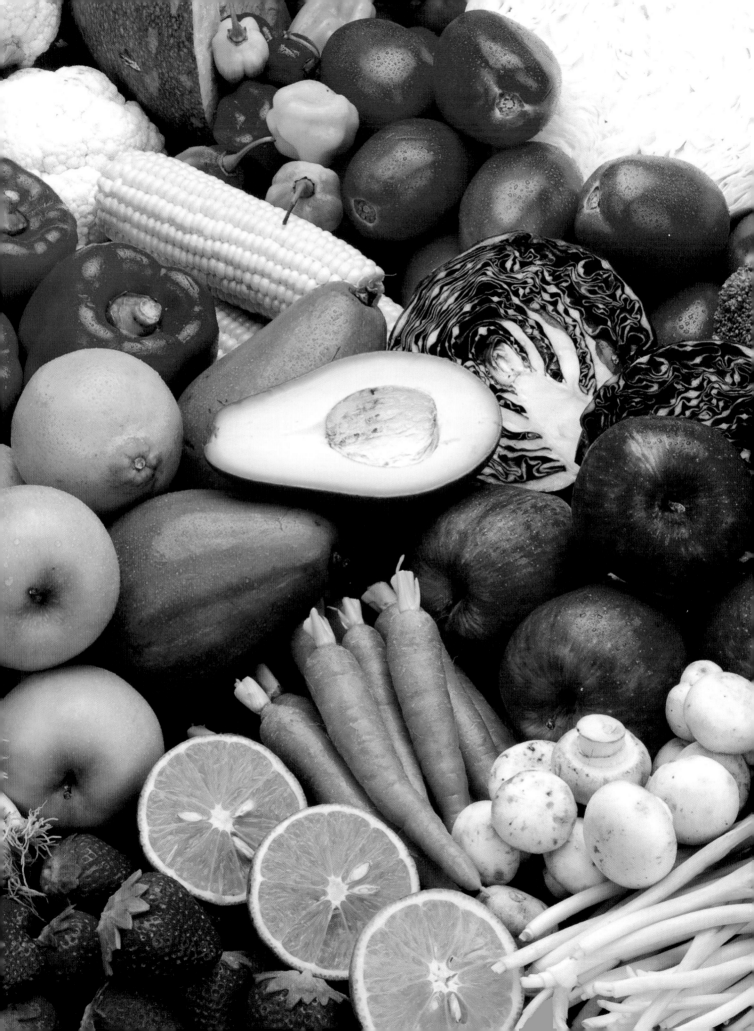

Nutrition throughout the life cycle

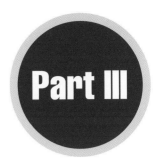

Part III

Chapters

45 Nutrition in pregnancy and lactation

Aim

1 To describe the nutritional needs of pregnancy and lactation

Physiological preparation for pregnancy and lactation occurs during normal growth and development. Nutritional status will influence the capacity to support the pregnancy to a successful outcome (Figure 45.1).

Nutrition at conception

Nutritional status at the time of conception is critical for early fetal development.

Fertility is affected by *body weight* and is optimum within the BMI range of 18.5–24.9 kg/m²:
- Women with a BMI of <18 may experience amenorrhoea and risk of ovulatory failure.
- Obese women may develop ovulatory failure.
- An elevated waist-to-hip ratio (>0.8) is associated with decreased fertility.

Weight normalisation is frequently all that is needed to help infertile women to conceive.

Folic acid supplementation around the time of conception reduces the incidence of neural tube birth defects (NTD). Because of this, it is now recommended that all females who could become pregnant should be taking 400 µg/day of folic acid from at least 3 months before conception until week 12 of pregnancy. Realistically, this intake can only be met from supplements because dietary sources do not contain sufficiently high levels and also because the bioavailability of natural folates is lower than that of folic acid. Because at least 50% of pregnancies are unplanned, compliance with this advice tends to be low. As a consequence, the USA, Canada and >60 other countries have introduced mandatory fortification of flour (and/or other cereal products) with folic acid. As a result of this measure, NTD rates in these countries have fallen substantially.

No alcohol should be consumed at all by women trying to get pregnant or who may be pregnant.

Adequate nutrient stores are vital to sustain implantation and organ formation in the first weeks of pregnancy, as the placenta (which acts as the 'nutritional gatekeeper' for the fetus) is not fully functional until the third month of pregnancy.

Nutrition during pregnancy

Several adaptations occur in the mother's body to increase the efficiency of nutrient provision for both the mother and the fetus.

Energy needs and weight gain

The typical increase in weight during pregnancy is 11–16 kg, but this figure may vary depending on the pre-pregnancy BMI of the mother. Gains in the second and third trimesters should average 0.4 kg/week for normal weight women, less (0.3 kg/week) for overweight women and more (0.5 kg/week) for women who are underweight:
- During pregnancy, excessive weight gain is associated with a large baby and an increased risk of complications at delivery. Excessive weight gain should be managed by professional dietary advice. However, weight-loss diets are not recommended.
- Low weight gain carries the risk of a low-birth-weight baby, with possible long-term health implications.

The extra energy costs of pregnancy are estimated to be about 310 MJ (77 000 kcal). To help cover the increased energy needs, physiological adjustments occur to the mother's metabolic rate, which increase the efficiency of energy utilisation. The remainder of the increased energy requirements are met by a reduction in physical activity and an increase in food intake.

In general, it is better to monitor weight gain rather than specify precise energy needs. However, an additional 340 kcal/day is

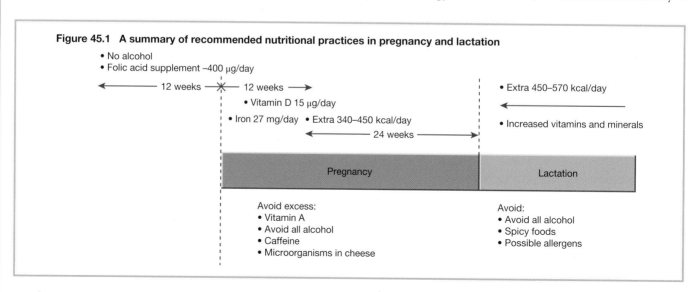

Figure 45.1 A summary of recommended nutritional practices in pregnancy and lactation

- No alcohol
- Folic acid supplement –400 µg/day

← 12 weeks → ✳ ← 12 weeks →

- Vitamin D 15 µg/day
- Iron 27 mg/day   • Extra 340–450 kcal/day

← 24 weeks →

- Extra 450–570 kcal/day

- Increased vitamins and minerals

| Pregnancy | Lactation |

Avoid excess:
- Vitamin A
- Avoid all alcohol
- Caffeine
- Microorganisms in cheese

Avoid:
- Avoid all alcohol
- Spicy foods
- Possible allergens

Table 45.1 Population groups who may be at risk of not meeting nutritional needs in pregnancy.

Group	Reasons for risk	Action/advice
Teenagers	Own needs for growth still high May deny pregnancy, be reluctant to adjust diet/behaviour	Ensure high dietary quality Focus on adequate weight gain, calcium, iron and folate intakes No alcohol or smoking
Overweight/obese	Increased risk of complications, including preterm delivery, hypertension, and gestational diabetes mellitus (GDM)	Keep gain within recommended levels Ensure dietary quality, advise exercise Use slowly absorbed carbohydrates and regular meals to manage GDM
Vegetarian/vegan	Potential for lower nutrient intakes	Ensure balanced/varied diet to provide a range of micronutrients Long-chain PUFAs, vitamin B_{12}, iron, zinc, calcium and vitamin D may be particular issues
Low income	Poorer reserves at start of pregnancy, lower micronutrient intakes, less weight gain, and higher risk of low birth weight	Advise on cheaper sources of nutrient-rich foods, such as fortified breakfast cereals, wholegrain bread, tinned pulses, fruit and vegetables, and small amounts of meat and tinned fish

recommended during the second trimester, and an additional 450 kcal/day is recommended during the third trimester.

Iron needs

Expansion of the blood volume requires additional iron. Iron can be provided from:
• Body stores (however, up to 50% of women may have low or no stores)
• Cessation of menstruation
• Increased iron absorption in the gut
• Iron supplements
• Dietary intake (see Table 45.1)

Calcium and vitamin D needs

Calcium requirements increase during the third trimester of pregnancy. Additional calcium can be provided by:
• Remodelling of the bone, facilitated by oestrogen, prolactin and increased levels of active vitamin D
• Increased absorption

Vitamin D levels must be adequate for effective calcium utilisation. Pregnant women are advised to take a vitamin D supplement to achieve an intake of 15 µg/day, especially during winter months, or when skin is regularly covered for cultural reasons.

In teenage pregnancies, intake of rich calcium sources such as milk, dairy products, nuts, pulses, bread and tinned fish should be increased to meet requirements.

Calcium is also important for the maintenance of normal blood pressure in pregnancy.

Other nutrients

• *Long-chain PUFAs* are needed for development of the brain and retina. Requirements can be met by increasing consumption of oily fish. Some can be synthesised from α-linolenic acid, found in oils (soya, rapeseed and walnut), green vegetables and meat from grass-fed animals.

• Requirements for *protein* and *B vitamins* (except folate) increase in proportion to energy needs. Therefore, women eating to appetite from a balanced diet should meet these requirements.
• *Iron*, *potassium*, *magnesium*, *calcium*, *iodine*, *vitamin A* and *riboflavin* have been found to be low in some diets in pregnant women.

At-risk groups

Some groups of women need special nutritional attention (Table 45.1).

Lactation

The mother's nutritional status is unlikely to affect the volume or macronutrient content of her milk during the first few weeks of lactation. However, poorly nourished women will not be able to sustain the same macronutrient content in milk for prolonged periods.

Potentially harmful substances such as alcohol, drugs and allergens that may be passed to the baby through the milk should be avoided altogether.

Although human milk is the ideal food for almost all babies, many women choose not to breastfeed. Additional health promotion and education information are needed to increase breastfeeding rates (see Chapter 46).

Advice for women planning to conceive

• Avoidance of excessive vitamin A (retinol) (especially in liver and liver products) – potential teratogenic effect.
• Complete avoidance of alcohol – teratogenic effect – can cause fetal alcohol spectrum disorder.
• Cessation of smoking.
• Avoidance of excessive amounts of caffeine (>300 mg/day).
• Avoidance of foods that may contain harmful microorganisms, such as unpasteurised milk or cheese.
• A healthy balanced diet, including plenty of fruit and vegetables to provide micronutrients and sufficient iron intake and fish consumption to provide PUFAs.

46 Nutrition in infants, toddlers and preschool children

Aims

1 To describe the nutritional content of human and formula milk in relation to the nutritional needs of infants
2 To explain the process of complementary feeding of infants
3 To consider the nutritional needs of preschool children

The challenge in meeting the nutritional needs of infants arises from their:

- Limited capacity for food due to the infant's size and the immaturity of the digestive and excretory systems
- Relatively high demand for nutrients to fulfil the needs for growth
- Total dependence on another person for the provision of food

Growth rates

Growth rates in infants are highest in the first 6 months of life, during which time body weight doubles from birth weight. Over the next 6 months, the rate of growth slows down so that at 12 months of age, the body weight is about three times the birth weight. Body weight doubles again between the ages of 1 and 5 years.

Standard growth charts are useful to check that growth is progressing appropriately. Rates that rise too steeply or fall below the expected trajectory need attention and explanation.

Nutrition in infants

Breastfeeding is the preferred method of feeding infants for its nutritional and immunologic benefits and subsequent enhanced growth and development of infants and toddlers. Therefore, the nutritional composition of breast milk is the optimum food for infants, this is the reference for both nutrient requirement values for this age group and the composition of formula milk alternatives.

Breastfeeding

The composition of breast milk is perfectly balanced for human consumption, ensuring that it is readily digested and absorbed (Table 46.1). All other milks, including unmodified cow's milk, are not ideal for infant consumption. Cow's milk contains higher proportion of casein compared to whey protein and is deficient in vitamin C and iron.

Table 46.1 Factors in breast milk aiding digestion and absorption.

Factor	Effect on digestion and absorption
High lactose content	Promotes calcium absorption Supplies galactose for brain development
High whey protein content	More readily digested than casein
Non-protein nitrogen	Includes taurine, urea and growth factors, which may be utilised in the colon
Lipid profile	Contains lipase and bile salts to facilitate fat digestion
Specific binding proteins for vitamins and minerals	Facilitate absorption

Human milk also contains *protective factors* that are critical in the early weeks of an infant's life when its own defences are undeveloped (Table 46.2). These protective factors are not found in formula milk. Exclusive breastfeeding is recommended for 0–6 months old with nothing else being given, even water.

The actual composition of breast milk (Table 46.3) varies between mothers, between feeds and even during a feed in the same mother.

Table 46.2 Protective factors occurring in human milk.

Protective factor	Functionn
Secretory immunoglobulin A	Protects mucosal surface against antigens Primes immune system
Macrophages, lymphocytes, lysozyme	Engulf bacteria Secrete immunoglobulins and lymphokines
Lactoferrin	Binds Fe and compete with bacteria for Fe
Bifidus factor	Stimulates growth of bifidobacteria and lactobacilli, reducing the pH

Other benefits of breastfeeding

Apart from the nutritional advantages, there are other benefits of breastfeeding for both the mother and infant:
- For the infant, there are less risk of infection, especially gastrointestinal and respiratory infection, and improved cognitive development.
- For the mother, there is a period of anovulation (which may help with birth spacing) and reduced risk of premenopausal breast cancer.
- Bonding between mother and baby.

Formula milk

Infant formula is designed to meet the complete nutritional needs of infants up to 4–6 months of age and is subject to strict regulations. Formula milk can be derived from cow's milk or soy (for infants who are allergic to components of milk).

Cow's milk formula can be classified as:
- 'Casein dominated' when based on the entire protein fraction
- 'Whey dominated', containing the dialysed whey protein

Table 46.3 Macronutrient composition of mature human milk compared with whey-dominated infant formula (per 1000 mL).

Nutrient	Human milk	Infant formula
Energy MJ (kcal)	2.95 (700)	2.8 (670)
Protein (g)	11–13*	15
Fat (g)	42–45	36
Carbohydrate (g)	70	72

*The actual protein content of human milk is uncertain.

Nutrition at a Glance, Second Edition. Edited by Sangita Sharma, Tony Sheehy and Fariba Kolahdooz.
© 2016 John Wiley & Sons, Ltd. Published 2016 by John Wiley & Sons, Ltd.

Further modifications include the addition of lactose, maltodextrins, vegetable oils, long-chain fatty acids (DNA, arachidonic acid), taurine, carnitine, nucleotides, vitamins and trace elements and reduction in the levels of electrolytes, calcium and phosphorus.

Specialised products are available for low-birth-weight and preterm babies, and babies with metabolic or absorption disorders.

Older infant or follow-on formulas are also available for use beyond the age of 6 months. These products are modified (e.g. with extra iron) and as such are better than cow's milk. However, there is little evidence that they are superior to the continued use of ordinary formula, together with complementary feeding.

Complementary feeding

The WHO recommends exclusive breastfeeding until the age of 6 months, at which complementary feeding should be started at this time, with breastfeeding continuing to the age of 2 years or beyond.

To achieve normal developmental goals, suitable foods need to be introduced at an appropriate pace to match the infant's digestive and metabolic capabilities:
- Introduction of complementary foods too early may give rise to allergic reactions due to the immaturity of the gut.
- Delayed introduction may miss the developmental 'window' when the ability to chew first occurs and may result in growth faltering due to nutritional needs not being met.

Throughout complementary feeding:
- An infant may take some time to become accustomed to new flavours and textures, so new foods need to be tried several times.
- Feeding must always be supervised to avoid danger of choking.
- Foods containing iron and calcium should always be included.
- A low-fat or high-fibre diet; added salt and sugar; nuts (choking); honey, soft-boiled eggs, pate and mould-ripened cheese (microbial contamination) should not be given.
- Energy density of the foods should meet the infant's energy and nutrient requirements. Commercially prepared foods can be more energy dense than home-made meals.

The WHO recommends that infants receive iron-fortified foods at 6 months of age and vitamin A supplementation in countries with high rates of vitamin A deficiency or high under-5 year mortality.

Infants fed strictly regulated formula rarely need additional supplements because the formula is fortified with all essential nutrients. A child following its growth centile and developing a broad appetite for various foods is a good indicator of successful complementary feeding.

recommendations and provides items from all food groups. When in line with dietary recommendations, family food should form the basis of the diets of toddlers and preschool children (Table 46.4).

Table 46.4 Some issues that may arise in preschool children.

Issue	Possible strategy/advice
Food refusal, fussy eating, narrow range of foods eaten	Parents/carers to provide example, eat with family, introduce foods gradually, keep trying with new foods, do not offer a range of alternatives for disliked foods
'Grazing' between meals – limits appetite at mealtimes	Restrict between-meal food availability; eating is an 'event' and not a passive accompaniment to other activities
High consumption of fruit juice and soft drinks	Risk of effect on appetite and dental health: offer only water, diluted fruit juice and milk
Low-fat/high-fibre diet perceived by parents as 'healthy'	Ensure child is able to consume sufficient to meet needs; growth pattern critical. Low-fat products inappropriate before age of 2 years. Gradually increase whole foods during this period, as appetite allows
High level of snack food consumption – cakes, biscuits, crisps, confectionery, sweets	Offer alternative snacks – fruit, scones, yogurt, toast + spread, breakfast cereal
Foods used as rewards	Use alternative rewards, not food related

Children in this age group may be looked after by parents, but an increasing number may go to day-care facilities, where they receive some food. Guidelines exist for the provision of healthy food for snacks and lunch in nursery or day-care units.

Nutritional principles to be addressed include:
- Achieving the dietary recommendations for this age group.
- Low-fat diets are not recommended.
- Attention to nutrient density; especially at risk are calcium, iron, zinc, vitamin A and vitamin C.
- Avoidance of excess amounts of non-milk extrinsic sugar or fatty foods.

Reasons for introducing additional foods after 6 months are:
- Provision of more energy and nutrients to meet growth needs
- Provision of iron, as supplies from birth become depleted
- Developmental stimulation: hand to mouth, facial and oral development, essential for speech
- Able to cope with digestion, absorption and excretion of other foods
- Development of social skills, eating with the family
- Acquisition of taste discrimination

Nutrition in toddlers and preschool children

Between the age of 1 and 5 years, a child moves from a diet dependent on milk for many nutrients and containing up to 50% of its energy as fat towards one that meets the dietary

---

A suggested scheme for progressive complementary feeding at 6 months

Stage 1
Smooth puree (generally as single item), for example, non-wheat cereal (to avoid development of gluten allergy) and puréed cooked vegetables

Stage 2
Mashed and lumpy food, for example, minced meat, fish, cooked vegetables and fruit

Stage 3
Finger food (from about 9 to 12 months), for example, rusks, fingers of toast, pieces of hard cheese, fruit or vegetable
Drink in a cup to be introduced as suckling declines: milk, water and very diluted fruit juice

47 Nutrition in school-age children and adolescents

Aims

1 To describe nutritional needs during childhood and adolescence
2 To consider how these needs can be met and the problems that may arise

Growth rates

Growth and development occur over a long period of time in humans, from conception to late adolescence. Mean growth is relatively constant during childhood and averages 4.5–6.5 lb (2–3 kg) and 2.5–3.5 in (6–8 cm) per year. During puberty, on average:
- Girls increase by 20 cm (height) and 20 kg (weight).
- Boys increase by 30 cm (height) and 30 kg (weight).

Growth velocity is vulnerable to faltering if nutritional intakes do not keep pace with demands.

Nutritional needs

Dietary recommendations reflect the change in body size and composition. During childhood, the majority of nutritional needs are the same for boys and girls and increase only slightly between younger (4–6 years) and older (7–10 years) children.

Once into adolescence, there are much greater nutritional demands, reflected in increased recommended levels, which should be met by increased intakes from all food groups (Table 47.1).

There are guidelines that recommend optimal dietary intakes for children and adolescents. For example, the Canadian Food Guide recommends that adolescents should consume:
- Sources of carbohydrates high in starch – six servings for females and seven servings for males per day
- Fruits and vegetables – seven servings for females and eight servings for males per day
- Milk and dairy products – three to four servings for females and males per day
- Meat and alternatives – two servings for females and three servings for males per day

Fatty and sugary foods should be limited and only consumed when other food groups have been adequately provided. Variety reduces the risk of omitting particular nutrients.

Body composition

- Between the ages of 4 and 6, there is a second, rapid increase in percentage of body fat known as *adiposity rebound*. Heavier children may experience adiposity rebound at an earlier age, which may be associated with a higher risk of later nutrition-related non-communicable diseases (NR-NCDs).
- In boys, the percentage body fat starts to fall during the pubertal growth spurt, but in girls, it continues to increase, resulting in the average 10% fat content differential between the sexes seen in adults.
- A critical fat mass is essential for menarche in girls. The hormone leptin is proposed as the link between nutritional status and the initiation of menstruation.
- Lean body mass increases throughout childhood but particularly in males during puberty.
- Changes in height require bone growth to be maintained. As weight increases during puberty, the bones increase in strength and undergo their most rapid period of mineral accretion.

School meals

In school, food provided for children must:
- Sustain their ability to concentrate and learn
- Contribute to an overall balanced diet and meet nutritional requirements
- Help teach them about food, nutrition and the social aspects of eating

Many countries around the world provide meals for students.

Table 47.1 Main nutritional needs in adolescence.

Nutrient	Reason for increased need	Additional points to note
Energy	Synthesis of new tissue is energy demanding. Increased body size results in an increase in metabolic rate and energy needs for activity	Needs are greater in boys than girls, linked to larger overall size
Protein	Synthesis of new tissues	Intakes generally high in developed countries. Restricted diets may be inadequate
Fats	Unsaturated fatty acids needed for membranes. Cholesterol synthesis increases for synthesis of sex hormones	Diets containing large amounts of 'fast foods' may not contain sufficient unsaturated fats
B vitamins	Cofactors for metabolic and synthetic reactions	Needs increase in line with energy (for thiamin and niacin) and protein (pyridoxine)
Iron, copper, folate and vitamin B_{12}	Required for expansion of blood cell mass to support extra tissues. In girls, onset of menstruation increases iron requirements	Poor iron status may result in impairment of cognitive function
Calcium and vitamin D	Needed for skeletal growth	Additional nutrients also required for the skeleton include vitamins A, C, and K, phosphorus, magnesium, potassium, and zinc

Nutrition at a Glance, Second Edition. Edited by Sangita Sharma, Tony Sheehy and Fariba Kolahdooz.
© 2016 John Wiley & Sons, Ltd. Published 2016 by John Wiley & Sons, Ltd.

In the USA, the National School Lunch Program endeavours to provide healthy food alongside health education so students can also make healthy choices outside of school. Students, however, are still lacking in their nutritional profile as many do not meet the requirements for vegetables, fruit and wholegrain intakes and most consume excess amounts of sodium and empty calories from added fats and sugars.

School lunches in Finland are renowned for their quality and provision to all students. Finland boasts the longest-running school lunch programme in the world, which began in 1948. All school lunch meals are prepared using local ingredients and follow the Finnish dietary guideline of the 'plate model' in which half of the plate is vegetables, one-quarter is proteins and the remaining quarter is carbohydrates.

In Japan, school lunches are given to all elementary and junior high school students and provide well-balanced, nutritious foods that meet the food-based dietary guidelines developed by the Japanese government. School meals in Japan aim to decrease overall sodium intake and increase fruit, vegetable, small fish and seaweed intake, which represent nutritional concerns in the school-age population there.

Table 47.2 Summary of nutrition standards for foods available in schools.

Nutrient	Guideline (per portion)	Examples
Energy	≤200 calories	• Individual fruit cups
Fat	≤35% of food energy	• Fresh fruit and vegetables – apples, bananas, baby carrots, broccoli
Saturated fat	<10% of food energy	• 100% fruit juice
Trans fat	Zero trans fat (≤0.5 g per serving)	• Wholegrain, low-sugar cereals
		• 8 oz serving of low-fat or fat-free yogurt
Sugars	≤35% of food energy	• 8 oz serving of low-fat or fat-free milk
Sodium	≤200 mg	• Wholegrain bread or crackers
		• Low-sodium vegetable juice
		• Low-sodium, wholegrain fruit and nut bars

Adapted from Institute of Medicine 2009.

Case study: Improving the nutritional quality of school meals

In recent years, the nutritional quality of school meals has come under heavy criticism for having:
• Too much fat
• Too much saturated fat
• Too much non-milk extrinsic sugar
• Too much salt
• Too few fruit and vegetables

New initiatives

In order to address the problem, strategies were developed *to engage all the major participants* in school meal provision. These strategies included:
• The creation of new standards for school meals, and snacks with food- and nutrient-based guidelines (Table 47.2)
• Engagement of parents, schools and local authorities

• Restriction on certain foods and drinks within schools
• Improving school kitchens and upgrading of training and qualifications for catering staff
• Inclusion of school food provision as part of the national school inspection process
• Advice on additional meal provision within the school, such as breakfast and after-school clubs
• Advice for parents on the content of packed lunches

Other targets for improvement included type and quality of foods sold in tuck shops and vending machines, dining room environments and provision of water.

Initiatives were also created to encourage children's involvement with food, including growing food in school allotments and cookery clubs.

By enhancing children's interest in food and knowledge about nutrition and by improving the variety and quality of food provided in schools, the aim is to reverse some of the deterioration in the dietary habits of school children and ultimately halt the increase in obesity and associated health problems.

48 Nutritional challenges in infants, children and adolescents

Aims

1 To describe issues associated with poor nutrition in infants, children and adolescents

2 To identify practices that may lead to poor nutritional status

These age groups are vulnerable to poor nutritional status because:

• Nutritional needs relative to body size are greater than in adulthood.

• There is a smaller margin for error with nutritional intakes.

Low birth weight

Low birth weight (LBW; <2500 g) may arise because the baby:

• Is born preterm

• Has suffered intrauterine growth retardation (IUGR) and is small for gestational age (SGA)

Such infants have high nutritional requirements but only limited capacity and developmental ability to receive required nutrition. Enteral feeding (preferably a nasogastric tube) may be considered to provide adequate nutrition, until sucking and swallowing reflexes are sufficiently developed for breast- or bottle feeding.

Feeding LBW babies

1 Mothers who deliver prematurely usually produce breast milk with a higher energy and protein content than term milk, providing greater nutritional, immunological and developmental benefits to the premature infant. Preterm breast milk is also better tolerated by the infant and allows for easier establishment of feeding and reduced risk of complications. Preterm infants may display higher developmental scores when supplied with their mother's breast milk compared to term infants.

2 If breast milk is not available, *preterm formula* may be used, which is more nutrient dense than standard formula milks as it contains more protein and minerals. Vitamin supplements, including vitamins A, C, D and folic acid, may also be needed. Iron supplements are usually not recommended as these may act as pro-oxidants.

3 Very small babies may need to be fed intravenously, but enteral feeding starts as soon as possible.

Growth faltering

Growth in infants and young children, usually recorded as weight, should progress along a centile line on standard growth charts. If the growth pattern crosses from one centile line to another, indicating change in weight, the reason for this should be established to prevent any potential health issues and enable early intervention:

• An infant that was undernourished in the womb may show increased growth velocity and *catch-up* growth.

• Infants of diabetic mothers are often born very large (>4.5 kg) and may exhibit *catch-down* growth during their first year. Once removed from the oversupply of nutrients in the womb, their growth rate may decrease.

Other reasons for growth faltering are summarised in Figure 48.1. With appropriate intervention, a child should exhibit 'catch-up' growth and return to its growth centile.

Overweight and obesity in children

The prevalence of overweight and obesity has been increasing rapidly among children around the world, in line with the general trend of increasing obesity across all age groups. The *causes* of this increase in children are multifactorial but are likely to include:

• Reduced levels of physical activity (more sedentary leisure activities, less effort used in daily travel, reduced open play space and poor quality environments)

• Passive overconsumption (increased energy consumption without increase in the energy expenditure) due to increased snacking on energy-dense foods and drinks (a process fuelled by advertising)

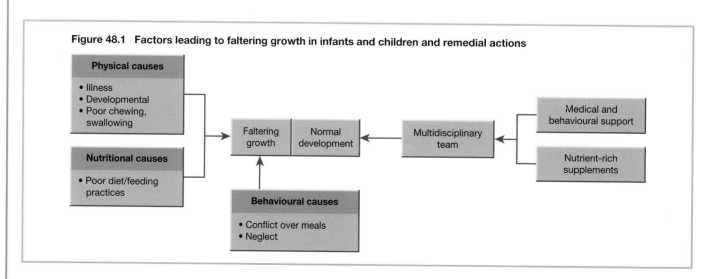

Figure 48.1 Factors leading to faltering growth in infants and children and remedial actions

Nutrition at a Glance, Second Edition. Edited by Sangita Sharma, Tony Sheehy and Fariba Kolahdooz.
© 2016 John Wiley & Sons, Ltd. Published 2016 by John Wiley & Sons, Ltd.

• Reduced consumption of freshly prepared meals due to the increased availability and consumption of manufactured and processed foods, which often contain more energy per unit weight

Overweight and obesity in children are difficult to define precisely. Various child BMI references, similar to growth charts, have been derived by age and sex. International child BMI classification systems have been developed from various reference populations and include the World Health Organization (WHO), Centers for Disease Control and Prevention (CDC) and International Obesity Task Force (IOTF) systems. The CDC defines overweight in children as having a BMI between the 85th and 95th percentiles for age and sex, and children are considered obese if their BMI is equal to the 95th percentile or higher. The WHO defines overweight and obesity in children ages 5–19 years using standard deviations, where a BMI between one and two standard deviations above the mean for a given age is considered overweight and two or more standard deviations above the mean is considered obese.

Preventing/managing excess weight gain in older children

Preventing excess weight gain and early intervention in overweight are key aspects for health professionals and should involve balance in energy intake and output. Common approaches include:

Reducing energy intake by:
• Providing foods with high satiety value
• Providing regular meals
• Reducing snacks/drinks containing 'empty calories'
Increasing energy output by:
• Encouraging movement and physical activity
• Reducing sedentary pastimes
• Involving the family in physical activity

Iron status

Iron deficiency is common in children throughout the world. Teenage girls represent a particularly vulnerable population as they require adequate iron stores due to menstruation and in anticipation of childbearing needs when they reach adulthood. Iron deficiency anaemia affects preschool and school-age children worldwide. In the USA, many toddlers experience iron deficiency. In the UK, some young children and adolescents suffer from iron deficiency anaemia, and many more have low stores and poor iron status; up to half of adolescent girls have intakes well below recommendations.

Age-specific advice regarding sources of dietary iron is vital for improving iron status in this population. Iron supplements may be recommended if dietary intakes cannot be increased.

Causes of low iron status

• Reserves present at birth are depleted by 4–6 months, and breastfeeding alone is insufficient to provide high iron needs for growth; iron must be supplemented in the weaning diet.
• In the first year, diets that exclude meat and fortified cereals or formula milk may lead to poor iron status.
• Fussy eaters are vulnerable. Carers may need advice on enhancing iron absorption.
• Needs remain high throughout growth to produce haemoglobin and iron-containing enzymes and for menstruation from puberty.

Table 48.1 Potential risks to nutritional status of children as a result of poorly constructed vegetarian/vegan diets.

Possible threat to nutrition	Possible solution
Lower nutrient density, need to eat larger volumes of food to reach energy needs; problem in young children and children with small appetites	Plan nutrient-rich snacks at regular intervals throughout the day
Avoidance of meat, with no planned substitutes included – risk of low energy and absence of iron, zinc, B vitamins, vitamin D	Ensure meat alternatives included, for example, pulses, meat replacements based on soy
	Include fortified cereal grains and starchy foods to meet energy and nutrient needs
Low intakes of essential fatty acids	Include some green vegetables and seed oils in the diet
Exclusion of dairy products reduces calcium intake	Use calcium-fortified soy products
	Ensure alternative sources of calcium included, for example, spinach
Low-nutrient snacks and soft drinks provide empty calories	Avoid these in favour of more nutrient-dense snacks, for example, dried fruit, nuts and milk

Consequences of low iron status

• Anaemia, characterised by pallor, tiredness, apathy, breathlessness, poor appetite and poor growth
• Effects on cognitive development, poor attention span and lack of interest in learning, resulting in diminished achievement in school

Vegetarianism

Vegetarian diets may be introduced to children by their parents, or alternatively, as children become more independent, and especially in adolescence, they themselves may choose to become vegetarian.

A well-balanced vegetarian diet can provide all the necessary nutrients required for growth and development, but if there is insufficient knowledge or inadequate planning to select a balanced intake, deficiencies can occur (Table 48.1).

Dieting and eating disorders

Many teenage girls experience dissatisfaction with their body image and body weight and attempt to address this by dieting. At any one time, approximately 30% of teenage girls are actively dieting, while the majority will have dieted at some point during their adolescence. A wide variety of diets are popular within this population, and often these diets are only adhered to for relatively short periods of time. These diets do very little to encourage healthier eating habits as they do not educate individuals about the fundamentals of healthy eating.

These extreme dieting behaviours can lead to disordered eating. Some teenage girls employ more drastic measures, such as use of diuretics, laxatives or self-induced vomiting, to lose weight in the short term. The most common forms of clinically diagnosed disordered eating are **anorexia nervosa** and **bulimia nervosa**. Anorexia is up to 10 times more common in girls than boys, and it is assumed that this is due to different pressures related to body image ideals. Disordered eating is more likely due to psychological, rather than physiological, factors. Treatment should involve not only dietary intervention but also psychotherapy.

49 Nutrition and early origins of adult disease

Aims

1 To describe the evidence for a link between fetal development and later risk of disease

2 To consider the implications of these findings for maternal nutrition

An observation that coronary heart disease (CHD) rates during the 1970s in the UK followed a similar geographical distribution to infant mortality rates at the beginning of the 20th century gave rise to the suggestion that the experience of the fetus in the intrauterine environment plays an important role in determining that individual's subsequent risk of developing a variety of diseases in adult life.

Early evidence

Initial evidence in the UK was obtained from birth and early growth records from the first decades of the 20th century, as well as records charting neonatal body proportions such as length, head and abdominal circumference and placental weight. Epidemiologists then traced many of these people and recorded their current state of health or, where appropriate, their cause of death.

Across the range of birth weights, there were:

• A statistically significant correlation between lower birth weight and an increased risk of death from cardiovascular disease (CVD)

• In survivors, a higher risk of type 2 diabetes and its markers and greater levels of other CVD risk factors (such as hypertension,

raised blood lipids and increased levels of blood clotting factors) in those whose birth weight had been lower. Risk was potentiated by having a high adult BMI. Similar trends also began to emerge in other countries (Table 49.1).

Overall, present evidence suggests that for CHD and stroke, there is a 40% difference in risk between those individuals who had the highest and lowest birth weights. This difference persists even when other factors commonly associated with CHD have been taken into account. Studies have also linked low birth weight with the development of asthma and chronic obstructive pulmonary disease (COPD).

Programming

Studies in animal physiology have for many years reported the existence of 'programming', whereby different organs develop at specific stages of gestation. If a physiological insult occurs at this specific time period, development will be affected, and the organ or tissue will not be able to recover later.

In addition, cells and tissues exhibit *plasticity*, being able to adapt to particular circumstances. These *adaptations* enable a fetus to survive in adverse conditions, but the cost, in terms of long-term biological functioning of the individual, is their *potential susceptibility to disease*. This has been termed the *thrifty genotype*, which ensures survival in the womb and continued survival in an anticipated environment of deprivation. However, where the

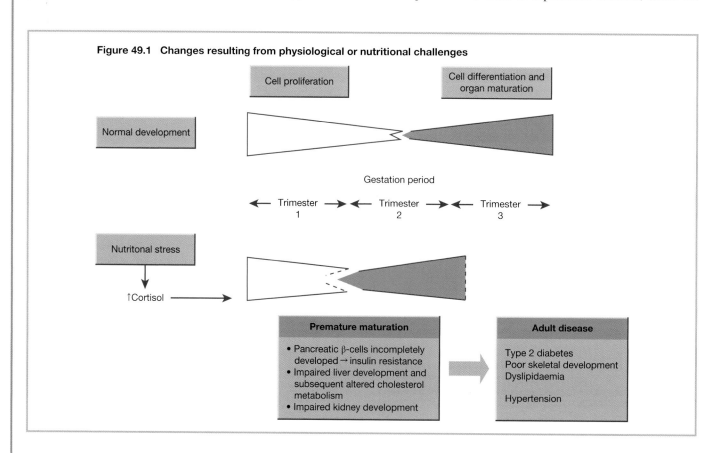

Figure 49.1 Changes resulting from physiological or nutritional challenges

Nutrition at a Glance, Second Edition. Edited by Sangita Sharma, Tony Sheehy and Fariba Kolahdooz.
© 2016 John Wiley & Sons, Ltd. Published 2016 by John Wiley & Sons, Ltd.

Table 49.1 Summary of studies on early origins of adult disease

Region (year)	Exposure	Associated adult health issues
USA (1990s)	Environment (e.g. diet and living conditions) during infancy and early childhood	CHD
Norway (1970s)	Poverty and resultant deprivation either during fetal development or early infancy	Morbidity and mortality in middle age due to arteriosclerotic heart disease
South Africa	Low birth weight	Hypertension and impaired glucose tolerance in young adults (without manifesting standard risk factors such as obesity and excess visceral adiposity)

postnatal environment is nutritionally plentiful, these adaptations become a handicap and may lead to disease.

Developmental consequences

Birth weight is a very crude measure of fetal development in the womb. A reduced birth weight can arise from slower development of many different tissues; equally, a normal birth weight may mask disproportionate development of different parts of the body.

Variations in body proportions are believed to indicate different rates of fetal development at different stages of gestation. Different patterns of disproportionate growth have been identified, including:
- Shortness (poor overall increase in length)
- Thinness (low muscle bulk, low ponderal index – weight/height³)
- Large head in relation to trunk (brain growth protected)
- Small abdominal circumference (poor organ development)
- Disproportionate infant weight in relation to placenta (uneven partitioning of nutrients)

In broad terms, it is possible to summarise the changes that appear to result from physiological insults or challenges at different stages of pregnancy (Figure 49.1):

1 Inadequate nutrition at *all stages* of pregnancy results in increased stress either to the mother or the fetus and leads to raised cortisol levels, which affect the development of key organs. In particular, a series of changes can result in an increased tendency to *hypertension*:
- Maturation of the nephrons in the kidneys is adversely affected.
- Reduced elastin in blood vessels result in stiff arterioles.
- Endothelium-dependent relaxation of blood vessels is impaired due to low levels of nitric oxide production.

2 In the *second trimester*, poor nutrient supply results in relative insulin resistance and the utilisation of amino acids for energy. This results in poor skeletal muscle development, which persists into postnatal life, and can be linked to later insulin resistance, poor glucose tolerance and the development of *type 2 diabetes*.

3 In the *third trimester*, poor nutrient supplies can result in 'brain sparing', with changes to blood flow diverting nutrients to the brain at the expense of the trunk. This results in poorer development of the liver and its associated products. Consequences include altered ability to control blood cholesterol levels and blood clotting factors, resulting in increased risk of *dyslipidaemia* and *CHD*.

Links to maternal nutrition

The ability of the mother to provide nutrients to the fetus depends on:
- Her own development and ability to sustain good uterine blood flow
- The quality of the placental development and blood flow in the umbilical cord
- The growth of the fetus, which plays a part in regulating its own nutrient supply

All of these factors can be affected by nutritional status, and any constraint will adversely affect fetal growth and development. Evidence supporting this includes:

- *General food shortage* affecting women in a previously well-fed population (the Dutch Hunger Winter) has resulted in CHD, obesity, hyperlipidaemias and type 2 diabetes in the offspring as adults. The type and severity of disease varied depending on the mother's stage of pregnancy when the famine occurred.
- Women with *low BMI*, low weight gain and low triceps skinfolds have offspring with higher blood pressure by adolescence and increased risk of insulin resistance and dyslipidaemia as adults.
- *Folate* may be a key nutrient in early pregnancy diets, due to its role in controlling gene expression. Ensuring adequate intakes of green vegetables in women on poor diets increased birth weights.
- *Calcium* supplementation reduces blood pressure in offspring, but shows no effect on birth weight.

Practical implications

These findings emphasise the crucial importance of girls and young women being nutritionally prepared for pregnancy, so they can fully sustain the nutritional and physiological demands:
- Diets during pregnancy should ensure an adequate supply of all nutrients.
- Babies who are born small should have particular attention paid to them. As they progress from childhood to adulthood, these individuals (initially through their parents) should be targeted for advice to maintain normal body weight and avoid overweight.
- It is the concurrence of a low birth weight, rapid growth in childhood and later overweight in adulthood that imposes the greatest risk of disease.

Possible mechanisms

Many of these mechanisms have been developed from studies in animal models, but they are believed to apply also in humans. Ethical considerations make such studies in humans difficult:
- During early fetal development, cells normally undergo periods of proliferation followed by cell differentiation. Under normal circumstances, this leads to organs that are the correct size and fully developed.
- The balance between proliferation and differentiation is controlled by the hormone cortisol, which initially is released by the maternal adrenal cortex and towards the later stages of pregnancy is augmented by fetal release (mostly after week 23).
- In the early stages of pregnancy, maternal cortisol readily passes across the placenta into the fetal circulation.
- Prematurely high levels of cortisol during this period will lead to organs maturing before they are fully formed (Figure 49.1).
- Maternal undernutrition (particularly low protein and energy intake) represents a physiological stress to the mother, and her response is to increase production of cortisol by the adrenal cortex.
- The placenta produces the enzyme 11-β-hydroxysteroid dehydrogenase (HSD), which inactivates cortisol and protects the fetus from excess maternal cortisol levels.
- The enzyme is most effective in the later stages of pregnancy.
- If the mother experiences stress associated with undernutrition in the early months of pregnancy, the fetus is likely to receive abnormally high levels of cortisol, which may interfere with the normal programming of organ development.

50 Nutrition in older adults

Aims

1 To describe the physiological changes that occur during ageing and their impact on nutrition

2 To consider how nutritional vulnerability in older adults may be identified and their nutritional needs addressed

Increases in the number of people aged over 65 years, and a sharp rise in those aged over 80 years, mean that the over-65 age group in many Western countries will soon account for one-quarter of the total population.

The ageing process

Ageing results from the interplay between genetic programming, lifestyle and nutrition. Both lifestyle and nutrition are within an individual's control and thus can be modified to enhance longevity. In recent decades, it has been noted that the biological changes associated with ageing are occurring later than in the past, such that chronological age may now be up to 10 years ahead of biological age. This is thought to be at least partly due to better nutrition and lifestyle choices.

Physiological changes associated with ageing

Many physiological changes occur during ageing, albeit at different rates and to different extents in individuals (Table 50.1). Of particular concern is the development and progression of *sarcopenia*, the age-related loss of muscle mass, strength and function. Sarcopenia causes decreased mobility, which has a significant impact on older people's quality of life and their ability to live independently. Inactivity contributes to the rapid progression of sarcopenia, which can be attenuated by physical activity and weight-bearing exercises.

A recent phenomenon is the development of *sarcopenic obesity*, which is the occurrence of declining lean body mass in older people who also have excess fat mass. The simultaneous presence of sarcopenia and obesity is a cause for concern because excess weight contributes to decreased physical activity, which in turn accelerates the progression of muscle loss.

Factors affecting nutritional status in older adults

Medical conditions can impact on nutritional status in older people in a number of ways, either due to the disease itself or to its treatment. Examples include:
- Reduced mobility – due to musculoskeletal, neurological, circulatory or respiratory conditions or excess weight
- Impaired cognitive function and dementia
- Psychological illnesses – including depression (also reactive depression following bereavement), mental illness and alcoholism

Social factors may also affect food intake in older people; these include educational level, financial status, type of housing, access to shops and facilities, awareness of appropriate meal composition and cooking skills.

The following help to achieve good nutrition in older people:
- Physical activity – this *maintains energy needs* and appetite, ensuring adequate food intake. It also maintains muscle mass, which supports independent living, activities of daily life and the ability to provide oneself with food.
- Social interaction – this *encourages eating* and maintains an interest in food.
- Selecting *a wide variety* of foods, including all food groups in appropriate amounts.

Assessment of nutritional status in older adults

The older adult population encompasses a wide range of ages and a large variation in physical and mental health status. This makes it difficult to set standards of 'normality' against which individual

Table 50.1 Physiological changes associated with ageing and their impact on nutrition.

Physiological change	Potential consequences for nutritional intake
Reduced lean body mass, associated with culturally determined sedentary lifestyle	Lower BMR, smaller energy needs, poorer nutrient intake
Loss of sensory acuity – taste, smell, hearing, vision	Reduced enjoyment of food, inhibits desire for eating
	Less confidence in obtaining and preparing food may limit quantity and variety of food intake
Quality of dentition; dry mouth with reduced saliva flow	Lack of teeth or poorly fitting dentures have a detrimental effect on the quality and quantity of food intake. Some food groups may be excluded
	Poor oral hygiene causes sores and ulcers, making eating painful
Reduced kidney function	Affects ability to concentrate urine or deal with low fluid intakes
	Risk of dehydration, and subsequent state of confusion, including disregarding food intake
Gastrointestinal tract changes, including secretion of hormones, enzymes and acid, reduced motility	Prolonged satiety caused by slow movement along tract and raised levels of hormones (CCK), reduce appetite
	Reduced acid secretion may affect absorption of minerals from food
	Slow motility may result in constipation, affecting appetite and tendency to use laxatives, which may reduce nutrient absorption
Reduced immune system efficiency, lower T-lymphocyte production; may also be stressed by chronic disease states	An adequate intake of a wide range of nutrients is needed to sustain the immune system
	Poor immune status increases risk of infection with consequent poor food intake

Nutrition at a Glance, Second Edition. Edited by Sangita Sharma, Tony Sheehy and Fariba Kolahdooz.
© 2016 John Wiley & Sons, Ltd. Published 2016 by John Wiley & Sons, Ltd.

assessment results can be compared. It is therefore more effective to adopt a *combination of screening tools*, including:
• Assessment of current health status – presence of disease, mental health, medications, dentition and weight changes
• Social and psychological factors – living alone, level of independence, bereavement, alcohol dependence, mobility, interest in food, ability to buy a variety of foods and food choice
• Food intake and anthropometric measurements
• Haematological measurements
• Biochemical measurements

Nutritional requirements

Because of the diversity in this age group, information about nutritional requirements remains speculative and is often extrapolated from data based on younger adults. To alleviate some of the uncertainties, many health agencies divide the group into two separate age categories: 51–70 and >70 years.

Energy requirements in older adults are likely to be lower due to a reduction in metabolic rate and reduced physical activity. However, the energy cost of activities, including walking, may be higher than in younger adults because of mobility issues.

Protein requirements are similar or slightly higher than for younger adults, while **vitamin and mineral requirements** may also be higher or at least the same due to less efficient absorption and metabolism.

A number of nutrients appear to be less well supplied in the diet of this group, and intakes fall below recommended levels (Table 50.2). In addition, there is likely to be low biochemical status of these nutrients, with consequent implications for health. Because older people tend to have lower caloric requirements and the same or increased requirements for vitamins and minerals, **nutrient-dense foods** should be consumed to meet these requirements. There should also be an emphasis on **complex carbohydrate** consumption to ensure adequate fibre intake, which is essential to alleviate constipation, a serious concern in this population.

Adequate **water** intake is also crucial for older adults because a proper fluid balance is essential for maintaining normal physiological functions. Changes in body composition during ageing, especially a reduction in lean body mass, reduce the body's water holding capacity. Additionally, older adults experience an increased risk of dehydration due to anxiety about incontinence, impaired thirst sensations and functional declines resulting in the inability to obtain fluids.

Care for the older adult

Care provisions exist in many countries for older people who become nutritionally at risk, including:
• Community meals – delivered to people's homes or provided in lunch clubs and sheltered accommodation.
• Residential and nursing homes – these provide accommodation and care for more vulnerable and frail older people, who are more likely to have additional clinical problems that contribute to a poorer nutritional status.

Standards and guidelines are in existence to ensure that the provision is appropriate; however, studies have indicated that these are not always met.

Survival mechanisms

Survival is attributable to having good 'maintenance and repair' systems within the body to deal with changes as they occur and limit damage that leads to ageing and disease:
• These systems are supported by nutrition, which provides energy, protein and the vitamins and minerals necessary to maintain homeostasis; most notable are the antioxidant nutrients that limit damage caused by free radicals.
• In parallel, avoiding factors that cause damage is also important. For example, toxins such as alcohol, smoking, drugs, excessive intakes of salt, sugar and fat, as well as environmental contaminants like pesticides, additives or preservatives, should be limited as far as possible.

Other health issues in older adults

• The majority of older adults are not undernourished, and in common with other age groups exhibit an increase in the prevalence of overweight and obesity and associated health problems.
• Thus, type 2 diabetes, cardiovascular disease and cancers are the main causes of morbidity in this age group and should be addressed by healthy eating and lifestyle interventions in younger adults.

Table 50.2 Key nutrients that may be at risk in older adults.

Nutrient	Who is at risk of poor intake	Possible health consequences
Energy/protein	Inactive, poor appetite, frail elderly, institutionalised, post-trauma	Poor general nutritional intake – all nutrients low Weight loss, low plasma albumin, poor wound healing, depressed immune status High risk of mortality
B vitamins (including folate, B_6, B_{12}, thiamin and riboflavin)	In cases of atrophic gastritis; heavy drinkers; poor diet, especially low intake of milk, green vegetables	Raised levels of homocysteine, link with cardiovascular disease and Alzheimer's disease Impaired cognitive function Megaloblastic anaemia
Vitamin D	Housebound/institutionalised	Consequences for bone health, immune system and muscle strength Increased risk of bone fracture and loss of independence
Iron	Where there is poor dentition and low meat intake; use of non-steroidal anti-inflammatory drugs (NSAID), causing gastric blood loss. Institutionalised	Poor iron status
Vitamin C	Lower socioeconomic groups; institutionalised	Less resistance to infection, poor wound healing
Potassium	Low fruit and vegetable intakes – associated with poor dentition	Low status, linked with high salt intakes, contributes to hypertension. Also poor muscle strength
Zinc	Low food intake, especially little meat	Depressed immune function, increased susceptibility to infection, poor wound healing Reduced taste acuity

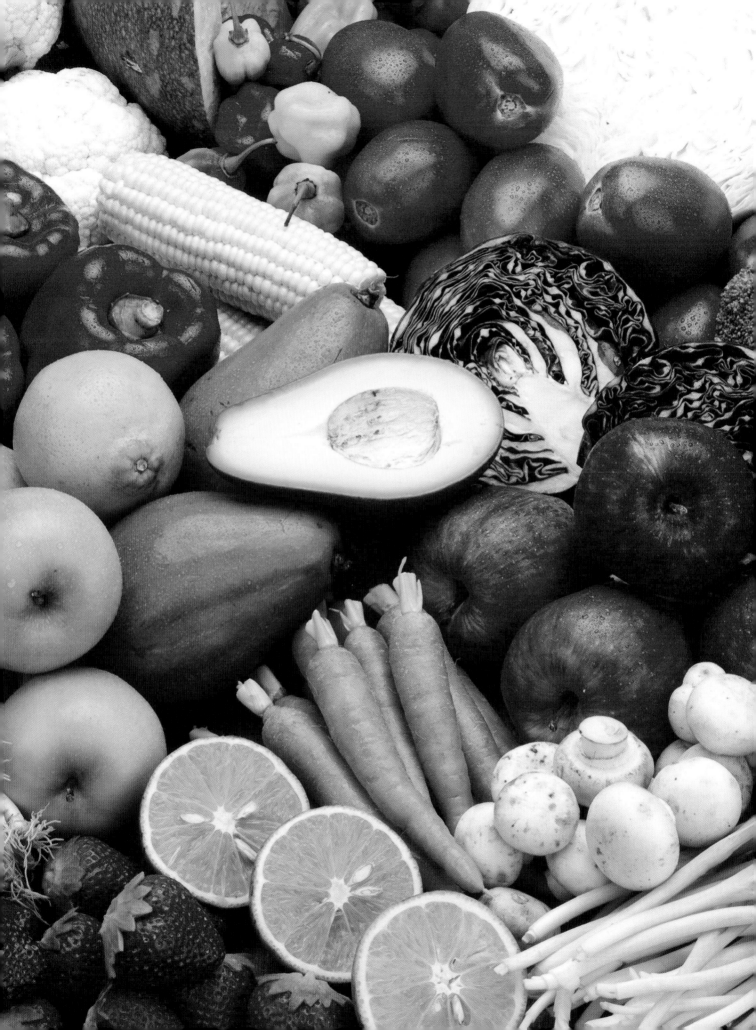

The role of nutrition in key organs/systems

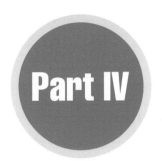

Part IV

Chapters

51 Nutrition and the gastrointestinal tract I

Aims

1 To review the general functions of the gastrointestinal (GI) tract
2 To consider some disorders of the GI tract that can have an impact on nutritional status
3 To consider the interdependence of the upper GI tract and nutritional status

Food enters the mouth at the start of the GI tract, and as it makes its way along the tract, an enormous variety and complexity of products are converted into simple nutrients, which are then absorbed across a very large surface area composed of villi and microvilli.

To carry out its role efficiently, the GI tract itself must be supplied with energy and nutrients. Nutritional deficiencies that affect cell division (e.g. folate, vitamin B_{12}, riboflavin and niacin) will rapidly impact the GI tract, as the cells here have a short life-span and undergo continuous replication.

General functions

In addition to the processing of foods, the GI tract fulfils a number of other important roles, including regulation of feeding behaviour and the provision of protective and barrier functions. These are summarised in Table 51.1.

Because of the diversity of roles carried out by the GI tract, a number of disorders (including coeliac disease, Crohn's disease, ulcerative colitis and inflammatory bowel disease) may have an impact on its overall function. These are summarised in Table 51.2.

Interrelationship between nutrition and functionality of the upper GI tract

The mouth

The teeth and jaws initiate the physical breakdown of food by the action of mastication (chewing), while saliva helps lubricate the food for swallowing. Saliva also contains α-amylase and proteolytic enzymes that begin to break down small amounts of starch and protein and help the development of taste during chewing. In addition, lingual lipase (secreted by the tongue) begins the process of fat digestion:

• **Teeth** are important for chewing, and although edentulous subjects (i.e. people without teeth) can grind food with their gums, studies of older adults without their own teeth show that nutritional intakes are poorer.

• Nutrients of importance for healthy teeth include **calcium**, **phosphorus** and **protein**, while **fluoride** increases strength and resistance to decay. Intake of **fermentable carbohydrate** in

Table 51.1 A summary of the roles of the GI tract and consequences if these are compromised.

Role of GI tract	Specific functions	Impact on overall health if role is compromised
Processing of food	Ingestion, chewing, swallowing Digestion, absorption Excretion of waste material	Nutritional deficiencies, which are likely to affect the function of the GI tract as well as other parts of the body
Regulation of feeding behaviour	Signals arise from the mouth, stomach and small intestine; include chemical and neural signals	Overall food intake may be poorly controlled if signals are absent
Protective and barrier function	Low stomach pH is bactericidal	Produces a balance of responses, to neutralise harmful organisms but maintain beneficial flora
	Mucus coating	Inappropriate antibody responses to foods must be avoided
	Innate immune system secretions, including lysozyme, antibacterial enzymes, mast cells and macrophages	If these fail, hypersensitivity may develop, with chronic GI conditions
	Adaptive immunodefences, including production of immunoglobulins and antibodies Secretion of cytokines and interleukins	

Table 51.2 Disorders of the GI tract that may affect digestion and absorption.

Disorder	Aetiology	Symptoms/treatment
Coeliac disease	Sensitivity to gluten in cereals; may be diagnosed in infancy or not appear until later in life	Atrophy of villi of the small intestine, resulting in malabsorption and potential malnutrition if not treated. Improved by following a gluten-free diet
Crohn's disease (CD)	Inflammatory condition affecting terminal ileum and colon but with normal areas between sites. Some genetic links but triggered by environmental factors, increased by smoking	Diarrhoea or constipation. Low-grade chronic fever. May be associated with anaemia, vitamin B_{12} deficiency Treated with anti-inflammatory or immunosuppressive drugs May have some success with probiotics
Ulcerative colitis	Similar to CD but confined to the colon and continuous. Does not extend through bowel wall	Diarrhoea; other symptoms similar to CD. Risk of development of colon cancer Treatment as for CD
Irritable bowel syndrome (IBS)	No obvious pathology, may exhibit increased motility, sensitivity to specific foods, altered bowel flora	Pain or discomfort relating to the GI tract, bloating, but with no obvious pathology Treatment varies with individual and may include behavioural therapy, food elimination and probiotics. Increased fibre intake is of benefit in some cases

Nutrition at a Glance, Second Edition. Edited by Sangita Sharma, Tony Sheehy and Fariba Kolahdooz.
© 2016 John Wiley & Sons, Ltd. Published 2016 by John Wiley & Sons, Ltd.

forms that adhere to the teeth (especially if consumed between meals) is a major contributory factor to tooth decay and ultimately loss of teeth.

- The **sense of taste** allows food to be recognised and decisions to be made about its palatability and consumption. Gastric secretions begin as a result of reflexes triggered by eating. Taste sensitivity is affected by nutrient deficiencies, most notably **vitamin A** and **zinc**. Some drugs also affect taste and therefore possibly food consumption.
- **Saliva flow** can diminish with ageing as well as with drug treatment and disease, and artificial saliva may be used to help with chewing and swallowing in these situations.

The stomach

Food is liquidised in the stomach by pressure and a churning action and released at a controlled rate into the duodenum. This rate is controlled by neural and hormonal signals arising in response to nutrient levels in other parts of the gut. Important elements in this response include the regulatory peptide hormones **cholecystokinin** (CCK), **neurotensin**, **peptide YY** (PYY) and **glucagon-like peptides** (GLP).

Key components in the secretions in the stomach are **hydrochloric acid**, **proteolytic enzymes**, **intrinsic factor** and **mucus**. Gastric juice is very acidic (typically pH 1.0), but the presence of food rapidly elevates the pH to approximately 4.5. Gastric acidity serves to:
- Provide the correct environment for the activation of proteolytic enzymes (pepsins) that start the process of protein digestion
- Solubilise the divalent minerals in the diet (especially calcium and iron)
- Prevent the conversion of nitrates to nitrites, which form carcinogenic nitrosamines
- Release protein-bound vitamin B_{12} for later attachment to intrinsic factor and absorption

Reduced gastric acidity will therefore interfere with the absorption of some minerals and of vitamin B_{12}. For example, use of antacid indigestion remedies will raise the pH and therefore limit the solubilisation of minerals.

Excessive **alcohol intake** also damages the gastric mucosa, resulting in chronic gastritis, and affecting normal digestive processes and therefore nutritional status.

52 Nutrition and the gastrointestinal tract II

Aim

1 To consider the interdependence of the lower GI tract and nutritional status

The small intestine

The small intestine is the major site of digestion in the GI tract. Digestion in the small intestine is brought about by bicarbonate and enzyme secretions from the pancreas and enzymes located in the microvilli that make up the brush border.

Bile, which is manufactured by the liver and stored in the gall bladder, is carried to the small intestine via the common bile duct and enters the duodenum at the ampulla of Vater. Bile acids are required for the emulsification of fats and micelle formation, so failure of bile production or secretion will compromise fat digestion and result in the presence of fat in the faeces (steatorrhoea). This may occur due to liver disease or blockage of the bile ducts preventing the release of bile.

Figure 52.1 Summary of the physiological/nutritional aspects of gastrointestinal function and nutrition-related pathology

Physiological/nutritional function		Nutrition-related pathology

Mouth

- Mastication → food breakdown
- Saliva → – Early digestion
  – Facilitates taste
  – Maintains oral health

Poor dentition → food incompletely masticated

Stomach

- Food mixing
- Release of HCl →
  – Activates proteolytic enzymes
  – Activates intrinsic factor
  – Facilitates vitamin B_{12} release
  – Reduces the formation of nitrites
- Release of mucus

- Reduced HCl release (e.g. in elderly)
  – Reduces vitamin B_{12} uptake and some minerals
- Excess alcohol intake
  – Damages gastric mucosa

Pancreas

- Release of bicarbonate and enzymes

- Pancreatic insufficiency
  – Protein and fat malabsorption leading to steatorrhoea
  – Loss of Ca^{2+} and Zn^{2+}

Liver

- Release of bile salts

- Bile salt deficiency
  – Reduced fat digestion (steatorrhoea)

Small intestine

- Elaborate microvilli
- Enzyme release
- Solute transport (uptake)
- Major site for water absorption

- Damaged microvilli
  – Disrupted solute/mineral uptake
  – Reduced water uptake

Large intestine

- Bacterial fermentation
  – Mostly carbohydrates releasing short-chain fatty acids

- Dry compacted faecoliths
  – Reduced peristalsis and increased transit times
  – Diverticulosis

Nutrition at a Glance, Second Edition. Edited by Sangita Sharma, Tony Sheehy and Fariba Kolahdooz.
© 2016 John Wiley & Sons, Ltd. Published 2016 by John Wiley & Sons, Ltd.

Absorption

Absorption is a key function of the small intestine, and under normal circumstances, a mixture of passive and active transport mechanisms operates to absorb the products of digestion.

Absorption is facilitated by the presence of a very extensive network of villi and microvilli on the surface of the small intestine, which increases its surface area enormously. Damage or flattening of these villi due to **coeliac disease** and other malabsorption states has serious consequences for absorption.

Failure to absorb specific nutrients can also occur for other reasons; examples are shown in Table 52.1.

Water absorption

Water absorption is another critical function carried out in the small intestine. Each day, some 8 L of water (from digestive secretions as well as food intake) is reabsorbed here, and only about 100 mL of water per hour enters the large intestine.

Water follows the absorption of solutes, principally glucose and sodium, but gene studies suggest that specific water transporters may also be involved. If solutes are not absorbed, water remains in the intestine and moves along to the large intestine, where it will result in osmotic diarrhoea. Malabsorption of sugars, for example, **lactose**, artificial sweeteners such as **xylitol**, and **lactulose** (a synthetic disaccharide used as a laxative), can all have this effect.

The large intestine

Undigested or unabsorbed food residues, as well as endogenous substances, reach the large intestine together with approximately 1–1.5 L of water. Water reabsorption occurs here along with the absorption of solutes such as short-chain fatty acids and with the active transport of sodium. Some water absorption may be under hormonal control.

Any breakdown of residues in the colon occurs largely by the action of bacteria. This includes:
- Proteins, which are broken down to volatile amines
- Carbohydrates, which are mainly broken down to **short-chain fatty acids** (acetic, propionic and butyric acids), carbon dioxide, hydrogen and methane
- Phytochemicals and hormone residues, which may be broken down here, together with bile acids that escaped absorption in the ileum

Long-chain fatty acids that reach the colon are generally not fermented and therefore result in steatorrhoea.

Butyric acid is an important nutrient for the colonocytes, so its synthesis is critical for the health of the colon.

The recognition that the large intestine contains a bacterial flora that may have beneficial effects has led to the development of foods containing **probiotics**. These are intended to rebalance the bacteria to a more beneficial profile and eliminate less desirable strains such as *Escherichia coli* and *Clostridium difficile*.

The physiological and nutritional relationships along the GI tract are summarised in Figure 52.1.

Pancreatic insufficiency

All three macronutrients (proteins, fats, carbohydrates) are digested by pancreatic enzymes. Pancreatic insufficiency therefore will have a profound effect on nutritional status. This is likely to include:
- Generalised macronutrient undernutrition, predominantly relating to protein and fat malabsorption
- Fat-soluble vitamin malabsorption
- Steatorrhoea, which also causes loss of calcium from the body due to its binding to fatty acids
- Zinc deficiency due to absence of zinc-binding protein to facilitate absorption

In **cystic fibrosis**, where pancreatic secretions are blocked by mucus, ingestion of enzymes to digest food is necessary to prevent nutritional deficiency, and macronutrient intakes larger than normal are required to compensate for the reduced digestion efficiency.

Colonic bacteria and micronutrients

There is still uncertainty about the nutritional significance of any synthesis of vitamins by the colonic bacteria and their availability to the body:
- Vitamin K synthesised here may be of some significance to the body.
- B-vitamin synthesis may only be of use to the colonocytes themselves and not be available to the whole body.

Minerals that had been trapped in dietary fibre matrices may be released here, but it is uncertain whether they are absorbed for whole body use.

Table 52.1 Summary of the absorption of nutrients from the small intestine and some reasons for failure.

Nutrients	Mechanism of absorption	Possible reasons for failure
Fat-soluble vitamins	Absorbed with fat digestion products. Require fat in the diet and normal fat digestion	Pancreatic or biliary insufficiency
Water-soluble vitamins	Generally absorbed by sodium-dependent active transport mechanisms	May become saturated by high intake
Folate	Polyglutamates must be split by a zinc-dependent enzyme (conjugase), then reduced and methylated prior to absorption	Excess amounts of alcohol interfere with conjugase activity and therefore reduce folate absorption
Vitamin B_{12}	Requires binding to intrinsic factor (produced by parietal cells in the stomach) for absorption	In pernicious anaemia, autoantibodies are produced against intrinsic factor or the parietal cells
		Bariatric surgery, atrophic gastritis, gastric ulcers, excessive consumption of alcohol
Iron and zinc	Require carrier for absorption	Rapid movement of intestinal contents
	Enterocyte binds the transported mineral to a protein, from which it is released into the circulation only as required. Unabsorbed mineral is lost when cells are sloughed off at the end of their life cycle	Mineral not solubilised
		Competition for carrier
Calcium	Carrier activated by vitamin D	Inadequate vitamin D status
Endogenous secretions	Many nutrients are secreted as part of the digestive process and are recycled by absorption with ingested GI contents	

53 Nutrition and the brain I

Aims

1 To consider the nutritional requirements for brain development
2 To describe the nutrients needed for brain function

The brain relies on adequate nutrition for its development, maintenance and function. At the same time, the brain is also essential for the control of food intake and, as such, determines the nutritional status of the whole body (see Chapter 54). In addition, behaviour may be related to the supply of nutrients to the brain.

Much of the discussion about the brain also applies to the spinal cord, which together form the central nervous system (CNS). The peripheral nervous system may also be affected by some of the nutritional factors discussed.

Growth of the brain

The most rapid period of brain growth occurs from mid-gestation to 18 months after birth. At birth, the brain accounts for 10% of body weight, whereas an adult brain weighs about 1.4 kg and comprises 2% of body weight.

Different components of the brain grow at different rates and have *critical periods* when growth is most rapid and vulnerable to adverse influences.

Nutritional links in brain development

Although brain *development* may be protected to some extent in fetal life by diversion of nutrients to the brain, there may be long-term consequences for brain *function* (Table 53.1). The role of excess intake of alcohol during pregnancy in the aetiology of fetal alcohol syndrome has already been discussed (see Chapter 28).

One of the most significant changes in brain composition after birth is a reduction in water content and increase in lipid content, emphasising the importance of lipids.

Nutritional requirements of the brain

Energy: Supply of glucose

The energy needs of the brain are normally met by glucose, which is transferred across the blood–brain barrier by a glucose transporter that is not responsive to insulin. This transport system has a capacity some 10 times greater than the actual daily transport of glucose. Active uptake of glucose by the neurons of the brain is matched to their needs by alterations in blood flow. Up to 20% of the body's oxygen requirement is used by the brain.

Protein

The brain requires protein for its own structure, but protein synthesis in the brain does not appear to be related to dietary protein intake, other than in very early life. However, levels of amino acids in the blood determine their uptake by the various transporters that carry these across the blood–brain barrier (Table 53.2).

Table 53.1 Summary of the potential associations between early nutrient intake, brain development and possible long-term consequences for brain function.

Nutrient	Role/effect of excess/deficiency
Generalised undernutrition	Potential to recover some of the deficit with good nutrition, possibly up to 18 months Neuronal networks may not be as extensive, affecting long-term cognitive performance and behaviour
Lipids	Approximately half of the lipids are present in myelin; adult amounts are present by the age of 4 years Long-chain PUFAs are required for development; breastfed infants receive higher levels in milk. Some formula milk is fortified with these fatty acids
Vitamin A	Excess intakes are teratogenic to the brain
Folate	Low levels can result in neural tube defects, including anencephaly
Copper	Needed for synthesis of myelin
Iodine	Deficiency results in cretinism and serious learning disabilities
Iron	Severe iron deficiency in infancy results in long-term reductions in cognitive performance
Alcohol	Intake during pregnancy can result in fetal alcohol syndrome, with developmental changes to organs including the brain, and behavioural and cognitive abnormalities

Table 53.2 Transport of amino acids across the blood–brain barrier.

Main direction of transport	Examples of amino acids carried	Function in the brain
From blood into the brain (Mainly essential amino acids)	Tryptophan	Tryptophan used to synthesise serotonin
	Phenylalanine Tyrosine	Phenylalanine and tyrosine used for catecholamines
	Histidine	Histidine used for histamine synthesis
	Arginine	Arginine used in the production of nitric oxide
	Lysine Methionine	
From the brain to blood (Mainly non-essential amino acids)	Glutamate	Glutamate is a major neurotransmitter; mainly transported out of the brain to prevent excessive excitatory effects
	Aspartate Alanine Glycine Cysteine	Other amino acids may also have excitatory transmitter or cotransmitter roles, and the brain requires a mechanism to prevent excessively high levels being reached

Nutrition at a Glance, Second Edition. Edited by Sangita Sharma, Tony Sheehy and Fariba Kolahdooz.
© 2016 John Wiley & Sons, Ltd. Published 2016 by John Wiley & Sons, Ltd.

Table 53.3 Role of fatty acids in brain structure and function.

Fatty acid	Role in the brain	Specific function
Linoleic acid and α-linolenic acid	Included in membranes as part of phospholipid molecules, which also contain choline	Influence the fluidity of the membrane and functions of associated molecules, such as transporters and receptors
Docosahexaenoic and arachidonic acids	Used in production of prostaglandins and leukotrienes	Regulate second messenger molecules
Balance of *n*-3 and *n*-6 acids		May be associated with mental health

Table 53.4 Role of vitamins in the brain.

Vitamin	Role within the CNS/peripheral nervous system	Consequences of deficiency/protective role
Thiamin	Metabolism of glucose	Deficiency – Wernicke's encephalopathy, with loss of vestibular function, poor nerve conduction, mental confusion. May lead to Korsakoff's syndrome with loss of short-term memory and degeneration of the midbrain, thalamus and cerebellum. Peripheral neuropathy affecting nerve fibres
Riboflavin	Oxidation–reduction reactions	Needed for monoamine oxidase synthesis, no evidence of neurotransmitter abnormalities in deficiency
Niacin	Oxidation–reduction reactions	Pellagra associated with depression and dementia, but mechanisms of this are unclear
Pyridoxine	Role as cofactor in many amino acid transformations	Role in synthesis of many neurotransmitters; deficiency may lead to depressed mood and, rarely, seizures
Folate	Involved in DNA synthesis, key role in development	Developmentally linked to neural tube defects. Also associated with depression in adults, mechanism unclear
Vitamin B$_{12}$	Methylation reaction within the nervous system for myelin synthesis	Demyelination of nerve axons and ultimate degeneration. May also protect axons from damage due to toxins
Vitamin C	Cofactor for dopamine β-hydroxylase for noradrenaline synthesis; antioxidant	May be associated with depression; suggested to protect blood vessels in the brain from free radical damage and maintain cognitive function
Vitamins B$_6$, B$_{12}$, folate	Required for metabolism of homocysteine	High plasma levels of homocysteine may be associated with development of dementia
Vitamin A	Essential role in the retina	Night blindness
Vitamin E	Antioxidant role	Protects fatty acids in neuronal membranes; deficiency may be associated with peripheral nerve degeneration; suggested role in protection against Parkinson's disease and Alzheimer's disease

Table 53.5 Role of minerals in brain function.

Mineral	Role within the CNS/peripheral nervous system	Consequences of deficiency/protective role
Iron	Iron-dependent enzymes needed for neurotransmitter synthesis; possible role in myelination	Effects on cognition and behaviour. High levels may contribute to oxidative damage
Copper	Needed as cofactor, for example, for dopamine β-hydroxylase, used to synthesise noradrenaline	Neurodegeneration seen in Menkes disease, a rare genetic disorder with very low copper levels. High levels may contribute to oxidative damage

Fatty acids

Fatty acids are required for the synthesis of neuronal cell membranes (Table 53.3).

Vitamins

Water-soluble vitamins are needed to serve as cofactors for a number of key reactions (Table 53.4).

Minerals

Minerals are involved in cofactor roles, in electrical conduction and in ionic channels (Table 53.5).

Food intake and the brain

- *Glucose transport* into the brain is not affected by intake of carbohydrate or energy supply.
- *Hypoglycaemic episodes* can occur when a large dose of insulin is given or an intake of readily absorbed carbohydrate (e.g. carbonated drink with a high GI) triggers an insulin reaction, reducing glucose levels drastically. This may also happen when alcoholic drinks are consumed on an empty stomach. This can result in confusion, coma and death.
- Overnight fasting, not followed by a balanced breakfast meal, may also result in low blood glucose levels. This has led to the belief that *eating breakfast* helps maintain concentration levels in the morning. It is particularly promoted for children, whose attention span in school is likely to be affected.
- *Alcohol ingestion* reduces glucose transport into the brain, which could explain the depressant effect of alcohol on the CNS.
- During *starvation*, the brain adapts to the use of ketone bodies (derived from fat breakdown for energy) by inducing a ketone body transporter across the blood–brain barrier.
- Blood ketone levels can also be elevated by very high-fat diets, and such *ketogenic diets* have been used successfully by some therapists to treat seizures, as they are believed to reduce neuronal excitability, especially in children. However, adherence to the diet is difficult.

54 Nutrition and the brain II

Aims

1 To consider the role of the brain in the control of food intake
2 To review the potential role of nutrition in behavioural aspects of brain function
3 To consider eating disorders

Role of the brain in control of food intake

The **hypothalamus** plays an integrative role in the control of food intake. Elements that are involved include the following:
• Information originating from the mouth, senses, stomach and intestines is conveyed to the hypothalamus via both nervous and chemical signals.
• Numerous **gut peptides** play key roles in regulation of hunger and feeding. Some of these are also found in the brain.
• Metabolic activity in the liver and end products released from it into the circulation contribute further to regulation.
• One of the key signals is via **leptin**, a hormone produced predominantly from adipose tissue that acts on the hypothalamus to induce satiety.
• In addition, neurotransmitters acting within the brain are thought to regulate preferences for particular macronutrients. **Serotonin** may influence the balance between carbohydrate and protein intakes. Noradrenaline and opiates are also believed to have a role.
• Disturbances of neurotransmitter release, whether of endogenous (e.g. in disorders of brain function) or exogenous origin (e.g. by drugs), are likely therefore to affect food intake.

Drugs that affect release of neurotransmitters (e.g. **serotonin reuptake inhibitors**) are used to help with weight loss. However, other drugs that are prescribed for the treatment of mental illness may have an effect on neurotransmitters involved in food intake and thereby cause increases or decreases in food consumption.

Role of diet in behaviour and disease

The role of diet in the function of the brain and in everyday behaviour, disordered behaviour and disease is of great interest. Research into these links is continuing and some areas are summarised in Table 54.1.

Much work is still needed on the nutritional needs of normal brain function; such studies are complicated by the ethical issues involved and the complexity of human behaviour.

Eating disorders

In disordered eating, food intake patterns may appear to be outside the rational control of the subject and may be seen as part of a mental health disorder.

Most generally, there may be a preoccupation with slimming diets, or fad eating, which coexists with restrained eating, and is associated with a *fear of fatness*.

Recognised eating disorders may form a continuum from the most restricted eating, as seen in **anorexia nervosa**, through binge–purge behaviour, as seen in **bulimia nervosa**, to **binge eating** characterising some cases of obesity (see Figure 54.1). Specific diagnostic criteria exist for the better recognised conditions of anorexia nervosa and bulimia nervosa.

Anorexia nervosa

This represents the most severe deficit, with extremely low energy intakes over a period of time, resulting in extreme weight loss. Energy intake may be further reduced by *self-induced vomiting* and use of *laxatives*. Weight loss may be accelerated by high levels of energy expenditure. Micronutrient status is also likely to be poor, although requirements may be reduced. Consequently, there are physiological changes typical of starvation that affect all systems of the body. Most notable are changes to:
• Gastrointestinal tract (poor motility, delayed gastric emptying, bloating, constipation, anatomical damage due to vomiting and overeating in binges)
• Musculoskeletal system (loss of muscle and demineralisation of bone)
• Endocrine system (depressed activity of reproductive system hormones, high levels of cortisol, low levels of thyroid hormones – leading to low metabolic rate and hypothermia)
• Central nervous system (may have poor memory and concentration, depression, irritability, some evidence of reduction in brain substance)

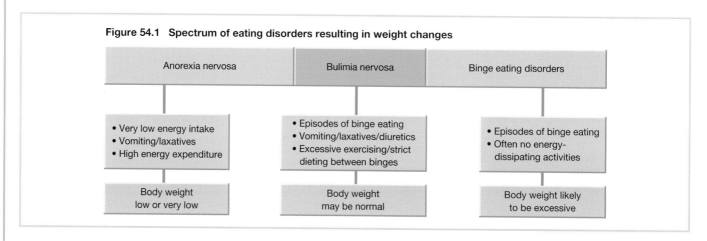

Figure 54.1 Spectrum of eating disorders resulting in weight changes

Anorexia nervosa	Bulimia nervosa	Binge eating disorders
• Very low energy intake • Vomiting/laxatives • High energy expenditure	• Episodes of binge eating • Vomiting/laxatives/diuretics • Excessive exercising/strict dieting between binges	• Episodes of binge eating • Often no energy-dissipating activities
Body weight low or very low	Body weight may be normal	Body weight likely to be excessive

Table 54.1 Some suggested dietary links with brain function.

Behaviour/disease state	Suggested dietary links/evidence
Mood	Evidence suggests that carbohydrate intake may elevate mood due to increases in brain serotonin levels Carbohydrate 'craving' and 'addiction' described, but evidence is equivocal
Stress-induced eating	Associated with higher intakes of either protein-rich or carbohydrate-rich foods May be related to release of catecholamines or levels of sex hormones in women during phases of menstrual cycle
Depression	Possibly related to low levels of *n*-3 fatty acids in the diet; some supplementation trials have shown benefits, but evidence is still equivocal Low folate, iron and selenium statuses have all been linked with depression
Attention deficit hyperactivity disorder (ADHD)	Relationship with *n*-3/*n*-6 fatty acid imbalance suggested but more trials are needed
Autism	Some suggestions of a link with gluten sensitivity; more evidence needed
Alzheimer's disease/other dementias	Current evidence suggests a link with raised homocysteine levels. Also link with antioxidant status However, results from supplementation trials with B vitamins or antioxidant nutrients have failed to replicate epidemiological findings High levels of some metals (e.g. iron, copper, zinc, aluminium) have been proposed as contributing to oxidative damage
Disruptive/antisocial behaviour	Trials on prisoners and offenders have suggested that an improvement in overall nutritional intake, by removal of refined carbohydrates and inclusion of more balanced nutrient-rich meals, is rapidly followed by less antisocial behaviour Such studies have also been performed in schools, using mineral and vitamin supplements, in which increases in IQ were reported. Further work is needed

- Cardiovascular system (reduction in size of the heart, lower blood pressure, poor circulation to periphery, cardiac arrhythmias)
- Blood (fewer red and white blood cells, reduced immunity)

The condition is characterised by a disturbed body image, and any treatment requires a **multifactorial approach** addressing both the requirements for food and the underlying psychological causes.

Bulimia nervosa

This is characterised by episodes of *binge eating*, during which energy intakes are very high, averaging at least 2000 kcal. These are generally accompanied by the use of *laxatives*, *diuretics* and *self-induced vomiting*. The episodes are triggered by 'loss of control' in the majority of cases. There may also be excessive exercising and strict dieting between these episodes. Body weight may be in the normal range, and the typical features of starvation absent. Food intakes may be relatively normal outside binge episodes.

The bingeing, vomiting and purging result in damage to the gut, teeth and salivary glands, as well as causing electrolyte imbalances (especially of potassium) and the risk of dehydration. Other minerals affected include calcium, magnesium, phosphate and sodium.

Kidney damage has been reported from overuse of diuretics.

Binge eating disorder may be differentiated from bulimia nervosa as it lacks the compensatory energy dissipating mechanisms. It is therefore more likely to be associated with obesity and thus the accompanying health problems.

As with anorexia nervosa, treatment of both bulimia nervosa and binge eating requires behavioural approaches.

55 Nutrition and the eye

Aims

1 To describe the role of nutrition in the structure and function of the eye
2 To consider the consequences of nutritional deficiencies on eye function

The eye as a sensory receptor provides visual information enabling us to obtain and enjoy food. The **visual appeal of foods** is important to encourage consumption. Individuals who have visual impairment are potentially disadvantaged in terms of their ability to control their food intake.

Adequate nutrient supplies are vital for the eye during development and in maintaining its integrity and function, and a loss of function in older age may be caused by a failing supply of protective nutrients.

Structure of the eye: Introduction to nutritional links

The eye is supported by the choroid, which supplies nutrients via the blood. The sclera encases the inner eye and rests within a fat-lined socket, supported by muscles that allow the eye to move. **Thiamin deficiency** may cause paralysis of these muscles and affect eye movement. The fat provides a supportive cushion and a lack of it, in **starvation**, may result in potential damage to the eye on impact.

Retinal function and nutrition

The essential light-sensitive area of the eye is the *retina*, which lines the interior of the inner eye. The retina contains two families of specialised cells called *rods* (about 100 million) and *cones* (about 3 million). The rods and cones contain light-sensitive pigments that consist of opsin proteins associated with 11-*cis*-retinal (derived from retinol). Rhodopsin, found in the rods, is more sensitive to a lack of retinol than is iodopsin, the pigment in the cones.

The sequence of events that occur in the photosensitive cells of the retina is shown in Figure 55.1.

The time taken for rhodopsin to be sufficiently resynthesised for night vision is known as the *dark adaptation time*. Individuals who are deficient in **vitamin A** have poor dark adaptation and may be unable to see clearly in the dark (*night blindness*).

Optic nerve neuropathy

Vitamin B$_{12}$ deficiency in individuals infested with fish tapeworm, and in heavy smokers and drinkers, has been reported to cause demyelination of the optic nerve and impaired vision. Cyanide

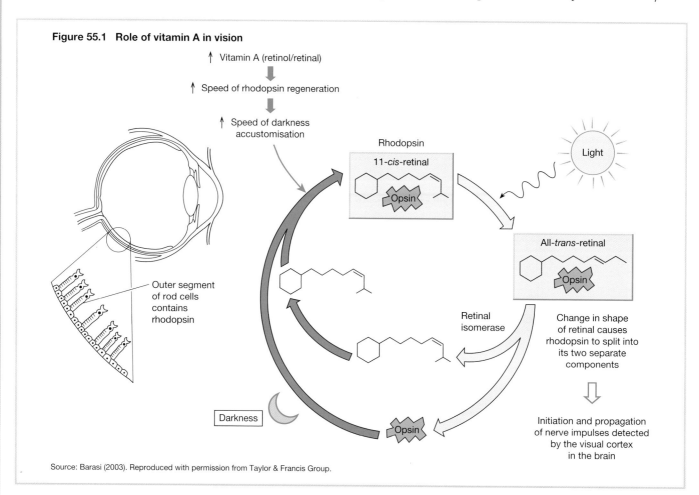

Figure 55.1 Role of vitamin A in vision

↑ Vitamin A (retinol/retinal)

↑ Speed of rhodopsin regeneration

↑ Speed of darkness accustomisation

Rhodopsin
11-*cis*-retinal
Opsin

Light

All-*trans*-retinal
Opsin

Outer segment of rod cells contains rhodopsin

Retinal isomerase

Change in shape of retinal causes rhodopsin to split into its two separate components

Darkness

Opsin

Initiation and propagation of nerve impulses detected by the visual cortex in the brain

Source: Barasi (2003). Reproduced with permission from Taylor & Francis Group.

Nutrition at a Glance, Second Edition. Edited by Sangita Sharma, Tony Sheehy and Fariba Kolahdooz.
© 2016 John Wiley & Sons, Ltd. Published 2016 by John Wiley & Sons, Ltd.

toxicity (from cassava-based diets) may also cause damage to the optic nerve in situations where B_{12} is deficient, as this would normally limit the toxic effects of cyanide.

The macula

High levels of *carotenoid pigments*, such as **zeaxanthin** and **lutein**, are found in the macula:

• It is believed that they provide powerful *antioxidant protection* against the effects of reactive oxygen species generated by light entering the eye, which is focused on this area for central vision.
• There is also a very high oxygen tension within the retina, contributing to potential oxidative damage.

Retinopathy

Premature infants who are treated with hyperbaric oxygen may experience degeneration of the retinal arteries, or *retinopathy of prematurity*. This has been associated with **vitamin E deficiency**, and supplements may be protective to an extent.

Retinopathy may also occur as a result of damage to the blood vessels supplying the retina. This could be due to *hypertension* or to deposition of glycated proteins in the capillary walls in diabetes. The latter causes thickening and destruction of the capillaries, leading to blurred vision. *Diabetic retinopathy* is more likely the longer the duration of diabetes and with poorer blood glucose control.

The retina may also be damaged by *glaucoma*, which is an increase in pressure within the eyeball that ultimately damages the optic nerve. This may also lead to *age-related macular degeneration* (ARMD) and *cataract* formation.

ARMD

In this condition, abnormal material is deposited within the macula, which is situated between the retina and the choroid. This leads to gradual loss of central vision and ability to perceive fine detail.

ARMD is the leading cause of registered blindness in Western populations and increases with age.

Maintaining adequate intakes of antioxidants, particularly those carotenoids found in the macula, may prevent or delay the onset of ARMD. The condition is particularly common in smokers, whose intakes of lutein are lower than the population average.

Lutein cannot be synthesised by the body, so a dietary intake is required. Green leafy vegetables and orange/yellow fruits and vegetables are good sources.

The lens, cataracts and nutrition

Cataracts are the result of an increased opacity of the lens, often accompanied by loss of accommodation. The lens is exposed to ultraviolet light and oxidising products:

• Glutathione and glutathione reductase, which act as *antioxidants*, are present in high concentrations, but levels decline with age.
• Levels of reduced glutathione are maintained by *niacin, riboflavin* and *vitamin C*.

• Cataracts are more common in smokers, people with diabetes or taking certain medications (e.g. steroids) and those exposed to more direct sunlight. Protection against oxidative damage appears to be important.

The cornea and conjunctiva

The front of the eye requires protection since it is exposed to the external environment. The lacrimal glands secrete tears to lubricate the conjunctiva.

The integrity of the conjunctiva depends on normal epithelial cell differentiation to maintain barrier function and mucus secretion. These require an adequate *vitamin A* supply, and deficiency results in *xerophthalmia*, or dry eye. There is a failure of tear production and the eye lacks lysozyme to keep it clean. It is then more susceptible to bacterial infections, resulting in conjunctivitis and ultimately infection of the cornea, which becomes ulcerated and keratinised. If untreated, the condition leads to *keratomalacia*, with permanent scarring of the eyeball and blindness.

Zinc is concentrated in the cornea and deficiency may result in corneal oedema, conjunctivitis and xerosis.

Deficiency of **riboflavin** results in blockage of the sebaceous glands of the eyelids, which become inflamed and painful. There is also photophobia and excessive tear production, and new blood vessels may be produced on the cornea, leading to increased lens opacity. Riboflavin is believed to be important in facilitating oxygen supply to the front of the eye.

Wilson's disease, a genetic defect of **copper** metabolism, results in characteristic deposition of copper in the cornea (Kayser–Fleischer rings). Chelating drugs may be used in this condition to excrete excess copper from the body.

In *familial hypercholesterolaemia*, deposits of cholesterol are characteristic within the cornea.

The health of the eye thus requires good nutrition for its function, but may also reflect the state of health of the individual, as more general deficiencies or excesses are evident in the appearance of this organ.

Potential problems with the retinal cycle

• Retinol-binding protein is required to transport retinol to the eye. *Poor protein status* will affect the formation of rhodopsin.
• *A low-fat diet* may reduce the absorption of vitamin A.
• *Zinc deficiency* will compromise the visual cycle, as it is required for the synthesis of opsin and the conversion of retinol to retinal.
• The rods contain high levels of docosahexaenoic acid (DHA), an *n*-3 fatty acid that provides them with flexibility and contributes to their role in vision. Visual acuity is reported to be affected when diets *lack n-3 fatty acids* during key developmental stages.
• The retina contains substantial amounts of the amino acid *taurine*, which stabilises the cell membranes. Requirements are high in the newborn. Both taurine and *n*-3 fatty acids are present in greater amounts in human milk than in formula milk; some formula milks are now being fortified with both.

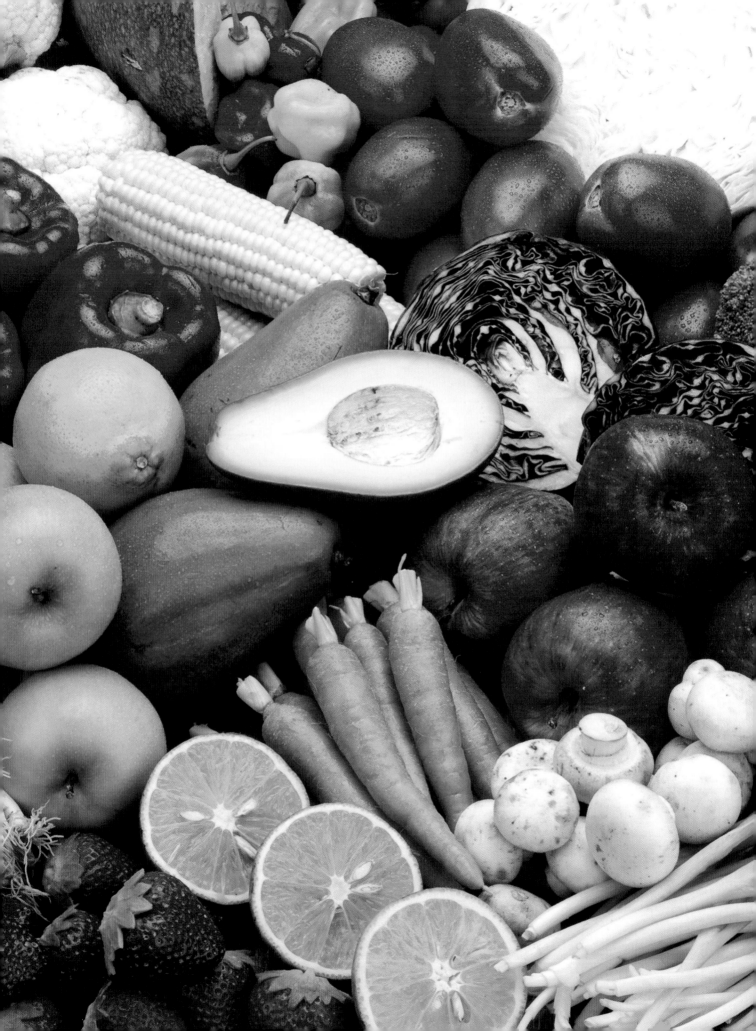

Nutrition-related diseases

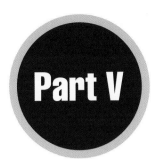

Part V

Chapters

56 Overweight and obesity: Aetiological factors

Aims

1 To define overweight and obesity and consider their prevalence
2 To consider the contributory factors in energy intake and energy output that lead to overweight and obesity

Definition

Overweight and obesity can be defined as an excessive accumulation of body fat. In men, healthy body fat may be 15% of total weight, while in women, this figure may be 25%, reflecting hormonal and physiological differences.

Excessive accumulations of fat may exceed 50% of total weight, contributing to major pathological consequences. Measuring body fat is not a straightforward process, although it is possible through bioelectrical impedance, hydrostatic weighing, dual-energy X-ray absorptiometry (DEXA) and other scientific methods (see Chapter 33 for more information). Several simple surrogate measurements are used to categorise overweight and obesity. These are:

- Body mass index
- Waist circumference
- Waist/hip ratio

Prevalence of overweight and obesity

Global prevalence has been rising steeply over the last 20 years in most countries, and there are now more overweight than undernourished people across the globe:

- Rates of overweight and obesity are increasing among children and adolescents.
- In general, obesity increases with age.
- Obesity is more prevalent in lower socioeconomic groups in Western countries, but in some parts of the world, such as India, it is seen more commonly among the more affluent groups.

Public health concerns regarding these trends relate to the parallel increase in risk of associated diseases:

- Obesity is directly responsible for some 6% of deaths in the Western world and reduces life expectancy by an average of about 9 years.
- The physical, metabolic and psychological consequences of obesity are also associated with substantial morbidity from cancer, cardiovascular disease and diabetes.
- External influences on energy intake.

Contributing factors in energy intake and output

Food availability

Both the quantity and the nature of the food available to people in many parts of the world have changed substantially in the last decades. Changes include:

- Greater choice, with more variety encouraging intake.
- Food on sale around the clock and availability of fast food.
- Improved preservation methods, so food can be always available.
- Many foods require little preparation, so can be eaten immediately.

Food quantity and quality

The rising incidence of obesity implies that energy intakes exceed expenditure (Figure 56.1).

Changes that play a part include:

- Increased consumption of convenience, ready prepared or 'fast' food, which has a higher energy density than typical traditional diets, resulting in 'passive overconsumption' of energy.

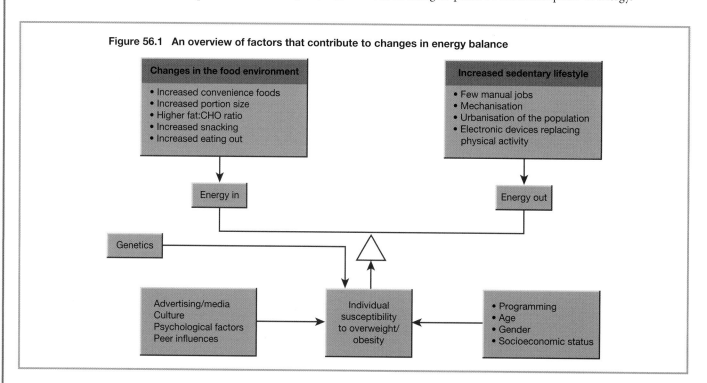

Figure 56.1 An overview of factors that contribute to changes in energy balance

Changes in the food environment
- Increased convenience foods
- Increased portion size
- Higher fat:CHO ratio
- Increased snacking
- Increased eating out

Increased sedentary lifestyle
- Few manual jobs
- Mechanisation
- Urbanisation of the population
- Electronic devices replacing physical activity

Energy in

Energy out

Genetics

Advertising/media
Culture
Psychological factors
Peer influences

Individual susceptibility to overweight/obesity

- Programming
- Age
- Gender
- Socioeconomic status

Nutrition at a Glance, Second Edition. Edited by Sangita Sharma, Tony Sheehy and Fariba Kolahdooz.
© 2016 John Wiley & Sons, Ltd. Published 2016 by John Wiley & Sons, Ltd.

• A trend to larger portion sizes becoming the norm, which also inadvertently increases food intake.

• People eating a rising proportion of their meals away from home; hence, the impact of the food industry on food quality and quantity becomes more pertinent to obesity trends.

Snacking and 'grazing'

There is a trend away from eating regular meals to a less structured food intake, typified by consumption of snack and convenience foods and soft drinks throughout the day, rather than eating to satiety at greater intervals. Such intakes tend to be high in fat and high-glycaemic carbohydrate, as well as being generally poor sources of slowly absorbable carbohydrate and micronutrients. The body's appetite control mechanisms are undermined in this way.

Psychological aspects

Attitudes and beliefs have a major impact on food intake. For any one individual, food intake could be affected by:

• Their mood and mental state
• Personality
• Self-image and culturally determined body images
• Socialised attitude to food
• External factors such as peer pressure, advertising and media influences

External influences on energy output

Increased mechanisation

Technological advances result in less need to use human muscle power to carry out energy-demanding manual tasks:

• There are now fewer occupations that can be classified as heavy manual work, and even tasks that were not very physically demanding have been lightened with robots and computer-driven technology. Fewer people have physically demanding jobs in agriculture, as urbanisation proceeds rapidly.

• Transport has become increasingly concentrated on the use of the car or other transportation, as opposed to walking and use of bicycles.

Leisure activity

Secular trends suggest reduced participation in active leisure pursuits:

• The widespread availability of computers and electronic home entertainment systems reduces outdoor leisure activities.

• Physical activity has for many become an item to schedule into the day, with a trip to the gym or swimming pool, rather than an intrinsic part of existence, as it was in the past.

• Increased urbanisation and road traffic, together with safety fears, may make outdoor activity less pleasant and compound the problem.

Individual susceptibility

Not everyone exposed to the same external influences on energy intake or output will experience weight gain. There is a heritable element, although this remains difficult to quantify and separate from environmental influences within families.

Genetics

In some inherited conditions, there is a clear link with obesity. Most notable among these are Prader–Willi and Bardet–Biedl syndromes.

For the great majority of cases of obesity, however, the rapid increase in incidence within a genetically stable population indicates that external factors play the major role. This does not exclude a genetic origin to susceptibility to obesity, which becomes expressed as a result of external changes.

Ethnicity

There are observed differences in patterns of weight gain between different ethnic groups, including body fat distribution and levels of adiposity at particular BMI values.

Vulnerable periods

Research from a number of areas suggests that there are periods during the life cycle when susceptibility to obesity may be programmed (in the fetus and infant) or be increased (during periods of rapid growth, including pregnancy and lactation). The latter may be linked to changes in levels of specific hormones. Age and gender are compounding factors, with patterns of weight gain in adult life differing between men and women.

Development of overweight and obesity

Weight gain occurs when the energy intake exceeds the energy output over a period of time.

This represents a *positive energy balance*, such that the energy supplied to the body as food is not used and is therefore stored in adipose tissue.

A reduction in energy intake, an increase in energy output, or both, are needed to remove the stored energy, create *a negative energy balance* and reduce body weight.

Control of energy balance

Physiological control mechanisms exist to regulate both energy intake and output. These are discussed further in Chapter 4.

For humans in modern society, both intake and output are subject to a variety of external influences. These interact with or override the internal regulatory mechanisms, creating a challenge to the maintenance of energy balance. In addition, the relative importance of these influences varies as a result of the underlying genetic make-up of the individual, dietary complexity and environmental variables.

57 Overweight and obesity: Consequences for health and chronic disease

Aim

1 To identify some of the major health consequences associated with obesity

There is a well-recognised relationship between the prevalence of overweight and obesity and rates of morbidity and mortality worldwide. Health risks are related to BMI in a J-shaped relationship (Figure 57.1).

At the lower end of the BMI range, usually below 18.5, risk increases due to the possibility of concurrent illness that causes loss of weight, such as cancer or complications of malnutrition. Above a BMI of 25 and especially above 30, there is a progressive increase in morbidity and mortality, associated with a range of factors. These are summarised in Table 57.1.

The metabolic effects associated with insulin abnormalities are discussed in Chapter 58.

Obesity and cardiovascular disease

Obesity is a major risk factor for cardiovascular disease (CVD), and data consistently show a higher incidence of disease with increasing BMI. However, obesity is also a risk factor in a number of the other conditions associated with CVD, such as dyslipidaemia, type 2 diabetes mellitus (and insulin resistance) and hypertension. It is therefore very difficult to separate the attributable risk to each of these comorbidities, as in addition their relative contributions may differ between individuals.

Overall, it is estimated that in subjects exhibiting the full spectrum of these conditions, CVD mortality is increased three-fold. Insulin resistance alone is responsible for about 18% of the variance in CVD risk. It is clear that the deposition of large amounts of fat within the body alters normal metabolic functions and results in a number of potentially harmful changes.

Table 57.1 Pathological consequences of overweight and obesity.

Type of effect	Examples of pathologies/consequences
Metabolic effects	Type 2 diabetes mellitus (impaired glucose tolerance, insulin resistance)
	Cardiovascular disease, including contributory abnormalities: hypertension, dyslipidaemia, clotting defects
	Cancers (colon, breast, endometrium, kidney and oesophagus) – associated with upregulation of cell growth or elevated hormone levels
	Hormonal dysfunction: menstrual abnormalities, pregnancy difficulties, anatomical changes
Mechanical effects	Musculoskeletal (including osteoarthritis in weight-bearing joints and back pain), resulting in disability
	Varicose veins, oedema
	Respiratory difficulties, including sleep apnoea and breathlessness
Surgical complications	Anaesthetic risk, poor wound healing, chest infections, thrombosis risk
Psychological/social effects	Tiredness, low self-esteem, depression, agoraphobia, isolation
	Unemployment, discrimination

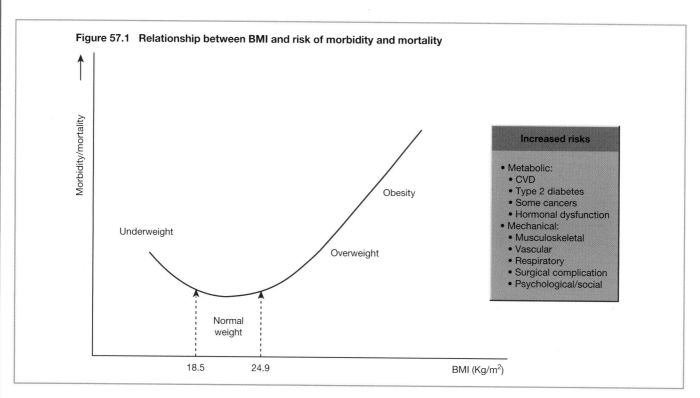

Figure 57.1 Relationship between BMI and risk of morbidity and mortality

Morbidity/mortality

Underweight

Obesity

Overweight

Normal weight

18.5   24.9

BMI (Kg/m²)

Increased risks

- Metabolic:
  - CVD
  - Type 2 diabetes
  - Some cancers
  - Hormonal dysfunction
- Mechanical:
  - Musculoskeletal
  - Vascular
  - Respiratory
  - Surgical complication
  - Psychological/social

Obesity and hypertension

There are several proposed mechanisms that offer an explanation for the high correlation between obesity and hypertension. These include:

• Increase in blood volume as a result of greater salt retention. This is attributed to an antinatriuretic effect of raised insulin levels.

• Changes in hormone levels affect blood pressure regulation. For example, cortisol production by adipose tissue increases, while leptin and angiotensinogen released from adipose tissue have direct hypertensive effects.

• Higher salt intakes and low levels of physical fitness may also contribute.

Obesity and cancer

Prevention of overweight is considered to be one of the strategies to prevent cancer. There is, however, a lack of clear evidence to support mechanisms by which excess weight may cause cancer.

It is proposed that in obesity:

• Receptors for insulin-like growth factor (IGF) are upregulated, as a consequence of metabolic changes in response to insulin. Growth of cells, especially tumour cells, which utilise glucose, is promoted.

• Hormone-dependent cancers, such as those of the breast and prostate, are promoted due to the conversion of androgens to oestrogens in adipose tissue.

It is very difficult to separate the effects of obesity from those of dietary factors that may have contributed to the obesity but at the same time also had a promoting effect on cancer development themselves. Nevertheless, weight loss and physical activity may be beneficial as preventive measures against cancer development in overweight subjects.

Other consequences of obesity

These are listed in Table 57.1 and relate to:

• The physical consequences of excessive weight on the skeleton and joints

• The consequences of increased effort by the respiratory muscles required to overcome resistance in breathing

• The consequences of higher body fat levels for anaesthesia and ventilation during surgery

• Poor peripheral circulation, resulting in slower wound healing

• Social consequences of overweight and obesity in terms of societal perceptions and effects on the formation and maintenance of personal relationships, if there is low self-esteem

These may have profound effects on the quality of life and the social experience of the affected individual and may have serious implications for levels of morbidity.

58 Overweight and obesity: Insulin resistance and metabolic syndrome

Aims

1 To consider insulin resistance as a major metabolic abnormality
2 To describe the metabolic syndrome and its diagnostic criteria

Metabolic effects of obesity

Insulin resistance (and possibly glucose intolerance/type 2 diabetes), dyslipidaemia and hypertension are the major metabolic consequences of obesity. Their coexistence characterises the *metabolic syndrome* (also known as insulin resistance syndrome or syndrome X). Generally, the syndrome is prodromic for (i.e. leads on to) type 2 diabetes mellitus.

Insulin resistance

The normal function of insulin is to act overall as an anabolic hormone, by targeting a number of tissues and either promoting storage of nutrients or preventing their catabolism (Figure 58.1).

Insulin levels normally rise after meals as glucose concentrations rise and are low in the postprandial state, when stored metabolites are used for energy.

When the response to insulin is muted, the condition is termed *insulin resistance*. In such subjects, a *higher plasma level of insulin is required* to achieve the same level of glycaemic control as in a normal subject.

Because insulin has a range of actions, resistance may affect all or only some of these, complicating the clinical picture.

Agreed criteria for diagnosis of metabolic syndrome

• Central obesity, with waist circumference above cut-off level for men (94 cm) and women (80 cm) (European figures)
 These also include **two** of the following:
• Raised serum triglycerides (above 1.7 mmol/L)
• Low high-density lipoprotein (HDL) levels (below 1.03 and 1.29 mmol/L for men and women, respectively)
• Systolic blood pressure above 130 mmHg, diastolic blood pressure above 85 mmHg or treatment for hypertension
• Fasting plasma glucose above 5.6 mmol/L or type 2 diabetes diagnosed

Benefits of weight loss

It is estimated that a 10% weight loss can achieve:
Blood pressure: reduction by 10 mmHg
Fasting blood glucose: reduction of up to 50% in newly diagnosed patients
Insulin levels and sensitivity: 30% lower fasting insulin levels and 30% increase in sensitivity
Progression to diabetes: 40–60% fewer developing diabetes
Lipids: fall of 10% in total cholesterol, 15% in low-density lipoprotein (LDL) cholesterol and 30% in triacylglycerols (TAGs) and 8% increase in HDL cholesterol
Mortality: 20% less from all causes and 30% less from diabetes-related disease

Features of insulin resistance

Mechanisms for insulin resistance have been studied extensively in animals, and findings include failure of second messenger signalling, presence of antagonists, a defect in a single cellular enzyme or cellular satiety due to overload with carbohydrate or fat.

However, in humans, it appears that over 75% of insulin resistance is attributable to obesity and low physical fitness.

The key elements of the metabolic abnormality are shown in Figure 58.2 and can be summarised as follows:
• Insulin resistance results in a *muted inhibition* of lipolysis of stored fat, with larger amounts of non-esterified fatty acids (NEFAs) released into the circulation. This is particularly detrimental in the visceral area, where the NEFAs arrive quickly in the liver via portal blood. It is for this reason that abdominal obesity is particularly involved.
• The NEFAs stimulate TAG synthesis in the liver and the *release of very-low-density lipoproteins* (VLDLs) into the circulation.
• Elevated VLDLs exchange TAGs with HDLs and LDLs, in exchange receiving cholesterol esters, producing small dense HDL.
• TAG-rich HDLs are broken down by hepatic lipase, resulting in a *reduction in levels of HDLs* in the circulation.
• TAG-rich LDLs also lose some of their TAGs in the liver by the action of hepatic lipase, becoming denser, due to a relative increase in the proportion of protein. These small dense LDLs are believed to be the most atherogenic lipoprotein particles and thus contribute to increased CVD risk.
• Clearance of chylomicrons and VLDLs from the circulation is also reduced as activity of lipoprotein lipase (LPL) in adipose tissue is insulin dependent. Persistence of these lipoprotein fractions contributes to dyslipidaemia.
• The circulating fats are eventually deposited in tissues, resulting in pathological alterations. Deposits can occur in adipose tissue, in hepatocytes and in skeletal muscle.

In addition to the above effects on fat metabolism, other consequences of insulin resistance include:
• High NEFA levels also inhibit glucose uptake and metabolism in tissues, resulting in *hyperglycaemia*. This in turn promotes increased insulin release, resulting in *hyperinsulinaemia*.
• Raised levels of insulin may independently activate the sympathetic nervous system activity and the hypothalamic–pituitary axis, resulting in *hypertension*.

Nutrition at a Glance, Second Edition. Edited by Sangita Sharma, Tony Sheehy and Fariba Kolahdooz.
© 2016 John Wiley & Sons, Ltd. Published 2016 by John Wiley & Sons, Ltd.

Figure 58.1 Main actions of insulin under normal conditions

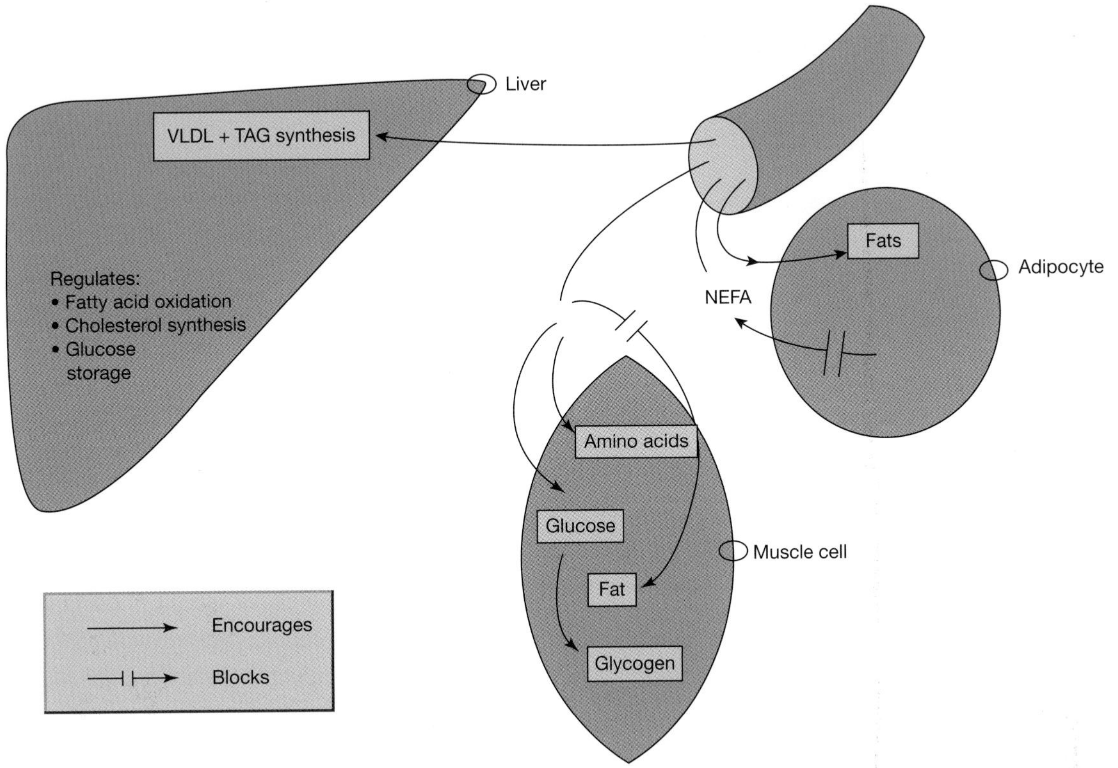

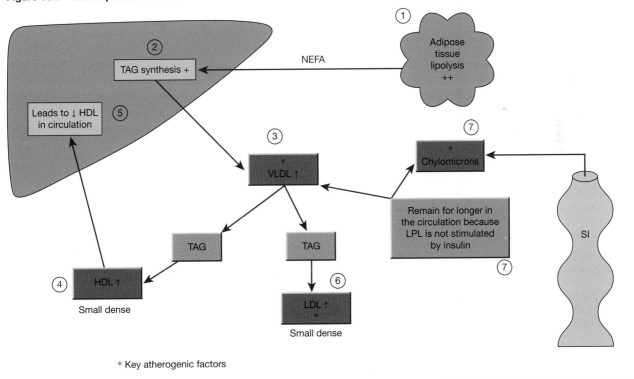

Figure 58.2 Consequences of insulin resistance for fat metabolism

* Key atherogenic factors

59 Overweight and obesity: Prevention and management

Aims

1 To consider ways of preventing overweight and obesity
2 To describe options to achieve weight loss and its long-term management

Prevention

Obesity has a multifactorial aetiology (discussed in Chapter 56), which should be addressed at various levels (Table 59.1).

Despite a clear understanding of what needs to be done, these approaches have not achieved the expected success. Reasons might include:

* Under-resourcing for individual action
* Inadequate monitoring of effectiveness
* Little surveillance to trigger early action on weight gain
* Insufficient coordination of initiatives
* Lack of understanding and treatment of underlying causes (e.g. psychological)
* Lack of cultural appropriateness

Non-surgical treatment

First-line treatment for overweight and obesity should be a *weight management programme* designed to:

* Help overweight individuals lose weight
* Maintain this weight loss with appropriate changes to *lifestyle* and *behaviour*
* Achieve a reduction in risk factors

Table 59.1 Approaches to prevention of overweight and obesity at the personal and societal levels.

Prevention at individual level	Prevention at community/ policy level: Action needed to facilitate individual change
Modify food choices to be healthier	Policies on labelling/easy availability of healthier choices
Reduce total energy intake to match output: moderate portion sizes	Food industry action on smaller portions
Regulate snacking/choose healthier snacks/drinks	Limit advertising of less healthy snacks, especially to children
Engage in more physical activity, reduce sedentary activities	Encourage walking/cycling and sport by attention to the environment, transport policies and safety measures on roads and in urban spaces
Early awareness of a need for action on weight	Policy of monitoring weight in children; availability of health checks and accessible evidence-based advice on weight management, with support
Clear guidance on the health risks of excess weight and the need for change	Regulation of poor-quality/ unsound advice

These programmes may be offered in primary care, by local dietitians or commercial slimming groups and health clubs.

A diet and lifestyle approach should be used, combining:

* Dietary measures
* Behaviour change
* Increased activity
* Psychological counselling

Dietary measures are based on healthy eating principles. These are discussed further in Chapter 60.

All dietary recommendations should be discussed with the individual and negotiated to take into account likes and dislikes to maximise compliance. Additional help may include:

* Shopping lists and menu plans.
* Diet plans.
* Fat content may be counted or specific points allotted to foods.

These are all techniques that may help with compliance and will suit particular individuals, but not others.

There are also many other 'slimming diets' available for consumers, discussed in Chapter 60.

Behaviour change techniques include:
* Setting realistic goals: overambitious targets are likely to be demotivating. These may be weekly or monthly rates of loss, a percentage of current weight or simply stabilisation, with no further gain.
* Support from family and friends: may also occur by a group or programme leader and include support to overcome obstacles and setbacks.
* Anticipating the barriers to progress: may include keeping a diary to identify triggers to eating, coping with difficult situations and establishing self-belief for success.

Physical activity provides an additional means of achieving a negative energy balance:

* In conjunction with dietary measures, activity contributes to weight loss and protects the lean body mass. This helps to maintain the metabolic rate, which decreases when energy intake is reduced.
* Vigorous activity also results in a post-exercise elevation of metabolic rate, further enhancing energy utilisation.
* Activity can increase fat utilisation and sensitivity to insulin and improve blood lipid profiles.
* Activity induces a feeling of well-being, which can improve the mood and self-image of an individual on a weight loss programme.
* Increased mobility and lung function may be additional benefits.
* Exercise on prescription, and referral to weight loss programmes and slimming groups, is becoming accepted within primary care.

Everyday activities make a worthwhile contribution to total energy output. Therefore, the simplest way of achieving an increase in activity is to incorporate more into the normal daily routine. This is more likely to be maintained than committing to a session in the gym.

Recommendations on the amount of activity are:
- For the general population for health: at least 30 min of moderate activity on at least 5 days of the week.
- To prevent weight gain, 45–60 min of moderate activity each day is recommended.
- For individuals who have lost weight, 60–90 min of moderate activity each day is needed to prevent regain.

Drug treatment and surgery should be considered only in more complex and severe cases.

Drug treatment

There are specific guidelines on the use of anti-obesity drugs.

Individuals should also have appropriate advice on diet and physical activity with behavioural strategy support.

There are a large number of over-the-counter formulations that claim to promote weight loss, but most of these have not been adequately evaluated for efficacy or safety.

Surgical treatment (bariatric surgery)

This approach is only used in cases of morbid obesity (BMI >40 or 35–40 kg/m^2 with comorbidities such as cardiovascular disease, metabolic disorders, severe psychological conditions related to diet). Two types of surgical intervention are used (Table 59.2):
- Restrictive surgery: designed to reduce the size and capacity of the stomach and induce an earlier feeling of satiety
- Malabsorptive surgery: designed to reduce the area of the small intestine available for absorption

With careful management before and after the procedure, outcomes are more favourable compared to non-surgical treatment, including greater reduction of body weight, waist circumference and plasma concentrations of triglyceride and glucose and greater chance of remission of diabetes and metabolic syndrome. However, the long-term benefit of bariatric surgery is currently not well examined. Appropriate consistent follow-up arrangements must be available for patients to manage complications. Malabsorption conditions arising from bypass operations are associated with nutritional deficiencies and require supplementation. The process of surgical treatment of obesity (pre- and post-operation and long-term follow-up) must therefore involve an interdisciplinary health-care team including physician, surgeon, psychologist, dietitian, nurse and social worker. Some examples of nutritional management for post-operative care include:
- Increased daily protein intake of 90–120 g to maintain lean body mass
- Long-term vitamin and mineral supplementation to compensate possible reduced uptake and absorption
- Continuous reinforcement of healthy dietary habits

Table 59.2 Overview of currently used surgical interventions for morbid obesity.

Name of treatment	Procedure	Comments
Malabsorptive surgery	Sections of GI tract bypassed to reduce surface area for absorption	Weight loss substantial and maintained
		Metabolic complications include vomiting, stenosis, dumping syndrome
		Patients need to be monitored
Jejunoileal	Bypasses a large area of small intestine (SI)	High risk of complications; rarely performed
Gastric bypass	Reduces stomach size and bypasses the duodenum	Reduced capacity and digestion
Biliopancreatic diversion	As above, but the jejunum also bypassed	More extensive effect on absorption
Restrictive surgery	Reduces the size of the stomach	Limits capacity for food, but not absorption
Gastroplasty	The stomach divided to make a smaller pouch (vertical division more successful)	Less weight loss than with gastric bypass
Gastric banding	Constricting band around the stomach limits capacity, may be adjusted to vary extent of restriction	

Overweight and obesity: Popular slimming diets

Aims

1 To identify the criteria relating to a safe diet designed for weight loss

2 To consider the types of commercially available diets for weight loss

The media promote 'diets', which are invariably focused on weight loss, such that the term 'diet' is synonymous in the public mind with eating less to achieve weight reduction. This is in contrast to the nutritionists' view that 'diet' refers to an individual's food intake.

The slimming industry

For many people, a slow and steady weight loss seems unsatisfactory, and 'quick fix' regimes are sought. In addition, those who have regained weight may look for a new approach. As a result, an ever-changing industry of slimming programmes has grown to fill this need. A poorly balanced slimming regime may lead to nutritional deficiencies.

Criteria for a nutritionally sound and safe slimming regime

A slimming regime should fulfil a number of criteria (Table 60.1) to be considered sound.

Healthy eating guidelines can underpin dietary advice for weight loss in a number of ways. These are summarised in Table 60.2.

Types of slimming diets

Various approaches are used by the slimming industry, from ones that are safe and based on good principles to others that can be viewed as potentially dangerous or at least misleading (Table 60.3):

1. Sensible healthy eating plans with reduced energy

A number of 'slimming' organisations have well-balanced diet plans and use systems such as points or exchanges that allow the individual to adjust their intake in line with a target energy allowance. Some include an exercise regime and provide group support through regular meetings. Generally, these are safe and meet essential criteria.

2. Diets that maintain satiety

The clear way to consume less energy is to eat less, but to ensure that this is acceptable, satiety needs to be maintained. This can be achieved by:

• Increasing intake of all plant foods. These can displace more energy-dense items, especially high-fat products, while providing bulk in the digestive tract, promoting satiety and avoiding hunger. This approach is used in many healthy diet plans and provides a sound framework for weight loss.

• Eating foods with a lower glycaemic index (GI) in place of high-GI foods slows down the absorption of glucose and the release of insulin. It is suggested that the high levels of insulin promote fat storage, making high-GI foods more 'fattening'. At present, there are insufficient data about the GI effect of mixed diets, as most studies have been done on single foods, so there is currently no evidence that this is a suitable diet to achieve weight loss.

Table 60.1 Summary of criteria for a nutritionally sound and safe weight loss regime.

Criterion to be fulfilled	Explanation	Comment
Nutritionally balanced	No major food groups should be excluded or eaten to excess; principles that underpin healthy eating should be evident	Avoids risk of deficiency or need for supplements
Biologically plausible	Should not make claims that run against known biological facts	May be difficult for consumer to recognise
Safe	Must not recommend levels of intake that endanger health	Should carry advice to check with doctor
Realistic	Results promised should be realistic	Misleading claims will be demotivating
Flexible	Diet should allow some personal choices to maintain motivation	Rigid eating regimes lead to abandonment
Sustainable	Diet should fit as much as possible into normal life; eating special and unusual foods may be a novelty, but does not fit easily into social existence	Special items increase costs and highlight 'dieting behaviour'
Physical activity	A sensible amount should be recommended to support dietary regime	Can improve self-image and help towards successful outcome

Table 60.2 Basic measures underpinning dietary advice for weight loss.

Dietary measure	Target change	Reasons for change/gain to be made
Reduction in total energy	2.4 MJ (600 kcal) or a 2–4-MJ (500–1000-kcal) deficit	To produce a negative energy balance
Lower total fat intake	To a moderate level	Monounsaturated fats should predominate
Starchy foods should be maintained	Include those with a lower glycaemic index	Maintain a steady blood glucose level, and avoid periodic hunger; a higher non-starch polysaccharide (NSP) intake will promote satiety
Fruit and vegetables	At least five a day	Provide micronutrients and low-energy, nutrient-dense intake. Useful snacks
Soft drinks	To be avoided	Provide energy and promote passive overconsumption

Nutrition at a Glance, Second Edition. Edited by Sangita Sharma, Tony Sheehy and Fariba Kolahdooz.
© 2016 John Wiley & Sons, Ltd. Published 2016 by John Wiley & Sons, Ltd.

Table 60.3 Evaluating types of slimming diets against criteria.

Type of diet	Balanced	Plausible	Safe	Realistic	Flexible	Sustainable
Healthy eating plans	Yes	Yes	Yes	Yes	Yes	Yes
Increasing plant foods	Possible	Yes	Yes	Yes	Possible	Yes
Eating low-GI foods	Possible	Little evidence	Yes	Yes	Possible	Possible
Lower fat diets	Yes	Yes	Yes	Yes	Yes	If not too extreme
Low-CHO diets	No	No	No	No	No	No
Food combining	No	No	Possible	Possible	No	No
Eating at certain times	Possible	No	Possible	Possible	No	No
Preload before meals	Possible	No	No	No	No	No
Avoiding allergens	No	No	No	No	No	No
Supplement-requiring diets	No	No	No	No	No	No
Eating one food only	No	No	No	No	No	No
Fasting/meal skipping	No	No	No	No	No	No

3. Diets that adjust macronutrient content

Low-fat diets. Fat in the diet is more energy dense than other macro-nutrients and is believed to be associated with 'passive overconsumption of energy', so reducing the intake of fat is a logical approach to follow. Many low-fat diets exist, where fat intake is 20–30% of total energy, with an increase in the content of complex carbohydrate.

This improves cardiovascular risk factors and may protect from other chronic diseases. Focusing on a reduction in fatty foods allows healthy eating to become established to help in longer-term maintenance. Combining a reduction in the percentage of fat with an overall lowering of energy intake produces better weight loss than simply replacing fat with carbohydrate.

Low-carbohydrate diets. These have been promoted, with the energy being made up from protein and fat. The most famous of these is the 'Atkins diet'. There is initial rapid weight loss as glycogen reserves and the associated water are lost. The lack of carbohydrate for metabolism results in ketosis, which causes nausea, dehydration and bad breath. Constipation is likely because of the low fibre intake.

The high fat intake is contrary to all healthy eating principles. Weight loss does occur, but this is attributed to the anorectic effects of a high-protein diet and the reduced overall energy intake. Low intakes of minerals and vitamins will, if not supplemented, result in deficiency.

4. Diets that prescribe meal composition or timing of meals

Food combining suggests that foods containing proteins should not be eaten with carbohydrate-containing foods, as they cannot be digested simultaneously. There is no scientific evidence for this. Weight may be lost because attention is being paid to what is eaten, and overall food intakes are likely to be reduced as a result.

Consuming foods only before a certain time in the day is proposed by another diet to allow the body to complete digestion before night-time. Again, the main effect of this is to limit overall food intake.

5. Diets that 'preload' the digestive system before meals

Eating a fruit before a meal to provide 'enzymes' and eating grapefruit to 'eliminate fat' are two suggested eating patterns, neither of which have any scientific base. In both cases, the preload is likely to reduce the food eaten at mealtimes.

Drinking water before meals to cause weight loss may promote a feeling of fullness at mealtimes and so reduce food intake. However, water is rapidly absorbed from the stomach, so would have a short-term effect.

6. Diets that avoid supposed 'allergic reactions'

These invoke claims that overweight is due to an allergic reaction by the body to food components that do not 'match', including eating different types of foods depending on blood group, or a mismatch of electric charges between the food and the individual. Both focus on elimination of entire food groups and are nutritionally dangerous without any scientific basis.

7. Diets that require supplements

A variety of these exist that are reported to boost energy, detoxify, improve cellular activity, etc. Unless there are clear medical reasons for poor digestion or absorption, these preparations will not help in weight loss.

8. Eating one food only

There are single-item, very-low-energy diet products that can be used for short-term rapid weight loss. The popular diets that advise consuming a single product, such as cabbage soup, have no nutritional credibility and are unsustainable.

Monotony and boredom restrict intake and the consumer learns nothing about a healthy balanced diet for future weight control. Serious risk of deficiency also exists.

9. Fasting/meal skipping

This may be seen as the easiest way of losing weight, but it is unsustainable and likely to result in a very erratic food intake with the risk of nutritional deficiency. Risks of dehydration in the short term and eating disorders in the longer term are possible.

Weight loss needs to be addressed by a public health approach with a higher rate of success than at present. Meanwhile, vulnerable individuals will continue to be exposed to unsound and unsafe slimming regimes. It would be helpful if at least the awareness of what to look for in a weight reduction programme was more widely recognised.

Principles of weight reduction

The scientific principle of weight reduction is straightforward:
- Energy intake must be less than energy output to create a negative energy balance, resulting in weight loss, as stored fat reserves are used for energy.
- Energy deficits of 500–1000 kcal (2–4 MJ) per day may be recommended, depending on body size and gender.

Weight loss is generally slow, ~0.5 kg/week, unless the energy deficit is great, when there is also likely to be significant loss of lean tissue.

When weight has been lost, the further problem of *maintenance* creates a challenge to individuals, who may gradually regain weight.

61 Underweight and negative energy balance

Aims

1 To consider reasons for underweight

2 To describe the body's response to a negative energy balance

A deficit of energy intake, in naturally occurring situations (e.g. famine conditions), is generally accompanied by an inadequate intake of nutrients. There are a number of contributory factors, which may also determine the metabolic consequences and any treatment that is attempted.

The most obvious consequence of the energy deficit is *loss of weight*, attributable to an imbalance between energy intake (which is reduced) and energy expenditure (which may be increased, unchanged or even reduced from a previous level).

In the majority of instances, there is an *adaptive physiological response* to minimise energy expenditure when intake is reduced and therefore facilitate survival.

Starvation

This is the most challenging situation, as energy intake falls to zero.

When no food is eaten, the body must adapt to utilise stored energy reserves. The largest of these is body fat, stored in adipose tissue, which can supply fatty acids for energy provision. However, the brain and red blood cells require a supply of glucose to function, and metabolic adaptations must occur to preserve carbohydrate and use it efficiently.

A number of neural and hormonal responses are involved; these include:

- Reduced sympathetic nervous system activity
- Lower levels of active thyroid hormone (T_3)
- Lower levels of insulin
- Leptin activity, which modulates the energy-sparing response

Adaptation to starvation

This develops over a period of time and involves changes to metabolism of substrates:

- Carbohydrate stores, as glycogen in the liver and muscle, are limited and may be completely exhausted within 24 h.
- Hepatic gluconeogenesis can generate glucose de novo, from glycerol (from lipids) and carbon skeletons of amino acids. There is an initial phase, lasting 3–4 days, of protein breakdown from skeletal muscle for energy.
- A fall in circulating glucose and insulin levels stimulates lipolysis; tissues use more fatty acids for energy and glycerol is directed to gluconeogenesis. Ketone bodies are produced by the oxidation of fatty acids in the liver.
- The brain adapts to the use of ketone bodies for energy, meeting some two-thirds of its energy requirements in this way. Small amounts of glucose are produced by gluconeogenesis. This adapted steady state may take up to 3 weeks to establish and can persist as long as fat reserves are available. This tends to be longer in women than in men and depends on the previous level of nutrition. As women have more body fat, this extends the survival period.
- Once fat reserves are depleted, structural proteins are broken down, and there is a rapid deterioration leading to death.

(See Figure 61.1 for a summary of this process.)

Adaptations of energy expenditure

These also occur and therefore contribute to minimising the energy imbalance:

- Resting metabolism – there is an early phase of increased metabolic efficiency; later metabolism uses less energy as a result of a smaller mass of active tissue.
- Thermogenesis – where no food is consumed, there will be no diet-induced thermic response; undernourished individuals have been shown to have a poorer thermogenic response on exposure to cold.
- Physical activity – observations of individuals who are starving, or in negative energy balance due to undernutrition, show that

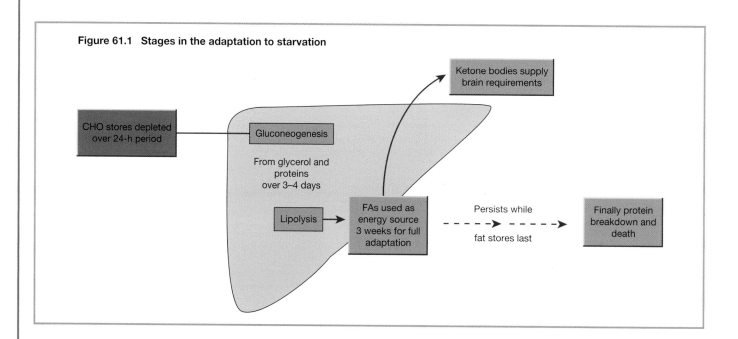

Figure 61.1 Stages in the adaptation to starvation

CHO stores depleted over 24-h period → Gluconeogenesis

From glycerol and proteins over 3–4 days

Lipolysis → FAs used as energy source 3 weeks for full adaptation

Ketone bodies supply brain requirements

Persists while fat stores last

Finally protein breakdown and death

Nutrition at a Glance, Second Edition. Edited by Sangita Sharma, Tony Sheehy and Fariba Kolahdooz.
© 2016 John Wiley & Sons, Ltd. Published 2016 by John Wiley & Sons, Ltd.

there is a reduced amount of physical activity undertaken. In addition, there is a greater ergonomic efficiency in activity. The post-exercise elevation of heat output is also diminished in undernutrition.

Altogether, these adaptations allow savings to be made in energy output.

Chronic energy deficits

For a large percentage of the population in the less developed countries of the world, chronic energy deficiency is a permanent feature of life. The adaptations that occur enable the body to survive but often at a cost to long-term health.

Energy deficit compounded by disease or trauma

The concurrence of a metabolic response to disease or trauma with energy deficit is likely to exacerbate the negative energy balance for a number of reasons:

• Injury, infection and fever increase the metabolic rate, in proportion to the extent of the physiological stress.
• Protein is catabolised from muscle for the production of acute-phase proteins by the liver, and nitrogen losses increase.

• The major hormones of the stress response are cortisol and catecholamines, which stimulate glucose production and increase energy expenditure.

This metabolic response may result in a serious loss of weight in an undernourished patient which, together with tissue wasting and anorexia, results in cachexia, with a high risk of mortality. This can occur in some chronic illnesses. The need for nutritional support must be assessed, and appropriate measures quickly introduced. This can be a major problem in hospital patients.

Causes of reduced energy intake

These might include:
• Poor food availability
• Inability to eat due to illness or following injury or trauma
• Intentional/deliberate restriction of food, either for a short term (e.g. to lose weight) or as a long-term behaviour (possibly associated with some form of eating disorder) or a political statement

Causes of increased energy expenditure might include:
• Heavy manual labour or physical activity
• Increased requirements for growth
• Fever/infection/post-traumatic response

62 Nutrition and cancer I

Aim

1 To describe the possible factors in the diet that may have a causative role in cancer

One in three people will be diagnosed with cancer in their lifetime. Specific types of cancer vary in prevalence in different parts of the world. This difference reflects the variety of environmental factors, including diet, that play a role in causation.

There is a growing burden of cancer deaths worldwide, associated with an ageing population. However, there are also differing trends in the rates of some cancers. For example, in the West, lung cancer rates have been falling in men but increasing in women, as smoking behaviours change. In Japan, there has been a rapid increase in colorectal cancer rates during the last 30 years, as diets become more Westernised.

What is cancer?

Cancer is a disorder of somatic cells, in which changes to the genetic material cause a normal cell to behave abnormally in form or function. The change that occurs may be inherited or may occur sporadically. The result is that the cell fails to function as it should, in not responding to regulatory signals that control its life cycle. As a result, it may divide inappropriately or fail to die (apoptose) at the end of its life cycle, with the result that a cluster of cells is eventually produced, forming a tumour.

Stages in the development of cancer have been identified, and mechanisms within these are still being studied. However, it is clear that movement through the stages is not inevitable, and repairs can be made that stop or slow down the process.

It is within these 'accelerating' or 'braking' mechanisms that the environment and diet can play a role. These are summarised in Figure 62.1.

Evidence on causation of cancer

A number of environmental factors, including diet, have been associated with the aetiology of cancer. However, providing sound evidence is sometimes difficult:

• Much evidence is based on *epidemiological studies* of populations (see Chapters 30 and 31), allowing the calculation of the relative risk of the disease, based on levels of exposure to a causative factor (e.g. diet). Epidemiology cannot provide proof of cause and effect, and associations may be confounded by other differences between populations. Studies of migrants who develop rates of cancer typical of their host country within a generation confirm the importance of environment.

• *Case–control studies* provide further information about exposure to causative factors, but the time course of cancer development can blur the relationship between exposure and diagnosis of cancer. Trials of interventions with putative preventive factors have been disappointing and have failed to confirm the protective roles of nutrients such as β-carotene or vitamin E. Reasons for this may include the use of a single nutrient supplement rather than whole food sources and the timing of the interventions.

• Very-large-scale *prospective cohort studies* are now under way, such as the European Prospective Investigation into Cancer and Nutrition (EPIC) ($n = 500\,000$) and the Multiethnic Cohort (MEC) ($n = 215\,000$), which have recruited participants who are being followed up, to identify cancer development and link this with earlier exposure to risk factors. Smaller cohort studies provide some evidence on diet and environmental associations, but with homogeneous cohorts, there are limits to the general application of the results.

• Findings from population studies are gradually being tested in *experimental situations* to elucidate mechanisms. For example,

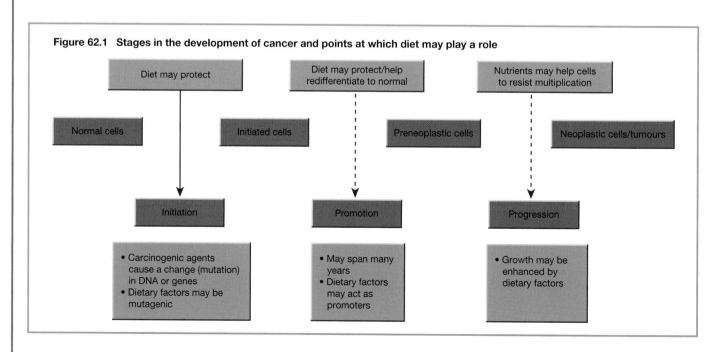

Figure 62.1   Stages in the development of cancer and points at which diet may play a role

Diet may protect

Diet may protect/help redifferentiate to normal

Nutrients may help cells to resist multiplication

Normal cells → Initiated cells → Preneoplastic cells → Neoplastic cells/tumours

Initiation
• Carcinogenic agents cause a change (mutation) in DNA or genes
• Dietary factors may be mutagenic

Promotion
• May span many years
• Dietary factors may act as promoters

Progression
• Growth may be enhanced by dietary factors

Nutrition at a Glance, Second Edition. Edited by Sangita Sharma, Tony Sheehy and Fariba Kolahdooz.
© 2016 John Wiley & Sons, Ltd. Published 2016 by John Wiley & Sons, Ltd.

an association between red meat intake and bowel cancer, observed by the EPIC study, has been tested experimentally. This has demonstrated that red meat consumption causes N-nitroso compound levels in faeces to increase and that there is an increase in DNA mutations of colonic cells with higher levels of these compounds.

Diet as a factor in cancer

It is estimated that an average of 30% of cancer is diet related: this ranges from a low level for lung cancer to 80% for colorectal cancer.

Difficulties in attributing causation to dietary factors occur because:
• Diets are extremely complex, and particular nutrients can occur in many different foods.
• Certain aspects of the diet co-vary in individuals, such that a high intake of one food, for example, meat, may be associated with a low intake of fruit and vegetables.
• Patterns of food intake obtained from food frequency questionnaires may not be sufficiently specific to demonstrate differences and relationships.
• Dietary records may contain errors, but more robust techniques are being developed that cross-check dietary records with blood concentrations and other biomarkers.

Nevertheless, information about the roles of diet suggests that it can:
• Be a source of preformed carcinogens or precursors (i.e. compounds that can be converted into carcinogens)
• Contain nutrients that affect the formation, transport, deactivation or excretion of carcinogens
• Contain nutrients that can be protective, by promoting the body's resistance to carcinogens and therefore increasing the resistance of cancer

Some evidence exists of a promoting effect of certain dietary factors in cancer (Table 62.1).

Avoidance of these foods or dietary components may help protect individuals against the development of cancer and should feature in advice (see Chapter 63).

Table 62.1 Dietary factors that may have a role in promotion of cancer.

Food or nutrients	Possible role in cancer promotion
Total energy intake	High energy intakes result in overweight and obesity, linked to greater incidence of hormone-related cancers: breast, endometrium and prostate. Also a positive association with cancers of the oesophagus, colorectum, pancreas and kidney
Fat intakes	Difficult to separate from the evidence on overweight. High fat intakes (especially of saturated fat) have been associated with lung, colorectal, prostate and breast cancers There is little evidence of specific risk from monounsaturated or polyunsaturated fats. Conjugated linoleic acid (CLA), found in dairy fat, may have a protective role, but evidence is equivocal
Alcohol	May potentiate the role of other carcinogens, increasing uptake or susceptibility of cells Intakes linked with cancer of the aerodigestive tract and liver; also evidence of an association with breast cancer, possibly through an effect on oestrogen metabolism Adequate intake of folate may offer some protection
Salt	Linked with gastric cancer; high levels of salt reduce gastric acidity, which in turn promotes conversion of dietary nitrates to nitrites and nitrosamines, which are carcinogenic Better methods of preservation have reduced the use of salt for this purpose, and there has been a parallel reduction in gastric cancer
Meat	Metabolic products in the colon arising from digestion of red meat are N-nitroso compounds, which have been found to cause DNA mutations. Thus, there is a possible mechanism for development of colorectal cancer. Processed meat and charred meat may also contribute by forming heterocyclic amines, which are broken down to carcinogenic products

63 Nutrition and cancer II

Aims

1 To describe possible factors in the diet that may have a protective role in cancer

2 To formulate dietary advice for prevention of cancer

Protective effects against cancer can be obtained from foods and nutrients, which act to repair damage or prevent promotion and subsequent progression to tumour development (Table 63.1).

Summary of evidence on diet and cancer

Although conclusive evidence of cause and effect from dietary factors is largely lacking in the causation of cancer, there is a substantial body of evidence that points to relationships between dietary components and increased or reduced risk. It should also be recognised that maintenance of physical activity and not smoking are key lifestyle guidelines that should be adhered to. These are summarised in Table 63.2 for the most common cancer sites.

There is evidence of a possible association for other sites and other dietary factors, but this at present is insufficient.

Advice on diet and lifestyle

The current evidence on cancer suggests that dietary change is important.

Following healthy eating guidelines, with particular attention to the following aspects, forms the cornerstone of dietary prevention of cancer:

- Maintenance of normal body weight
- Physical activity according to guidelines (at least 30 min on 5 days per week)
- At least 400 g/day of fruit and vegetables, including a variety of types
- Increased intake of plant foods rich in complex carbohydrates, for example, grains, cereals and pulses, to provide the main source of energy
- Minimal alcohol consumption
- Reduced intakes of red meat, fat and salt
- Avoidance of salt-preserved and processed foods
- Safe food preparation: avoidance of foods that are spoilt or potentially contaminated with moulds or bacteria.

Table 63.1 Dietary factors with a possible protective role in cancer.

Food or nutrients	Possible role in protection against cancer
Non-starch polysaccharides (dietary fibre)	Diets high in fibre confer some protection against colorectal cancer This may be effected in a number of ways: • More rapid removal of potential carcinogens by faster transit through the bowel • More beneficial nutrients available for the colonocytes • Healthier bacterial flora in a more acidic environment However, fibre intakes show high covariance with other beneficial foods, such as cereals, grains, fruit and vegetables, which may also have beneficial effects in other ways
Fruit and vegetables	There is consistent evidence that diets high in fruit and vegetables are associated with lower cancer rates and no evidence to the contrary It is believed that the antioxidants supplied by these foods play a protective role against damage to DNA and other molecules Other substances contained in fruit and vegetables may be important: these include various phytochemicals such as flavonoids, phytosterols, isothiocyanates, sulphur-containing compounds and phyto-oestrogens. A wide range of fruit and vegetables must be eaten to incorporate all of these
Folic acid	Evidence suggests that higher intakes of folate are associated with lower risk of cancer, particularly of the pancreas. The mechanism appears to be a protection against mutations of DNA
Calcium and vitamin D	An inverse relationship between calcium intake (as dairy products) and colon cancer has been reported. This may be due to binding in the gut of fats by calcium, thus reducing potential harm from fats and bile acids. However, a positive association has been reported between high intake of calcium and increased risk of prostate cancer Vitamin D may have an anticancer action in its own right and has been proposed to reduce risk of colon cancer

Nutrition at a Glance, Second Edition. Edited by Sangita Sharma, Tony Sheehy and Fariba Kolahdooz.
© 2016 John Wiley & Sons, Ltd. Published 2016 by John Wiley & Sons, Ltd.

Table 63.2 Summary of dietary and lifestyle factors for which there is strong or convincing evidence of an association with cancer.

Cancer site	Convincing/probable evidence of decreased risk	Convincing/probable evidence of increased risk
Aerodigestive system	Fruit and vegetables	Alcohol, smoking, tobacco
Stomach	Non-starchy vegetables, *Allium* vegetables and fruit	Salt, salted and salty foods
Colorectum	Physical activity, foods containing fibre, calcium, milk and garlic	Overweight/obesity, red and processed meat, total fat, alcoholic drinks, body fatness, abdominal fatness and adult attained height
Liver		Aflatoxins and alcohol
Lung	Fruits, foods containing carotenoids	Arsenic in drinking water and β-carotene supplements and smoking
Breast	Lactation and physical activity	Alcohol, obesity, adult attained height
Pancreas	Foods containing folate	Body fatness, abdominal fatness and adult attained height
Ovary		Adult attained height
Endometrium	Physical activity	Body fatness, abdominal fatness
Prostate	Foods containing lycopene and selenium	Diet high in calcium
Kidney		Body fatness
Skin		Arsenic in drinking water

Adapted from American Institute for Cancer Research 2007.

64 Diet and cardiovascular disease: Aetiology

Aims

1 To describe the development of cardiovascular disease
2 To identify the major risk factors involved in the aetiology of the disease

---

Definitions

Cardiovascular disease (CVD) includes coronary heart disease (CHD), cerebrovascular disease and peripheral vascular disease (PVD). All share the common features of thickening and hardening of the arterial walls resulting in a compromised blood flow.

Mortality rates

CVD is the leading cause of death in the developed world and accounts for approximately one-third of all deaths worldwide. Deaths from CHD comprise about half of the total and stroke deaths a further quarter:

• In general, death rates due to CVD are higher in industrialised countries but with substantial variation.
• In recent decades, death rates from CVD in many Westernised countries have been falling, but developing countries are experiencing rapid increases in these diseases as they undergo economic and nutritional transition.

Pathology

The fundamental lesion is the atherosclerotic plaque that develops within the arterial wall and its eventual rupture. These processes occur slowly and over a prolonged period.

The three main stages in the process are summarised in Figure 64.1:

1 The *vascular endothelium* is the key surface at which several contributory factors interact. The endothelium has many self-regulating properties, achieved through the production of nitric oxide, prostacyclin and other bioactive substances. Many of the risk factors cause dysfunction here. As a consequence, the endothelium becomes more permeable to lipids and proteins.
2 *Low-density lipoproteins* (LDLs) in the blood readily pass into the arterial wall to deliver cholesterol to the tissues. If they become oxidised, the cascade of events results in the formation of atherosclerotic plaque.

3 If the *plaque becomes unstable and ruptures*, activation of platelets and the blood coagulation cascade can result in clot formation (*thrombosis*) and a myocardial infarction (or ischaemic stroke in the case of its occurrence in the brain).

Risk factors for CVD

The pathological process comprises many elements, which may be exacerbated or ameliorated by 'risk factors'.

Two categories are identified: *irreversible* and *potentially modifiable* (behavioural) (see Figure 64.2).

Irreversible risk factors

• Genetic traits – include disorders of lipid metabolism.
• Male gender – higher risk than in premenopausal women; risk equalises later in life.
• Increasing age – progressive increase of risk.
• Lower socioeconomic status – associated with higher risk.
• Ethnicity – higher risk in some ethnic groups (e.g. from Indian subcontinent).
• Small for gestational age at birth – greater risk in later life.

Modifiable (behavioural) risk factors

These are related to diet and lifestyle factors and have been the focus of health education initiatives for many years. Many of these risk factors overlap, either in their consequences or in the causative factors (Figure 64.2).

Many of the risk factors have dietary components that contribute to or minimise the disease process. These are discussed further in Chapter 65:

• *Smoking* – contributes to endothelial dysfunction and increases oxidative stress, promoting oxidation of LDLs.
• *Physical activity* – an increased level of activity reduces the impact of many other risk factors. For example, physical activity reduces obesity, which is associated with insulin resistance, hypertension and abnormal blood lipids. Lipid profiles are normalised (including an increase in HDL levels), endothelial function and clotting-related factors are improved, and markers of inflammation decrease.

Modifiable risk factors offer an opportunity for intervention by health professionals, both as general health education and as targeted individual advice, to reduce the eventual risk of developing CVD. If CVD is already present, then more intensive advice or secondary prevention may be necessary.

Nutrition at a Glance, Second Edition. Edited by Sangita Sharma, Tony Sheehy and Fariba Kolahdooz.
© 2016 John Wiley & Sons, Ltd. Published 2016 by John Wiley & Sons, Ltd.

Figure 64.1 Summary of the risk factors, pathological process and consequences of the atherogenic process

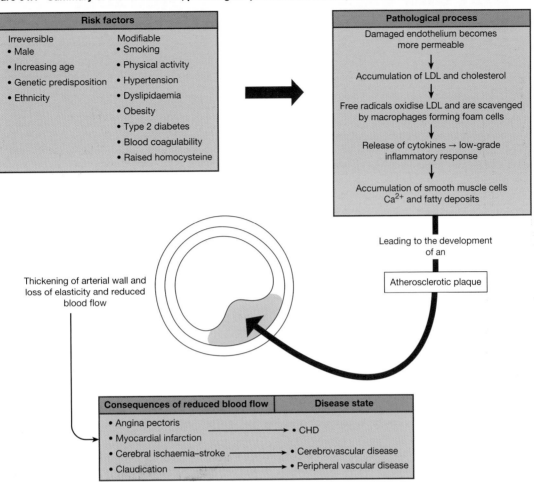

Figure 64.2 Interactions between the major modifiable risk factors for CVD

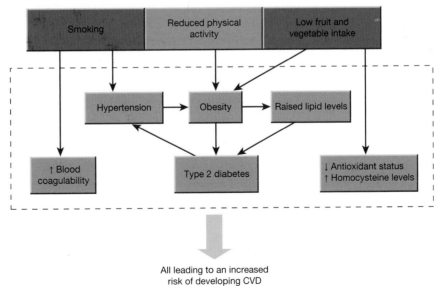

65 Diet and cardiovascular disease: Prevention

Aims

1 To describe the evidence for the dietary factors involved in each stage of the development of cardiovascular disease
2 To use this evidence to formulate practical dietary advice

The aetiology of cardiovascular disease (CVD) is multifactorial, with a number of risk factors influencing the development and progression of the disease.

From an understanding of the pathology of CVD (see Chapter 64), it is possible to identify dietary components that either contribute to or help to prevent the disease process. Although incomplete, current knowledge is used to advise on diets that reduce CVD risk.

Endothelial dysfunction

There is no 'gold standard' measurement for endothelial function, but vasodilatory capacity and assay of endothelium-derived products in plasma and urine are used as proxy indicators of function.

Many of the factors that affect the endothelium (see Table 65.1) also influence other stages of the pathological process.

Blood lipids

The *quantity* and *composition of dietary fats* are recognised as key determinants of the plasma lipid profile:

• Persistently elevated triglyceride levels alter the normal exchange of constituents between lipoprotein fractions, resulting in the formation of small dense LDLs and HDLs, which promote atherogenesis.

• Modifications to the proportions of consumed fats have been at the core of advice regarding dietary prevention of CHD since the 1970s.

The goal is to achieve *reductions in total cholesterol*, particularly that in the LDL fraction, and an *increase in HDL levels*. This advice reflects developments in knowledge and is summarised in Table 65.2.

Oxidative stress

The *oxidation of LDL particles* is a key stage in the pathology of CVD. LDL particles contain large amounts of polyunsaturated fats, which are vulnerable to oxidation. Markers of oxidative stress are increased in CVD.

Antioxidants are also present within the LDLs and can provide some protection against free radicals. The diet is an important source of exogenous antioxidants:

• *Fruit and vegetables* are the main dietary sources of antioxidants, and populations in which there is a high level of consumption of these foods have a reduced risk of CVD. An inverse association has been shown between plasma levels of antioxidants, including ascorbate and vitamin E, and CVD risk. However, intervention trials, using individual *antioxidant vitamins* alone or in combination, have failed to show evidence of benefit and in some cases produced negative outcomes.

• Plant foods contain many other compounds with antioxidant activity (e.g. flavonoids), but more information is needed about their precise chemical forms and concentrations in foods, their bioavailability and metabolism within the body and the likely plasma and LDL concentrations that can be reached when these foods are eaten before any conclusions can be drawn about their role as protective agents against CVD. Current advice is to focus on foods rather than specific dietary components and to increase consumption of fruit and vegetables to at least five portions (or 400 g) per day, thereby providing a range of antioxidants.

Table 65.1 Factors involved in endothelial function.

Factor	Suggested mechanism	Strength of the evidence
Dietary fat intake	Elevated levels of TAG-rich lipoproteins after meals have a pro-oxidant effect on the endothelium and may impair vasodilation	Consistent for harmful effect of atherogenic lipaemia
Fish oils	Especially docosahexaenoic acid (DHA), incorporated into membrane phospholipids, attenuates proinflammatory and prothrombotic activity	Evidence is consistent for reduction in fatal CHD
Antioxidant nutrients	Protect against free-radical damage, for example, resulting from hypertension, smoking and pro-oxidant products	Consistent evidence from laboratory and *in vivo* studies; benefits not shown in intervention trials
B vitamins and folate	Reduction of homocysteine (HCys) levels in circulation. HCys is believed toxic to endothelium, possibly through reduced response to acetylcholine	Reduction in vascular events in treatment groups and improved ECG; large trials of supplementation awaited
Alcohol	Increases HDL levels, which act as antioxidants. May also have anti-inflammatory effect	Moderate intakes lower CHD

Nutrition at a Glance, Second Edition. Edited by Sangita Sharma, Tony Sheehy and Fariba Kolahdooz.

Table 65.2 Practical advice on dietary fats to modify plasma lipids and the origins of such advice.

Dietary lipid	Effect on plasma lipids	Practical application
Total fat	High-fat diets generally associated with high CHD rates. Low-fat diets are shown to reduce LDL levels	Fat reduction to 20–35% of total energy is widely recommended
	However, replacement of fat with CHO may increase TAG levels; the effect can be counteracted with physical activity	More substantial reduction may limit compliance and may result in high CHO intakes, which increase VLDL levels
SFAs	SFAs with 14 and 16 carbons are particularly strongly related to raised LDL levels. Reduction in SFA intake reduces total cholesterol, LDL and HDL (less than LDL); effects on CHD well supported with evidence	Reductions in dietary sources of SFA generally agreed; target intakes normally 10% of total energy
Cholesterol	Increases levels of plasma cholesterol to varying extent in individuals. Absorption from diet is limited	Closely associated with SFA in the diet, and emphasis on reducing SFA also limits intake of cholesterol
		Eggs are cholesterol rich and intake may need to be controlled in susceptible individuals
n-6 PUFAs	Replacement of SFAs with n-6 PUFAs reduces LDL levels, with little change to HDL levels, resulting in improved lipid profile. May also help clearance of VLDLs in postprandial state	Substitution of SFAs with n-6 PUFAs recommended. Intakes above 10% of energy not recommended due to risk of peroxidation of double bonds
MUFAs	Replacement of SFAs with MUFAs reduces LDL levels, but not HDLs. Habituation to higher MUFA intake is associated with larger chylomicrons and attenuated factor VII activation (i.e. lower blood clotting tendency)	Substitution of SFAs with MUFAs is a beneficial dietary modification, especially in subjects with normal body weight where total fat reduction is unnecessary
Trans-fatty acids	Cause an increase in LDLs and reduce HDL levels, potential to contribute to CHD	Levels should be kept as low as possible;
n-3 PUFAs	Reported to improve the clearance of VLDLs from circulation and lower concentrations of small dense LDLs	Effects on lipid clearance seen at high doses only, greater than can be achieved with acceptable intakes from oily fish

Inflammation

An inflammatory state appears to exist in CVD, probably resulting from a generalised response to local factors associated with the atherosclerotic plaque.

Key indicators of this response are raised levels of C-reactive protein (CRP) and fibrinogen:

• *Obesity* is associated with raised levels of CRP, and levels fall on weight loss. However, it is unclear how and to what extent these findings are related to the inflammatory response.
• *Eicosanoids* derived from PUFAs play a part in inflammation, and those from the *n-6 PUFAs are pro-inflammatory*. Their synthesis is competitively inhibited by EPA and DHA present in oily fish, and the eicosanoids produced by the *n-3 PUFAs may be anti-inflammatory*.
• Additional effects of *n-3* PUFAs may include increased plaque stability and altered cytokine production. However, at present, it remains unclear how the *n-3* PUFAs exert the documented protective effect in CVD.

Haemostatic factors

The balance between *clotting tendency* and *fibrinolysis* determines the risk of thrombus formation. A large number of physiological factors have a role in these processes:

• *Obesity* has been associated with a raised concentration of fibrinogen and other markers of prothrombotic tendency. Weight loss and physical activity have a positive effect on these markers. Some of the contributors to a high energy intake may also affect thrombotic state; for example, heavy alcohol consumption and a high-fat diet both reduce fibrinolytic activity. However, moderate alcohol intakes may reduce fibrinogen concentration.
• Fibrinolytic activity is also improved by diets that promote weight loss, such as low-fat and high-fibre diets.
• *Fish oils*, providing *n-3 PUFAs*, attenuate the production of thromboxane A$_2$ and so suppress activation of platelets.

Other dietary factors impacting lipids

Other foods and nutrients that have been associated with effects on blood lipids include:
• *Soya*: Isoflavones are able to reduce plasma cholesterol. A reduction of 0.23 mmol/L with an intake of 25 g soya protein/day has been reported.
• *Dietary fibre*: Soluble fibre has been reported to reduce total cholesterol by 0.045 mmol/L for each gram of fibre. Population studies suggest that lower rates of CHD are associated with larger intakes of dietary fibre.
• *Alcohol*: Moderate intakes of alcohol (1–2 units per day) have been shown to reduce CHD in men (above 40 years) and postmenopausal women. Levels of HDLs are increased, but greater consumption increases triacylglycerol and CHD risk.
• *Plant stanols and sterols*: These reduce the absorption of dietary cholesterol and may also increase the activity of the LDL receptor and have a clear effect on reducing plasma cholesterol levels, especially in the LDL fraction.

Key dietary aspects

• Moderate total fat intake.
• Replace the saturated fats with polyunsaturated fats or preferably monounsaturated fats.
• Increase intake of *n*-3 polyunsaturated fats, preferably from oily fish.
• Consume at least five portions of fruit and vegetables per day.
• Eat wholegrain products to increase dietary fibre intake and provide additional micronutrients.
• If alcohol is included, consume in moderate amounts only.
• Maintain healthy body weight and remain physically active.

Summary

Taking all the stages of the pathological process individually enables a detailed breakdown of the associated dietary factors to be considered. However, many factors have effects across several components of the process, and these form the basis of dietary advice for prevention of CVD.

66 Adverse reactions to food and inborn errors of metabolism

Aims

1 To introduce the range of possible adverse reactions to food
2 To consider food intolerance and food aversion as adverse reactions to food

Food intolerance

Food intolerance is a generic name covering a range of *reproducible* responses to a specific food or nutrient. It includes allergic (either immunoglobulin E (IgE) mediated or non-IgE mediated), pharmacological and enzymatic reactions.

Allergic reactions

Allergic responses (usually to proteins in foods) are mediated by the immune system. The severity of the reactions varies between individuals and can involve a number of systems of the body, including the respiratory system, the skin, the blood vessels, the gastrointestinal tract, and the nervous system.

IgE-mediated reactions

Within a few minutes to a few hours after exposure to an allergenic food, IgE binding to the allergen triggers mast cells to release histamine and prostaglandins, causing the cascade of events including bronchoconstriction, vasodilation, oedema and abdominal pain (Figure 66.1). Any food can cause IgE-mediated allergic reactions, but the eight most common are egg, fish, milk, peanuts, shellfish, soy, tree nuts and wheat. A severe response to these foods may cause a major fall in blood pressure and result in anaphylactic shock, which requires immediate medical attention. Individuals who are aware of their risks for anaphylaxis are generally advised to carry epinephrine (adrenaline) to counter this reaction.

Breast milk provides immunoglobulin A (IgA), which protects the gut from potential food allergens until the infant's immune system matures. Children who are not exclusively breastfed are more vulnerable to allergic reactions to foods than those who are exclusively breastfed. Although children with allergies may grow out of most food allergies, those to peanuts, tree nuts, fish and shellfish may be retained in adulthood.

Risk factors for IgE-mediated food allergy include:
- Genetic predisposition
- Low birth weight
- Excessive hygienic practices among children, resulting in poorer immune system development
- Early cessation of breastfeeding
- Contemporary diets, which contain a higher proportion of *n*-6 fatty acids (pro-inflammatory) compared to *n*-3 fatty acids (anti-inflammatory)
- Early introduction of allergenic substances into the infant diet

Non-IgE-mediated reactions

Not all adverse reactions to food involve IgE- and histamine-mediated events. Other elements of the immune system, including T lymphocytes and scavenger cells, may become involved in reactions, which may take several hours or days to develop fully.

The most common example of a non-IgE-mediated reaction is coeliac disease, in which genetically susceptible people respond to gluten found in wheat, barley, rye and some varieties of oats. Exposure to dietary gluten leads to reductions in the number and complexity of villi lining the lumen of the gut, primarily in the small intestine. The resulting reduction in the surface area of the gut for absorption leads to malabsorption of nutrients. The condition may remain undiagnosed for a number of years until folate and iron deficiencies lead to anaemia or inadequate calcium and vitamin D absorption results in poor bone development or osteoporosis.

Traditionally, coeliac disease was confirmed following small bowel biopsy; however, more recently, serological tests for antibodies in blood have been developed. Besides coeliac disease, a

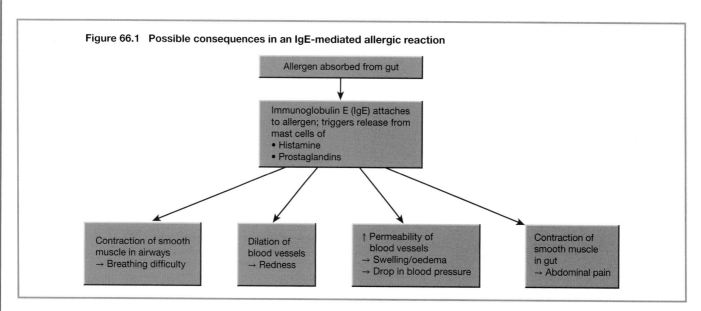

Figure 66.1 Possible consequences in an IgE-mediated allergic reaction

Nutrition at a Glance, Second Edition. Edited by Sangita Sharma, Tony Sheehy and Fariba Kolahdooz.
© 2016 John Wiley & Sons, Ltd. Published 2016 by John Wiley & Sons, Ltd.

number of other non-IgE-mediated allergic conditions have been investigated (but not necessarily confirmed) including:
- Urticaria and dermatitis
- Infant colic
- Irritable bowel syndrome
- Asthma
- Migraine
- Attention deficit hyperactivity disorder (ADHD)
- Rheumatoid arthritis

Attempting to identify foods that trigger symptoms in these conditions can be difficult as there is often inconsistency between subjects for trigger foods. Moreover, nutritional deficiencies can occur if a wide range of foods is found that seem to trigger symptoms, and these foods are then excluded from the diet. For these reasons, managing food intolerances requires careful dietary planning, and individual advice may be needed.

Inborn errors of metabolism

Inborn errors of metabolism are genetic disorders that involve enzyme defects and inability to metabolise certain nutrients. Inborn errors of metabolism and other genetically determined enzyme defects, principally affecting amino acid metabolism, require lifelong dietary modifications.

These may be responsible for food intolerances, causing unpleasant symptoms in certain people. Examples include:
- Phenylketonuria (PKU) involves reduced or absent activity of an enzyme, phenylalanine hydroxylase, and results in the accumulation of phenylalanine. Non-gastrointestinal symptoms such as cognitive delay, behaviour problems and fair skin and hair may present in people with PKU.
- Genetically determined absence of *alcohol dehydrogenase* in some populations results in the inability to metabolise alcohol.
- *Congenital lactase deficiency* is rare although the enzyme may disappear after infancy and compromise the digestion of milk and milk products. Disaccharide enzyme activities may be affected by drug therapies, binge drinking or chronic alcohol consumption. In these circumstances, symptoms of intolerance may occur, including bloating and diarrhoea, as a result of the bacterial fermentation of lactose.
- *Fructose intolerance* results in incomplete fructose metabolism, which leads to hypoglycaemia.
- Maple syrup urine disease (MSUD) is a deficiency of the *branched-chain alpha-keto acid dehydrogenase complex* resulting in an inability to break down branched-chain amino acids (leucine, isoleucine and valine). The deficiency gets its name from the characteristic sweet, burnt sugar smell of the urine caused by keto acid build-up as a result of the elevated branched-chain amino acids. If not treated with a special diet, cognitive function may be compromised.
- Deficiency of *cystathionine beta synthase* causes a condition known as homocystinuria, an inability to properly metabolise homocysteine. This results in the build-up of homocysteine and some of its metabolites in the blood and urine. It is an autosomal recessive inherited trait. The characteristic skeletal abnormalities and cognitive and vision impairments often do not present until the affected child is up to 3 years old. As a result, it is often required that newborns be screened with a blood test at birth.

Pharmacological reactions

Some foods contain pharmacological agents that may cause allergic reactions. However, the amounts needed are much greater than for the allergic reactions discussed previously. Examples include:
- Cheeses (Roquefort, Parmesan and mature Cheddar).
- Wine (and other fermented products).

- Bananas, yeast extract, avocados, chocolate, oranges and some fish products, which can contain biogenic amines such as histamine, tyramine, phenylethylamine and octopamine (depending on the food).
- Chocolate, tomatoes and strawberries can directly cause release of histamine.
- Caffeine can also trigger a pharmacological reaction in sensitive individuals.

Diagnosing allergic reactions to foods

Rigorous testing using strict criteria must be adopted before the existence of an adverse reaction to a food can be confirmed. This will involve:
- Excluding the food from the diet and noting that the symptoms disappear and that they reappear when the food is reintroduced.
- Taking great care if there is any suspicion of anaphylaxis; such testing must be done under clinical supervision.
- Taking a detailed history of diet and symptoms to identify possible triggers; testing of foods must be done using the double-blind technique, where neither the subject nor the tester knows when the food is being introduced, which can be difficult.

Tests for allergy include:
- The skin prick test.
- Assay of IgE levels.
- Intestinal biopsy or intestinal permeability may be carried out in the clinical setting.

Many tests are commercially available, but most have not been adequately validated and are not considered to be reliable in the diagnosis of food allergy. They may even represent a danger to the public in that they may result in misdiagnosis and the introduction of unnecessary exclusion diets, which in the case of children may be particularly hazardous. Dietary changes should ideally only be introduced under the supervision of a dietitian.

Food aversion

Food aversion is a learned response and not associated with a pathological response to a nutrient. In some cases, people believe there is a link between a food eaten and previous episodes of sickness or gastrointestinal upset.

Aversion reactions to food are not reproduced when the food is covertly presented. These responses are said to be of psychosomatic origin and may be significant (e.g. causing hyperventilation). Interestingly, studies have shown that in many patients such reactions are reduced following psychotherapeutic treatment. They may be of little nutritional significance in most subjects, unless the aversion extends to many foods or to foods that are important sources of nutrients.

Prevalence of food intolerance

Attempting to record the prevalence of food intolerance is notoriously difficult partly because of differences in definitions and also in methodologies. For example:
- Questionnaires may introduce bias.
- Diagnosis using challenge tests is time-consuming.
- Tests are often not very sensitive.
- The range of potentially allergenic foods is enormous.
- The time course of a response may be immediate or delayed, making it difficult to attribute to a specific allergen.

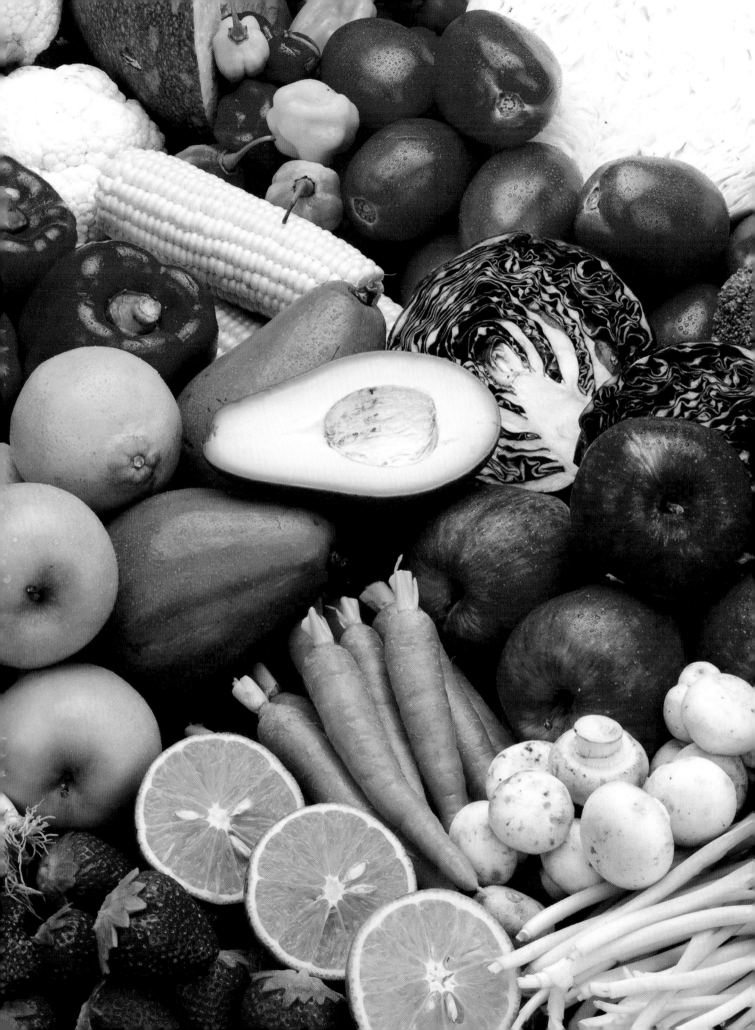

Public health and sports nutrition

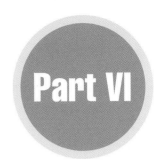

Part VI

Chapters

67 Nutritional genomics

Aims

1 To define nutritional genomics and the subcategories
2 To explore findings from current nutritional genomic studies
3 To introduce the application of nutritional genomics

Definition of nutritional genomics

Health or disease is a product of interaction between genotype and environment (e.g. diet, physical activity, etc.) (Figure 67.1). Nutritional genomics is the study of diet–gene interactions in relation to health outcomes. The term is a hypernym of two distinct fields: nutrigenetics and nutrigenomics. The importance of this new area has recently emerged, as it utilises innovative high-throughput technologies ('omic' technologies) such as genomics, epigenomics, transcriptomics, proteomics and metabolomics (Table 67.1).

Nutrigenetics investigates how genetic variances affect metabolism of nutrients or dietary components (Figure 67.2). This identifies individual susceptibility to diet-related diseases and allows personalised nutrition or dietary prescription to prevent or treat such diseases for individuals or sub-populations with certain genetic variances.

Nutrigenomics investigates how nutrients or dietary components affect gene expression (Figure 67.3) and may improve the quality of evidence for creating dietary recommendations at the population level.

Findings from nutritional genomic studies

Nutritional genomic research examines the mechanisms through which genetic variations affect utilisation of nutrients (Table 67.2), and nutrients are involved in gene expression (Table 67.3). Some nutrient–gene interactions involve single-nucleotide polymorphisms (SNPs), in which genetic variation is observed at one nucleotide. However, more complex relationships between nutritional stimuli and genetic responses and between genetic composition and nutrient metabolism also exist. For that reason, SNPs are more vigorously studied in relation to their interaction with nutrients or dietary components. Nutrients can act on any level of translation from genotype to phenotype.

Potential application of nutritional genomics

Integration of nutritional genomics into dietetic practice is at its infancy. With the 'omic' technologies, advanced understanding of diet–gene interactions may reveal the mechanisms of diet-related

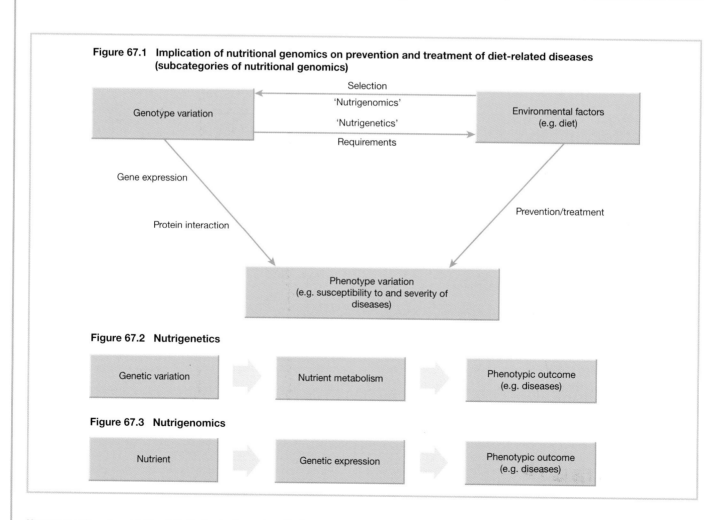

Figure 67.1   Implication of nutritional genomics on prevention and treatment of diet-related diseases (subcategories of nutritional genomics)

Figure 67.2   Nutrigenetics

Figure 67.3   Nutrigenomics

Nutrition at a Glance, Second Edition. Edited by Sangita Sharma, Tony Sheehy and Fariba Kolahdooz.
© 2016 John Wiley & Sons, Ltd. Published 2016 by John Wiley & Sons, Ltd.

diseases and transform the current concept of and ethics related to preventable medicine. Potential applications of nutritional genomics may include but are not limited to:

• Development of functional foods or beverages targeted to specific diseases or genetically predisposed individuals to prevent or manage diseases

• Effective address of current epidemiology of chronic diseases such as type 2 diabetes mellitus and cardiovascular diseases
• Stratification of populations based on genotypes and providing appropriate health care
• Integration of nutrigenomics and pharmacogenomics in disease therapy

Table 67.1 Definitions of high-throughput technologies.

Technologies	Definition
Genomics	Sequencing and mapping the genetic material (i.e. DNA) of an organism
Epigenomics	Investigating how DNA methylation regulates expression of DNA and subsequently produces functional proteins and phenotypic characteristics
Transcriptomics	Sequencing mRNA and investigating the effect of different stimuli on translation of mRNA into proteins
Proteomics	Examining formation, structure and function of proteins produced by gene expression
Metabolomics	Investigating non-protein metabolites present in the physiological system, which are produced by gene expression and resulting production and activity of proteins involved in certain metabolic processes

Table 67.2 Examples of findings from nutrigenetic studies.

Genetic variation	Metabolic and physiologic changes	Related disease	Suggested dietary therapy
5,10-Methylenetetrahydrofolate reductase (MTHFR) gene polymorphism: C/T	Reduced activity of MTHFR in TT carriers Accumulation of plasma homocysteine Reduced methionine level	Coronary heart disease Neural tube defects Premature cognitive decline Atherosclerosis	Increase folate in individuals with MTHFR-TT variant
Lipoprotein APOA1 gene promoter polymorphism: A/G	Increased and decreased plasma HDL in AA carriers and in GG or AG carriers, respectively, in response to high intake of PUFA		Increase PUFA in individuals with lipoprotein APOA1 promoter-AA variant
Angiotensinogen gene polymorphism: A/G	Increased activity of angiotensinogen in AA or AG carriers	Hypertension	Sodium restriction in individuals with angiotensinogen-AA or angiotensinogen-AG variant
HLA-DQ gene polymorphism: DQ2/DQ8	Uncontrolled activation of immune system and inflammatory response in heterozygotes	Coeliac disease	Strict exclusion of gluten
Phenylalanine hydroxylase gene mutation	Absence or reduced activity of phenylalanine hydroxylase Abnormally high level of phenylalanine Reduced plasma tyrosine	Phenylketonuria	Limited phenylalanine intake depending on the level of individual tolerance to phenylalanine

Table 67.3 Examples of findings from nutrigenomic studies.

Nutrient/dietary component	Changes in genetic expression	Result
Polyunsaturated ω-3 fatty acids	Downregulate expression of inflammatory mediator (TNF-α and IL-1) genes	Reduce inflammation by decreasing level of inflammatory mediators
Pomegranate polyphenols	Downregulate the expression of androgen synthesising genes	Inhibit the growth of prostate cancer cells
Cinnamon polyphenols	Downregulate the expression of the inflammatory genes in adipocytes	Reduce plasma free fatty acid and LDL cholesterol levels
	Upregulate the expression of the genes coding the insulin signalling pathway protein	Improve insulin resistance and reduce fasting glucose level

68 Nutrition transition

Aims

1 To describe the changes taking place in global dietary patterns and the major forces driving them
2 To consider the health implications of these changes

Over the course of the last 50 years, dietary patterns around the world have changed dramatically, first in industrial regions and later in developing countries. A pattern of 'Westernisation' of the diet has occurred practically everywhere, with traditional, largely plant-based diets being replaced by increased intakes of animal products, fats and oils, highly processed foods and added sugars and salt. At the same time, a shift towards more sedentary work and leisure patterns has also taken place. This phenomenon is known as the 'nutrition transition'.

The nutrition transition can be viewed as a series of adverse changes in diet, physical activity and health that occurs when a population moves, for example, from a predominantly rural, traditional lifestyle to an urban, industrial one. It is nearly always preceded by other transitions in that population, such as declining fertility rates, lower maternal and infant mortality, reduced mortality from infectious diseases and increased life expectancy. While it may have some beneficial effects, such as increased food availability and reduced prevalence of nutritional deficiencies, the major concern is that it is strongly associated with rising rates of obesity and non-communicable chronic diseases.

Trends in global food and nutrient availability

Data from the FAO food balance sheets show that since the early 1960s, per capita energy availability has increased substantially in most parts of the world (Table 68.1). However, the contribution of fat to total energy has also increased, and this increase has occurred primarily at the expense of carbohydrates. In South America, Southern Europe and East Asia in particular, the increase in dietary fat over a relatively short period of time has been quite dramatic.

These changing trends in dietary fat and carbohydrate reflect changes in the supply and utilisation of the various commodities in which they are found. Globally, cereals remain the most important source of dietary energy, but there has been a noticeable shift away from cereals, roots and tubers towards more livestock products and vegetable oils (Table 68.2). The reduced cost of vegetable oils is believed to be the main reason for the increased level of fat consumption worldwide.

Driving forces

The nutrition transition is being driven by a number of major factors related to changing population demographics, urbanisation, globalisation of food production, processing and marketing and technological innovations in communications.

Agricultural policies – Since World War Two, global agricultural policies have focused on providing cheaper sources of grains, animal products and vegetable oils. This has favoured a shift towards diets that are higher in sugars and fats.

Globalisation – With its focus on the freer movement of capital, technology, goods and services, globalisation has facilitated the spread of modern agricultural, food processing, marketing and distribution techniques, as well as fuelling the expansion of the global mass media and the ever-increasing demand for technologies that reduce energy expenditure in transportation, work and leisure.

Urbanisation – A large proportion of the world's population (especially the world's poor) now live in urban areas. Lack of land and the breakdown of traditional food sharing networks force urban dwellers to depend to a greater extent on market foods. Compared with rural areas, urbanisation is associated with greater intakes of animal products, fat, sugar and processed foods, especially in lower-income countries where food distribution systems are not as well developed as in higher-income countries.

Changing nature of work – Modern jobs tend to require less energy expenditure and may be less compatible with home food preparation, leading to a greater proportion of foods being prepared and/or eaten outside of the home. Increased participation of women in the workplace has accelerated this trend.

Rising incomes – Rising incomes tend to increase animal product consumption. In rapidly developing countries such as Brazil and China, consumption of animal products has risen dramatically in recent decades.

Transnational food corporations – Removal of trade barriers has given transnational food, beverage and fast-food companies access to an essentially global marketplace. To compete with them, local companies often copy their products or create processed versions of their own foods, thus further eroding traditional dietary patterns. Lower prices, larger portion sizes and aggressive marketing, especially to children, are inevitable consequences of this competition for market share.

Food distribution and retailing – With their temperature-controlled supply chains, supermarkets can provide animal food products that are less prone to spoilage and thus are safer to consume. However, supermarkets are also a major source of cheap, highly processed foods that are high in fats and oils and added sugars and salt and low in fibre and micronutrients. The poor in particular often depend on such products to obtain sufficient calories at low cost, at the expense of reduced overall dietary quality.

Mass media – Satellite broadcasting, the Internet and other technological advances in mass media now allow dietary, cultural and lifestyle trends in developed countries to be very rapidly disseminated to people in lower- and middle-income countries, affecting chronic disease patterns globally.

Marketing – As a result of the communications revolution, food marketers today have an unprecedented ability to market their products to billions of people, including children. Food products that are heavily marketed tend to be those that are energy dense and nutrient poor (e.g. confectionery, snack foods, soft drinks and alcoholic beverages).

Nutrition at a Glance, Second Edition. Edited by Sangita Sharma, Tony Sheehy and Fariba Kolahdooz.
© 2016 John Wiley & Sons, Ltd. Published 2016 by John Wiley & Sons, Ltd.

Table 68.1 A comparison of per capita energy availability and the percentage contribution of fat and carbohydrate to total energy supply in different regions of the world in 1961 and 2009.

Region	Energy (kcal/capita/day)		Fat (% of energy)		CHO (% of energy)	
Year	1961	2009	1961	2009	1961	2009
World	2189	2831	19.5	26.0	67.2	60.8
East Africa	1993	2103	13.5	16.0	73.0	72.2
Central Africa	2021	2227	16.1	19.4	72.5	69.0
North Africa	1948	3098	17.8	18.8	70.8	69.5
Southern Africa	2603	2914	20.0	24.9	67.0	60.1
West Africa	1893	2669	21.9	20.8	67.2	68.4
North America	2875	3659	34.4	38.1	49.4	46.2
Central America	2192	2974	19.9	26.0	68.1	61.3
Caribbean	1985	2636	18.7	22.2	69.8	65.3
South America	2306	2951	19.1	29.2	67.6	57.2
East Asia	1583	3000	9.9	28.3	77.8	57.1
South Asia	2002	2386	13.4	19.5	76.2	70.4
Western Asia	2479	3192	20.8	25.9	66.8	62.2
Eastern Europe	3114	3222	21.2	28.8	63.0	54.5
Northern Europe	3185	3385	37.3	36.5	48.5	47.3
Southern Europe	2830	3403	22.6	38.3	60.1	45.5
Western Europe	3034	3535	33.8	39.3	49.0	43.7
Australia and NZ	3062	3246	32.7	39.4	50.9	45.0

Table 68.2 A comparison of the percentage contribution of commodities to global dietary energy supply in 1961 and 2009.

Commodity	Contribution to dietary energy supply (%)	
Year	1961	2009
Cereals	49.3	45.6
Vegetable oils	5.2	9.8
Meat	5.0	8.1
Sugar and sweeteners	8.8	7.9
Starchy roots	8.0	4.8
Milk	5.3	4.7
Fruits	2.3	3.2
Vegetables	2.0	3.1
Alcoholic beverages	2.4	2.4
Pulses	4.1	2.2
Animal fats	3.3	2.1
Others	4.3	6.1

Implications of the nutrition transition

According to the WHO, chronic diseases will account for almost three-quarters of all deaths worldwide by 2020, and over 70% of deaths from ischaemic heart disease, stroke and diabetes will occur in developing countries. Obesity – a major risk factor for chronic disease – is already becoming a serious problem in Asia, Latin America and parts of Africa despite the continued presence of undernutrition. The burden of obesity is also shifting to the poorest sectors of society, who have the lowest access to treatment and the least power to effect change.

Countries with ageing populations and rising rates of obesity and chronic disease will face enormous challenges in terms of reduced economic productivity and spiralling health-care costs that will be difficult if not impossible to pay for. Moreover, because of the link between early nutritional insults and later adult disease, populations that are currently experiencing a high prevalence of impaired fetal and post-natal growth will face an even greater risk for chronic disease once those individuals reach adulthood.

In developing and middle-income countries, the coexistence of undernutrition and overnutrition in the same population (the so-called double burden of malnutrition) poses a serious challenge for the development of effective public health programmes.

Preventive strategies

The nutrition transition will result in increased rates of morbidity and premature mortality from non-communicable chronic diseases, as well as reduced quality of life for citizens and very high economic costs to society. Prevention will require an integrated approach that addresses the problem at a number of levels. Strategies should include:
* Efforts to vastly improve health and nutrition literacy among populations worldwide. All people need to have a better understanding of the role of nutrition in health promotion, and this education process should start at young ages. Additionally, professionals working in the fields of food science, marketing and medicine should have a far greater appreciation of the relationship between the modern Western diet and chronic disease risk and of their roles and responsibilities in reducing this risk.
* Tackling the obesity epidemic by creating food and physical activity environments that promote a healthy body weight rather than obesity. Dialogue with relevant industries (e.g. food producers, retailers, marketers, the media, transport authorities, planning agencies) may bring about positive changes, but regulatory, legislative and fiscal measures will probably also be required.
* Reforming agricultural and food policies so as to support the availability and affordability of healthy foods rather than energy-dense, nutrient-poor foods across all sectors of society.

Summary

A shift towards a more high-fat, high-sugar, energy-dense and highly processed diet that is low in complex carbohydrates and fibre is well underway across much of the world, and this trend is accelerating in lower- and middle-income countries. Combined with reduced physical activity, this transition will have major implications for non-communicable disease rates and will strain the capacity of even the richest countries to cope.

69 Promoting nutritional health: A public health perspective I

Aims

1 To recognise the multiple causes of poor nutrition
2 To describe the stages involved in developing a public health programme

For people to be able to maximise their nutritional health and so prevent disease and prolong life, scientific knowledge about nutrition should permeate all levels of society.

This is the realm of *public health nutrition*, which focuses on promoting good health throughout the population. In doing this, it uses a *biological and social science base*, together with a foundation of *epidemiology* and a *health promotion* approach.

UNICEF model of causation of malnutrition

Health is more than just the absence of disease. Rather, it encompasses:

- Both physical and mental health
- The ability of people to make choices to enable these to occur

Therefore, the societal framework is important, together with the policies that exist to shape it.

The UNICEF has developed a model (Figure 69.1) showing how disease and poor nutrition are not simply the result of the immediate food supply, but are a reflection of a number of *underlying causes* related to inadequate access to food, education, health care and sanitation, in addition to more *basic structural causes* in society including economic and political structures. Thus, changing people's food intake necessitates becoming engaged at all these levels if the solutions are going to be long lasting.

Aim of public health nutrition

Public health nutrition aims to find solutions to problems that will improve health. To reach this outcome, several logical stages must be completed.

Identify the problems

At the outset, it is necessary to identify the problems and their links with nutrition. This requires:

- *Data on the prevalence and incidence of disease*, patterns of morbidity and mortality and profiles of groups affected. This information may be collected routinely by health surveillance,

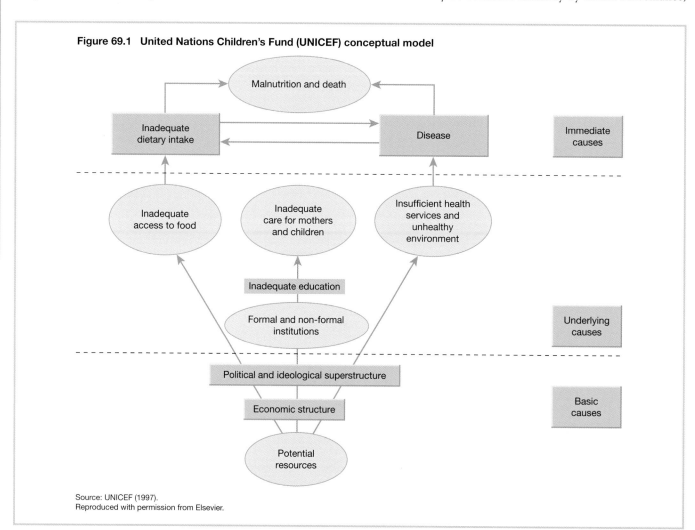

Figure 69.1 United Nations Children's Fund (UNICEF) conceptual model

Source: UNICEF (1997).
Reproduced with permission from Elsevier.

but its accuracy and penetration may vary. An independent nutritional assessment may be needed to establish this baseline information.

• *Scientific evidence*, based on a critical appraisal of the literature, that the problems identified have a plausible link with nutrition. This may be based on previous epidemiological studies.

• *Food intake patterns* from the population should support the association that particular nutrients or foods might have with the outcome. There should be a realistic assessment of how feasible it will be to alter these intakes to a more desirable level.

• *The constraints* that operate within the population should be identified, so that any goals and targets take these into account.

Broad aims and goals

For any public health intervention, broad aims and goals must be set so that specific improvements can be assessed against the baseline in evaluating the effectiveness of the intervention.

The broad aims may be part of a general policy, for example, to reduce the incidence of coronary heart disease over a period of time.

Clear objectives

Clear objectives must be established. There may be nutritional as well as other objectives, for example, relating to physical activity or food provision. Nutritional objectives may relate, for example, to the consumption of fruit and vegetables in the population.

Quantifiable targets

From the objectives, quantifiable targets should be set. For example, this might include a change in the sales of fruit and vegetables by supermarkets.

Any change must be measured against the baseline level, so tools to do this must be available from the outset. The targets set should be *specific*, *measurable*, *realistic* and *achievable*, as well as *worthwhile* for the overall aim. The time frame in which they are to be achieved must be clear.

Planning the programme

Once the aims have been refined into measurable targets, the programme can be planned in such a way that the targets can be achieved.

In aiming to alter the intake of specific food(s), the planning needs to consider all of the factors that apply to the current level of intake and whether it will be possible to change these. These include:

• The basic *factors affecting food intake*, such as the economic situation, or the degree of political support for the change

• Underlying factors such as the *level of education* of the main food purchasers and the potential to promote a change in intake through education

• An *awareness* or a *desire* for change among the population

• Other forces, such as *advertising*, or *other sectors with opposing interests* (e.g. commercial pressures from within the food industry)

Programmes may be aimed at different levels. They may target:
• Basic factors – through government policy on fortification or standards for school meals
• Underlying factors – by providing information on food labels to inform people about the 'healthiness' of foods or running cooking skills classes to enable people to take more control of their food intake
• Promotion of specific foods – such as fruit and vegetables – with targeted supermarket campaigns or school fruit schemes
   These approaches may also be *combined*. For example, to increase fruit and vegetable intake among children:
• School meals standards could include a requirement to serve fruit and vegetables at each meal.
• Cooking skills for preparation of vegetables and fruit could be taught.
• Children could be given fruit in school.

Implementing the programme

The final decision on implementing the programme may need to be pragmatic in terms of:

• Feasibility and anticipated effectiveness (based on previous knowledge)

• Acceptability to the target population (or individuals)

• Cost

Costs of all the stages of the project must be mapped.

Timescales for achievement of intermediate stages in the project must be set to ensure the work remains on track and allow achievement of targets and evaluation of the activity by the end date.

Evaluation

This assesses both the process (i.e. the delivery of the programme) and the impact (i.e. to what extent did it achieve its goals).

The whole process of public health nutrition intervention tends to be *cyclical*, as evaluation of one programme generally leads to the identification of further problems that can then be addressed by subsequent programmes.

Programmes may be affected by external factors that may have positive or negative influences on outcomes. These need to be taken into account in any evaluation (see Chapter 70).

Promoting nutritional health: A public health perspective II

Aims

1 To identify the barriers to implementing successful dietary change

2 To describe the relationship between food and nutrition policy and public health nutrition

Barriers to successful dietary change

Even with the best planned public health nutrition programmes, interventions may fail to make an impact on diet and produce no measurable change in dietary habits. This can occur for a variety of reasons:

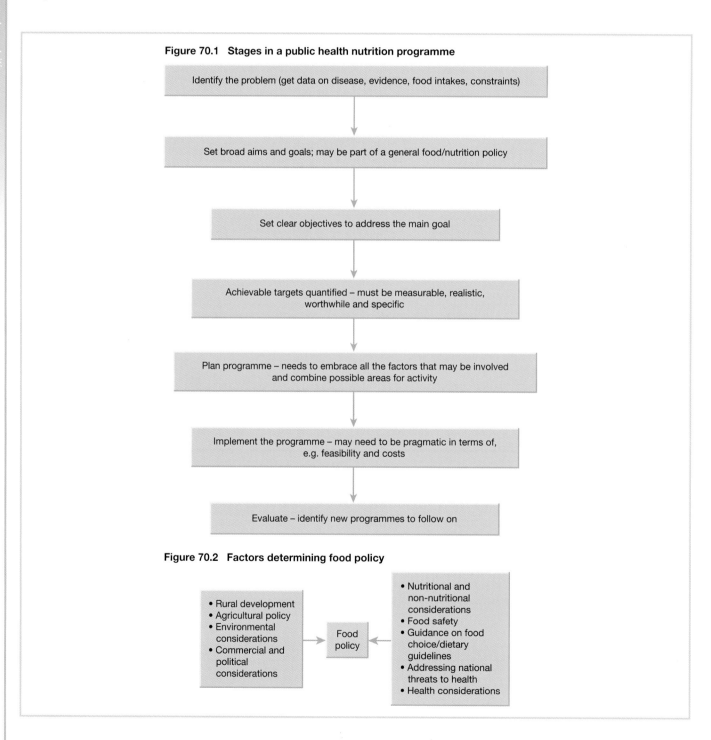

Figure 70.1 Stages in a public health nutrition programme

Identify the problem (get data on disease, evidence, food intakes, constraints)

Set broad aims and goals; may be part of a general food/nutrition policy

Set clear objectives to address the main goal

Achievable targets quantified – must be measurable, realistic, worthwhile and specific

Plan programme – needs to embrace all the factors that may be involved and combine possible areas for activity

Implement the programme – may need to be pragmatic in terms of, e.g. feasibility and costs

Evaluate – identify new programmes to follow on

Figure 70.2 Factors determining food policy

- Rural development
- Agricultural policy
- Environmental considerations
- Commercial and political considerations

→ Food policy ←

- Nutritional and non-nutritional considerations
- Food safety
- Guidance on food choice/dietary guidelines
- Addressing national threats to health
- Health considerations

Nutrition at a Glance, Second Edition. Edited by Sangita Sharma, Tony Sheehy and Fariba Kolahdooz.
© 2016 John Wiley & Sons, Ltd. Published 2016 by John Wiley & Sons, Ltd.

1 The intended subject did not receive the message: this may be because the medium for transmitting the message was inappropriate for the particular subject group. Identifying the most suitable channels of communication is an essential part of the planning process.

2 The message did not attract the attention of the target group: this may be because it was not presented in the most appropriate way to catch their attention or to maintain interest throughout the delivery (written, audio or oral or using social media).

3 The message was not correctly understood: either it was misinterpreted and incorrectly followed or was simply pitched at a level that was inappropriate for the capabilities of the subjects. Pilot testing is essential to ensure that messages will be understood.

4 Subjects found the message too complicated, forgot the information or did not believe it, because perhaps it contradicted commonly held beliefs in their culture or was not delivered in a way that inspired belief.

5 The message was received and understood, but did not result in behaviour change because of other constraints, for example, low income or lack of availability or unattractiveness of the food changes to be made.

6 Although the information received was acted on, it did not bring about the expected changes in health.

Unsuccessful health promotion activities may in themselves produce a negative perception because funding bodies may perceive that public health professionals do not produce an effective intervention.

It may also be negatively perceived by the potential subject group, who may become disillusioned and convinced that nutritional changes are difficult to implement and therefore ignore any future programmes.

This emphasises the need for careful planning to maximise the chances of success (see Figure 70.1).

Food policy

The field of public health nutrition operates within the organisational framework of a country's national food policy, the core aim of which is to ensure a safe, wholesome and nutritious supply of food to the population.

Food policy is informed by several influences (Figure 70.2), including the scientific evidence base, which comes from food and nutrition scientists. Also included within its remit are issues relating to agriculture, rural development, the environment and health. It is within the area of health that food safety regulations and nutrition are to be found.

Food safety is a major consideration of food policy, and with a global trade in food, the legislative and regulatory requirements regarding food safety are frequently reviewed. Because of the high profile and immediate risk that is associated with infringements of food safety, this aspect of food policy tends to have a high priority, at the expense of nutrition policy.

However, nutritional aspects of food policy are still highly relevant to people's health, as they can determine the food choices made by the population and their nutritional consequences.

• *Guidance about food choices* is one of the key aspects of nutrition policy. This is usually expressed in the form of dietary guidelines. The majority of countries now use food-based dietary guidelines, represented in some form of model, either a plate, pyramid or food circle (chapter 39). Foods to be eaten in greatest amounts are represented by the largest segment, while foods that should be eaten in smaller amounts form a lesser proportion of the model.

• The scientific basis of the dietary guidelines comes from the dietary requirements and reference standards that also exist in most countries.

National nutrition policy may also incorporate other interventions such as:

• Fortification of specific foods, such as flour, milk, spreading fats, baby foods and salt

• Recommendations on taking folate supplements when planning pregnancy

• Advice to avoid liver, which is rich in vitamin A, when pregnant

• Regulations regarding school meal standards

Nutrition issues also form a part of broader initiatives to improve health across the population and currently may focus on:
• Weight reduction, together with associated comorbidities such as diabetes and coronary heart disease
• Improving the diets of preschool children by attention to food in nurseries as well as programmes to help develop food and nutrition knowledge and culinary skills among mothers
• Improving access to health care, including better food in low-income areas
• Improving food in hospitals

All of the above initiatives require input from nutrition scientists to translate information from the research base into practical initiatives and carry these through. Public health nutritionists are ideally placed to carry out this role. Dietitians also possess these skills, and some of them also work in the community in health promotion activities.

71 Promoting nutritional health: The role of the dietitian

Aims

1 To consider the role of the dietitian in identifying and providing nutritional support and dietary modifications
2 To identify other roles of dietitians

Dietitians have a scientific training in diet and nutrition and are experts in translating scientific information about food and health into practical terms that can be understood.

The role of dietitians varies in different countries, but many are involved in clinical nutrition, which is the application of nutritional science for people with medical challenges. Clinical nutrition is likely to include other health professionals as well, such as doctors and pharmacists and several other therapists, in multidisciplinary teams.

Causes of nutritional problems

People with medical issues present a different nutritional challenge to those who are well. The three-stage model of potential threats to nutrition can be used to depict how issues with inadequate nutrition may arise (Figure 71.1):

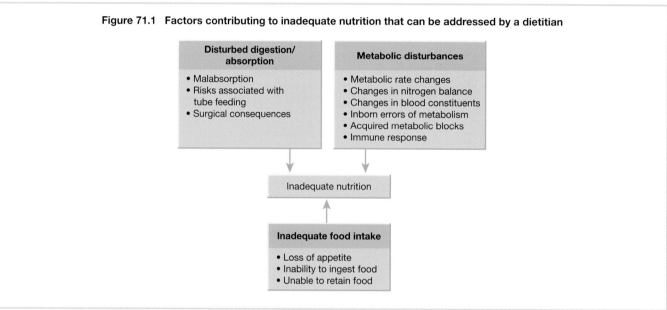

Figure 71.1   Factors contributing to inadequate nutrition that can be addressed by a dietitian

Disturbed digestion/absorption
- Malabsorption
- Risks associated with tube feeding
- Surgical consequences

Metabolic disturbances
- Metabolic rate changes
- Changes in nitrogen balance
- Changes in blood constituents
- Inborn errors of metabolism
- Acquired metabolic blocks
- Immune response

Inadequate nutrition

Inadequate food intake
- Loss of appetite
- Inability to ingest food
- Unable to retain food

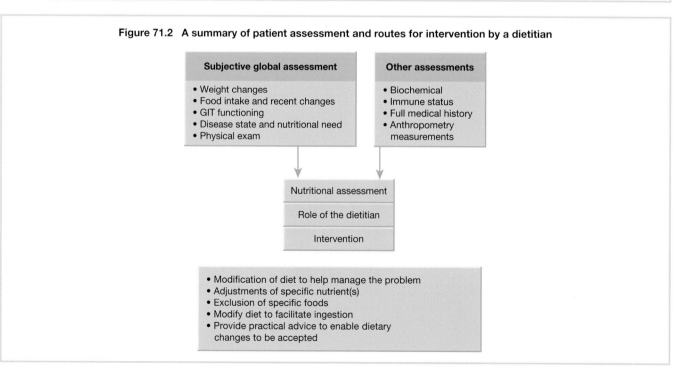

Figure 71.2   A summary of patient assessment and routes for intervention by a dietitian

Subjective global assessment
- Weight changes
- Food intake and recent changes
- GIT functioning
- Disease state and nutritional need
- Physical exam

Other assessments
- Biochemical
- Immune status
- Full medical history
- Anthropometry measurements

Nutritional assessment

Role of the dietitian

Intervention

- Modification of diet to help manage the problem
- Adjustments of specific nutrient(s)
- Exclusion of specific foods
- Modify diet to facilitate ingestion
- Provide practical advice to enable dietary changes to be accepted

Nutrition at a Glance, Second Edition. Edited by Sangita Sharma, Tony Sheehy and Fariba Kolahdooz.
© 2016 John Wiley & Sons, Ltd. Published 2016 by John Wiley & Sons, Ltd.

1 **Intake**: In healthy people, inadequate intake is the main area for concern, and this is often addressed by public health nutritionists. People with medical conditions may have additional challenges, due to loss of appetite, sickness and physical difficulties of ingestion (e.g. requiring tube feeding).

2 **Digestion and absorption**: In healthy people, the efficiency of digestion and absorption may be compromised by minor medical problems such as mild food poisoning or the use of indigestion remedies or laxatives. In acute or chronic medical conditions, much more serious problems can occur, including failure of enzymic secretions, malabsorption, blockages or surgical consequences.

3 **Metabolism**: Apart from increased needs during periods of rapid growth and during pregnancy or lactation, healthy people generally have few deficiencies associated with metabolic changes. In disease, however, major changes in metabolism can occur, including changes to metabolic rate, muscle wasting, blood loss, electrolyte imbalances and inflammatory states. All these changes can alter nutritional needs, and these are the main causes of potential deficiency that need to be addressed by clinical nutrition.

> **Identifying those in need of nutritional support**
>
> In order to identify the most appropriate response in any situation, it is necessary to screen patients and, if necessary, follow this up with a more in-depth nutritional assessment (Figure 71.2).
>
> Nutritional support must be timely, be provided by the most appropriate route and meet the ongoing needs of the patient. The intervention must be monitored, its effects evaluated across a number of indicators, and the results documented.

Dietetic intervention in disease states

In addition to nutritional support, which may be needed in a variety of patients, the dietitian also provides advice on modification of diets for many chronic disease states to improve health and quality of life. These include:
• Modification of basic healthy eating principles, for example, for the management of body weight, blood lipids and uncomplicated type 2 diabetes
• Adjustment of the dietary content of a specific nutrient, for example, fat, fibre, protein, salt, potassium or lactose, which may apply to a number of conditions
• Exclusion of particular foods that may be the cause of specific sensitivity, such as wheat (gluten content), milk, eggs or nuts, while ensuring the diet remains nutritionally adequate
• Alteration of the texture of foods to make eating and swallowing easier
• Providing practical advice and help for managing any dietary restrictions or modifications so they can be carried out in the home while always taking into account the patient's particular situation, likes and dislikes

Community dietetics

Dietitians also work in the community, where they can provide a clinical nutrition service within the primary care setting, as well as undertaking home visits to support patients.

In addition, community dietitians may take on some public health nutrition roles, such as providing nutrition education and health promotion to other health professionals, voluntary groups, schools and youth groups, local authorities and social services.

Sports dietitians

Sports dietitians provide specialist advice to athletes and other sports people, either on a one-to-one basis or working with teams and coaches. They may also train other sports professionals who work within the leisure industry.

Dietitians in the food and pharmaceutical industry

There are a number of companies that produce special dietary products for use in clinical settings. Dietitians are involved in the development of these products, using research evidence to guide new product development. They also advise hospital pharmacies and dietitians about the products that are available and their use.

Within the food industry, including the retail sector, dietitians may work on the development of new products, as well as providing consumer information about the range available. Dietitians also monitor nutritional standards for products that carry specific labelling information about suitability for people with medical conditions.

Freelance dietitians

Some dietitians provide a freelance service, using their knowledge of food and nutrition issues in the broadcast and written media, including newspapers and consumer magazines, and via the Internet, as well as providing consultancy for a range of companies and working in private practice.

Research dietitians

Underpinning the whole of dietetic practice is an evidence base that needs to be kept updated. This is the responsibility of all dietitians, who need to question and evaluate their practice. However, some dietitians work specifically in research and, in this way, add to the body of knowledge.

> **Importance of communication**
>
> The key to successfully modifying the diet of an individual is effective communication. Dietitians must be skilled communicators, and when giving dietary advice, they must take into consideration:
> • The individual's existing food choices and the factors influencing these (e.g. cultural)
> • Their motivation to change
> • How to communicate this, taking into account all aspects of the process, including verbal and nonverbal communication, and the individual's capacity to understand the messages
> • How to change the individual's behaviour by understanding the psychological aspects of behaviour and working with these to arrive at agreed strategies and goals
>
> In effect, the approach and outcome with every individual may be different.

Dietitians also need to consider the ethics of their practice and recognise the limits of what they can ask people to do in terms of dietary change or intervention and also when to stop.

Throughout all dietetic practice, evaluating the outcomes of any intervention is important. This requires dietitians to be reflective and consider how their own approach has had an influence on the interaction with the patient and to consider if in the future this can be modified for a better outcome. In addition, auditing the practice of a team of dietitians can show their overall effectiveness and indicate if changes need to be made.

72 Nutrition and sport I

Aims

1 To consider how energy is used in physical exercise
2 To determine the major energy substrates used during exercise

Increased physical activity requires energy to be supplied at an increased rate to active muscles. Although the energy requirement of a sedentary adult is approximately 7.5–11.5 MJ (1800–2800 kcal)/day, this can increase to as much as 36 MJ (9000 kcal)/day for extreme endurance athletes (e.g. cyclists competing in the mountain stages of the Tour de France). The energy needs of the majority of athletes will be more moderate, around 14.5–18 MJ (3500–4500 kcal)/day, depending on the sport and level of training.

Adenosine triphosphate

Adenosine triphosphate (ATP) is the fundamental molecule that, on breakdown to ADP, provides energy for all cells, including contracting muscle. ATP stores within the body are very limited and require continual replenishment, as the amount stored at any given time would only fuel about 2 seconds of exercise. The main routes for maintaining ATP stores are shown in Figures 72.1 and 72.2.

Importance of lipids as substrate

• Carbohydrate stores in the muscle (300–800 g) and liver (80 g) are limited. Therefore, carbohydrates cannot provide sufficient energy for extreme, high-intensity exercises or sustained endurance exercises. Fats, on the other hand, are stored mainly in subcutaneous adipose tissue and are present in much greater amounts (at least 5 kg in males and even more in females).

• Fats are more energy dense than carbohydrates (37 vs. 16 kJ/g dry weight); thus, the metabolism of one gram of fat delivers over twice as much ATP as can be obtained from one gram of carbohydrate. However, more oxygen is required to metabolise fats, and fats cannot be metabolised anaerobically (Figure 72.2).

Factors determining substrate use

The proportions of ATP derived from carbohydrate and fat depend upon a number of factors.

Duration and intensity of exercise (see Table 72.1)

Key issues in maximising energy supply are the following:
• Glycogen levels are crucial in enabling high-intensity exercise to be continued.
• Even relatively small amounts of energy from lipid breakdown during high-intensity exercise help to protect muscle glycogen stores and increase the time to exhaustion when stores are depleted.
• Maintaining blood glucose levels is essential, as reduction will impair accuracy and judgement in performance and contribute to fatigue. Dietary intervention to support blood glucose during high-intensity or long duration exercises is crucial for consistent performance.
• Levels of insulin, adrenaline and glucagon are important in determining which substrates are used in different circumstances.

Level of training

Training increases aerobic fitness. This has several benefits:
• Increased blood supply to the muscles, enabling faster delivery of oxygen

Table 72.1 Summary of the effects of duration and intensity of exercise on substrate use.

Level of exercise	Main substrate for muscle contraction	Comments
At rest/minimal physical exercise	Lipid metabolism	The CNS and RBCs require glucose for metabolism
Brief intense exercise (up to 10 s)	Anaerobic breakdown of ATP and phosphocreatine (PCr)	In muscle, PCr is found in concentrations about four times that of ATP and is used to recreate ATP during brief rest periods
Intense exercise (up to 90 s)	Anaerobic metabolism of glucose or glycogen to pyruvate, with net formation of two or three ATP units, respectively	Lactate later has to be reconverted to glucose Useful for short sprints before physiological adjustments have occurred
Medium-term intense exercise	Partly by anaerobic breakdown of glycogen or glucose, increasingly by aerobic metabolism	This yields more energy to sustain exercise
Light to moderate exercise	Lipid metabolism makes an increasingly significant contribution and CHO correspondingly less	Related to changes in hormone levels; adrenaline secretion stimulates lipolysis, and insulin is inhibited; may take 20 min to reach a steady state
Moderately high levels of sustained exercise	Lipids are the main energy substrate Depleted muscle glycogen eventually results in fatigue and terminates the exercise	Muscle glycogen stores are reduced and gluconeogenesis in the liver (predominantly from glycerol from fat breakdown or later amino acid residues from protein) becomes important to maintain blood glucose levels

Nutrition at a Glance, Second Edition. Edited by Sangita Sharma, Tony Sheehy and Fariba Kolahdooz.
© 2016 John Wiley & Sons, Ltd. Published 2016 by John Wiley & Sons, Ltd.

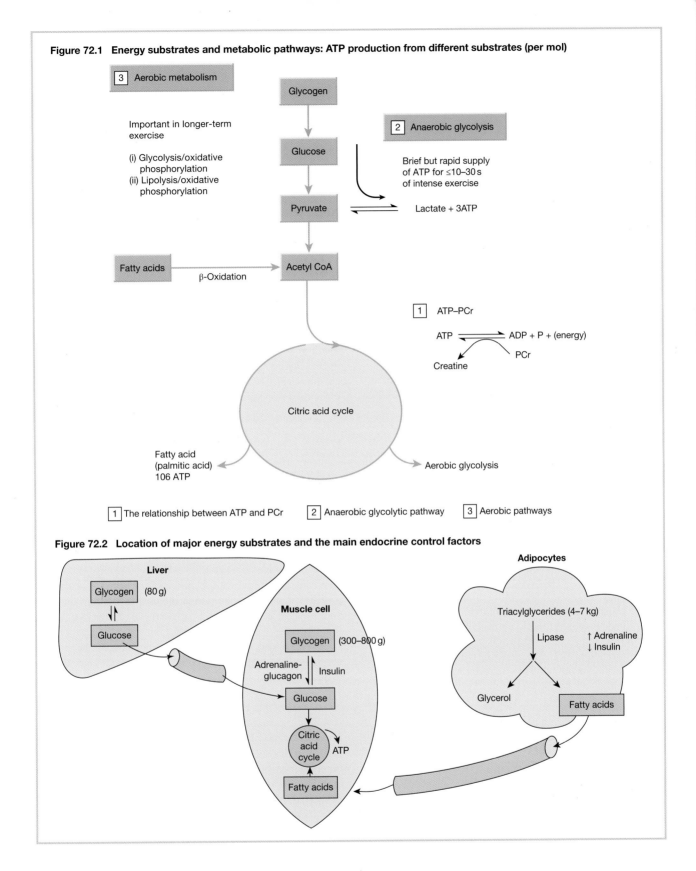

Figure 72.1 Energy substrates and metabolic pathways: ATP production from different substrates (per mol)

3 Aerobic metabolism

Important in longer-term exercise

(i) Glycolysis/oxidative phosphorylation
(ii) Lipolysis/oxidative phosphorylation

Glycogen

Glucose

2 Anaerobic glycolysis

Brief but rapid supply of ATP for ≤10–30 s of intense exercise

Pyruvate ⇌ Lactate + 3ATP

Fatty acids → Acetyl CoA
β-Oxidation

1 ATP–PCr

$$ATP \rightleftharpoons ADP + P + (energy)$$

Creatine ⟵ PCr

Citric acid cycle

Fatty acid (palmitic acid) 106 ATP

Aerobic glycolysis

1 The relationship between ATP and PCr   2 Anaerobic glycolytic pathway   3 Aerobic pathways

Figure 72.2 Location of major energy substrates and the main endocrine control factors

Liver

Glycogen (80 g) ⇌ Glucose

Muscle cell

Glycogen (300–800 g)

Adrenaline-glucagon ⇌ Insulin

Glucose

Citric acid cycle → ATP

Fatty acids

Adipocytes

Triacylglycerides (4–7 kg)

Lipase   ↑ Adrenaline ↓ Insulin

Glycerol   Fatty acids

• Increased levels of enzymes for aerobic metabolism, which increases the amount of fatty acids that can be metabolised for energy
• More rapid establishment of fat metabolism as energy substrate, thus providing better protection of carbohydrate reserves

Diet

The nature of an athlete's diet will significantly affect her or his ability to train and perform. This is discussed in Chapter 73.

Energy supply

Carbohydrates (in the form of glycogen and glucose) and fats (fatty acids) are the two main sources of energy. Protein makes a small (10–15%) contribution to total energy expenditure, generally towards the end of a period of endurance exercise.

73 Nutrition and sport II

Aims

1 To identify nutritional requirements for exercise and how these can be met
2 To consider some dietary supplements used in sport

Diet is a critical element of athletic training and performance (Table 73.1). The nutritional goals of athletes depend on their sport and may focus on increasing endurance, speed or power/strength. Actual body mass (and its control) may be important in certain sports, especially aesthetic sports (such as gymnastics) or where there are specific weight categories for competition (e.g. rowing, horse racing, weightlifting, bodybuilding, boxing and other combat sports).

Importance of carbohydrate in the general diet

A common feature of the dietary advice offered to athletes, either in training or in competition, is the need to increase or maintain carbohydrate (CHO) stores.

Length of time to exhaustion or duration of maximal effort can be increased by ensuring that glycogen stores are filled to their maximum capacity. This can be achieved by ensuring an adequate CHO intake (5–7 g/kg body weight/day for the training needs of average individuals and 7–10 g/kg body weight/day for endurance athletes). This is important for:
- Maintaining sufficient energy supplies for regular training
- Preparing for a competition/event

When preparing for competition, 24–36 h of rest with an adequate CHO intake will ensure that glycogen stores are replete.

Carbohydrate before exercise

Topping up glycogen stores is important in the hours leading up to exercise. A pre-exercise meal, rich in CHO of low and medium glycaemic index (GI) (~200–300 g), will ensure a steady release of CHO over several hours. The meal should preferably be low in fat and fibre to allow for easy digestion and have a low to moderate protein content.

In the last hour before exercise, high-GI CHO may be consumed, although this can lead to the release of insulin and inhibition of lipolysis during early exercise in a small number of athletes. Testing the effects of pre-exercise CHO ingestion is recommended to determine each individual's response.

Carbohydrate during exercise

Consuming CHO drinks during an event lasting more than 45 min is necessary to:
- Maintain blood glucose levels and brain function
- Provide additional fluid to prevent dehydration
- Delay the onset of fatigue

A CHO intake of approximately 60 g/h is recommended. The majority of CHO-containing drinks are isotonic and provide about 4–8 g CHO per 100 mL in a readily absorbable form, as well as electrolytes to facilitate CHO absorption.

Absorption of CHO is faster if the stomach already contains fluid; therefore, athletes are advised to start exercise with at least 300–500 mL fluid in their stomach.

Carbohydrate after exercise

After exercise, muscles need to be refuelled as rapidly as possible with glycogen to allow more exercise to be undertaken later that day or on subsequent days.

Glycogen synthesis in muscles is enhanced in the 2 h after exercise, so taking advantage of this by consuming high-GI CHO during this period allows more glycogen to be stored. An intake of CHO of 1–2 g/kg body weight/hour is suggested.

Refuelling diets should therefore contain high-GI CHO initially, in the form of snacks or drinks, followed by a meal of low- and medium-GI CHO to sustain the supply of glucose to the muscles over a longer period of time. Including protein in the meal enhances glycogen storage and may also benefit muscle repair and immune function, which can be compromised after exercise.

Protein needs in exercise

Protein does not contribute significantly to the energy supply in exercise. However, there may be an increase in protein requirement because:
- Muscle fibrils are damaged in exercising muscles, leading to an increased need for protein for repair.
- When athletes first start to train, the exercise causes hypertrophy of muscles, which increases protein needs to achieve a positive nitrogen balance.

Recommended protein intakes during training are 1.2–1.7 g/kg body weight/day, depending on the sport. In practice, this level of protein is typically consumed in the normal Western diet, making additional protein or protein supplements unnecessary to achieve these intakes.

Intakes above 2 g/kg body weight/day have not been shown to confer any advantage and could in fact limit performance by displacing CHO from the diet.

Vitamin and mineral needs in sport

A well-balanced diet supplies a sufficient amount of vitamins and minerals for training needs, but deficiencies in calcium, zinc and B vitamins can occur in athletes who train for extended lengths of time. Inadequate micronutrient intakes can hinder performance; for example, a reduction in VO_2 max (maximal oxygen consumption) has been observed when B vitamin and vitamin C deficiencies occur:
- B vitamins are required for energy metabolism, and as the rate of energy metabolism increases during training, the need for B vitamins increases, resulting in the potential for deficiency.
- Iron is crucial for optimal performance because of its role in transporting oxygen throughout the body (via haemoglobin) and in maintaining the oxygen holding capacity within muscles (via myoglobin). Low iron stores are common in athletes, particularly in young females, long distance runners, and those following calorie-restricted diets.

Nutrition at a Glance, Second Edition. Edited by Sangita Sharma, Tony Sheehy and Fariba Kolahdooz.
© 2016 John Wiley & Sons, Ltd. Published 2016 by John Wiley & Sons, Ltd.

Table 73.1 Summary of dietary principles in exercise and sport.

Nutrient	Advice	Reasons/benefits
Carbohydrate	Maintain intakes up to 7–10 g per Kg body weight per day during training and competition Attention to intake prior to, during and after exercise	Keeps muscle glycogen levels topped up and allows maximal performance Before exercise – tops up glycogen stores During exercise – protects blood glucose levels, delays fatigue After exercise – allows rapid replenishment of glycogen stores
Protein	Most athletes already consume sufficient protein in a mixed diet May need attention in vegetarian athletes or where food and energy intakes are very low (e.g. in low body weight sports)	Needed for muscle maintenance and repair Maintaining immune function
Fat	May need to consume upper recommendation for fat (35% of energy) in the diet if overall energy needs are high	Type of fat eaten should follow healthy eating advice. Fat-soluble vitamin intakes may be compromised by very low-fat diets
Minerals and vitamins	A balanced diet provides adequate levels Athletes with low overall dietary intakes may need supplements Particular attention to antioxidant nutrients	Female athletes may need additional iron if intakes are low Low body weight athletes risk low calcium status and may need to take supplemental calcium
Fluid	Essential to maintain hydration, habitual intake important	Fluid with electrolytes and CHO is useful to provide efficient absorption and maintain CHO levels during exercise

Fluid needs in sport

Fluid provides a mechanism for the body to dissipate heat during physical activity. To optimise performance, an appropriate body temperature must be maintained; therefore, consistent fluid intake is necessary. To ensure adequate water intake during exercise, individuals should consume enough fluid to match the amount lost as sweat. The best way to replenish water lost is to consume fluids containing electrolytes. This will increase the rate of absorption of water and replace any electrolytes lost during exercise.

Dietary supplements and sport

With the exception of energy intake, the evidence that normal dietary supplements enhance sporting performance is poor. Although free radical production increases during exercise, there is little evidence that vitamin C or E supplementation protects against oxidative damage. A very large number of ergogenic aids are marketed to and used by athletes, but for the vast majority, there is no clear evidence of improved performance.

Creatine

Creatine plays an important role in energy delivery to muscles and provides the majority of energy used during short-term, high-intensity exercise. Low-dose supplementation of about 5 g/day has been shown to provide greater benefits than the earlier practice of creatine loading, in which individuals consumed 20 g for 5 days. Supplementary creatine:

- Significantly increases muscle creatine levels
- May delay the onset of fatigue
- May improve high-intensity performance levels

Intermittent, short but intensive bouts of exercise appear to be improved most by creatine supplementation, while endurance events benefit least.

Caffeine

When ingested an hour before exercise, caffeine:

- Increases plasma fatty acid levels, which protect muscle glycogen stores
- Increases recruitment of muscle fibres
- Directly influences muscle contractility by assisting calcium transport
- Has beneficial effects on cognitive function, primarily psychomotor skill and attention

Even low doses of caffeine (5 mg/kg body weight) increase time to exhaustion when working at very high levels of activity.

CHO loading

Supercompensation of muscle glycogen stores can be achieved by a technique known as CHO loading. This is relevant where duration of exercise exceeds 90–120 min; time to exhaustion can be increased by 20%.

The technique involves a high CHO intake with tapered exercise and rest for 3–4 days prior to competition. A potential drawback of such supercompensation is that glycogen is stored with water (2.7 g/g glycogen). This can make the muscles feel heavy and requires the athlete to become accustomed to the sensation.

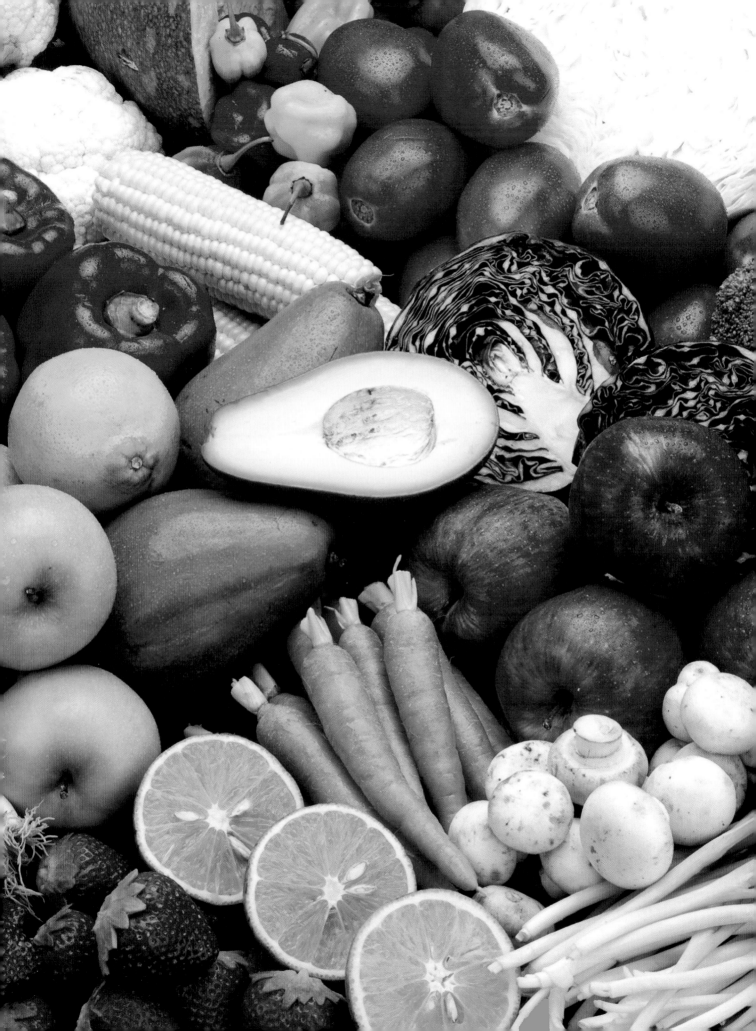

Foods, phytochemicals including functional and genetically modified foods

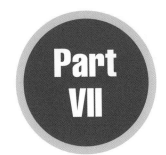

Part VII

Chapters

74 Functional foods

Aims

1 To introduce the concept of functional foods
2 To identify the major physiological targets for functional foods
3 To consider the requirements for successful functional food development

Functional foods are marketed as foods that provide health benefits beyond basic nutrition, thereby reducing the risk for chronic disease and helping to promote optimal health. Other terms such as nutraceuticals, designer foods, pharmafoods and vitafoods are sometimes used, but these are not as widely recognised by the media or consumers.

Over the past two decades, the growth in popularity of functional foods has been one of the dominant trends in the food industry. Factors driving this trend include ageing populations, rising health-care costs, consumers' interest in taking more responsibility for their health, the growing body of scientific evidence linking nutrition and health, technological advances in molecular biology, and bioinformatics and changing food regulations.

History

The concept of functional foods originated in Japan in the 1980s as a response to rising rates of non-communicable chronic diseases (e.g. cardiovascular disease, cancer, diabetes mellitus, osteoporosis) and rapidly escalating health-care costs associated with its ageing population. The Japanese Ministry of Health and Welfare initiated a regulatory system that allowed certain foods with documented health benefits to be designated as Foods for Specified Health Use (FOSHU). The first food product given FOSHU status was a hypoallergenic rice grain ('fine rice'). Since then, many hundreds of FOSHU products have been approved, targeting a wide range of health concerns.

Interest in functional foods began to grow in Europe, North America and elsewhere during the next decade as food companies began to realise the enormous opportunities they presented for turning basic commodities (and in some cases even processing by-products) into value-added products. Thus, the 1990s saw the emergence of a host of novel products such as plant stanol ester-enhanced margarines, n-3 fatty acid-enriched eggs, oat bran-enriched breakfast cereals, vitamin and mineral-fortified cereal bars, calcium-fortified fruit juices, fermented dairy products and sports and energy drinks containing probiotic bacteria. Since then, the functional food market has continued to expand – particularly the snack and beverage sectors – and a recent estimate placed the global market size at well over $40 billion.

Definitions

There is no official or universally accepted definition for functional foods. However, the basic concept is that a functional food:
• Is a conventional or everyday food and not a pill, capsule or any form of dietary supplement
• Is consumed as part of a normal diet
• Is composed of naturally occurring components
• Has positive effects on body functions beyond basic nutrition

Table 74.1 Examples of definitions for functional foods.

Source	Definition
Academy of Nutrition and Dietetics	'Functional foods are foods that provide additional health benefits that may reduce disease risk and/or promote good health'
Health Canada	'A functional food is similar in appearance to, or may be, a conventional food that is consumed as part of a usual diet, and is demonstrated to have physiological benefits and/or reduce the risk of chronic disease beyond basic nutritional functions'
EC Concerted Action on Functional Food Science in Europe (FUFOSE)	'A functional food is a food that beneficially affects one or more target functions in the body beyond adequate nutritional effects in a way that is relevant to either an improved state of health and well-being and/or reduction of risk of disease. It is consumed as part of a normal food pattern. It is not a pill, a capsule or any form of dietary supplement'
Commonwealth Scientific and Industrial Research Organisation (CSIRO)	'Functional foods are considered to be any food or food component that may provide demonstrated physiological benefits or reduce the risk of chronic diseases, above and beyond basic nutritional functions'
Institute of Food Technologists	'Functional foods describe foods and food components that provide essential nutrients often beyond quantities necessary for normal maintenance, growth, and development, and/or other biologically active components that impart health benefits or desirable physiological effects'
Journal of Functional Foods	'Functional foods are those containing various factors to ensure or enhance health'

• Imparts an enhanced state of health and well-being and/or reduces risk of disease

Some of the more widely referenced definitions for functional foods are shown in Table 74.1.

Development of functional foods

Generally speaking, a food product can be made functional by eliminating a deleterious ingredient, adding a beneficial ingredient, increasing the concentration of an ingredient known to have beneficial effects or increasing the bioavailability or stability of a beneficial ingredient.

Successful functional food development requires:
• Identification of foods/food components that have the potential to modulate target functions in the body in a way that is beneficial (i.e. reduces disease risk or creates an enhanced state of health/well-being)
• Identification of relevant biomarkers of such functions
• Development and validation of methods to measure how these biomarkers respond following consumption of the product
• For health claims, presentation to regulatory authorities of sound, consistent evidence from well-designed human intervention studies showing that the product is safe and effective

Nutrition at a Glance, Second Edition. Edited by Sangita Sharma, Tony Sheehy and Fariba Kolahdooz.

- Communication of product benefits to target consumers in a clear, credible and effective way
- Uncompromised taste, convenience and an acceptable price

Functional components

At present, thousands of bioactive components are under investigation, and some are already being utilised in the creation of functional foods. Much attention has focused on probiotic bacteria, prebiotics, vitamins, minerals, plant phenolics, plant sterols and carotenoids. Other components under investigation include dairy-based ingredients (e.g. conjugated linoleic acid, lactoferrin, milk-derived peptides, colostrum), fish and plant oil-based ingredients (e.g. EPA, DHA, α- and γ-linolenic acid), soy-based ingredients (e.g. isoflavones), proteins and related ingredients (protein hydrolysates, peptides, amino acids), creatine, caffeine, glucosamine and chondroitin. Increasingly, research is focusing on the recovery of bioactive components from food processing waste, seaweed, algae, wild plants, herbs and other unconventional sources. Non-nutrient bioactives are considered in more detail in Chapter 75.

Targets

Targets for functional food development include allergies and intolerances, athletic performance, blood glucose management, bone and joint health, cancer risk reduction, cardiovascular health, cognitive and mental function, energy metabolism, gut health, healthy ageing, immunity, inflammation, insulin sensitivity, maternal and infant health, men's and women's health, oral and skin protection and weight management.

Biomarkers

Functional foods typically carry health claims about the benefits they provide. However, in order to ensure that consumers can trust these claims, obtaining scientific support is essential. Product effectiveness can be demonstrated by measuring the response of appropriate biomarkers (see Table 74.2). Biomarkers should be scientifically well established and should accurately reflect the processes of interest. For some targets (e.g. cancer, cardiovascular disease, immune function, athletic performance), a large number of biomarkers are already available, which are validated to varying degrees. For others though, identification of valid biomarkers for use in human studies remains a challenge.

Regulation of health claims

In order to enhance consumers' ability to make informed choices, some countries have specific laws regarding the type of claims that can be made about food products. Health claims in the USA and Canada are overseen and regulated by the Food and Drug Administration (FDA) and Health Canada, respectively. In the European Union, harmonised rules governing the use of nutrition and health claims right across the EU have been introduced and a register of permitted claims established.

Criticisms of functional foods

Critics of the functional foods concept make the following points:
- Given the way functional foods are defined, practically all foods could be regarded as 'functional' in some way because virtually all foods contain at least some components that have been linked to a health benefit. The creation of a separate functional foods category appears essentially meaningless nutritionally; however, it has been extremely useful from a marketing perspective, and that, it is argued, is the real motivation.
- The claim that functional foods provide health benefits that go 'beyond basic nutrition' is difficult to sustain.
- Stating or implying that functional foods can provide an 'enhanced' state of health or well-being creates the impression that ordinary foods are only capable of providing a 'basic' standard of health. However, the health benefits claimed for functional foods are precisely the same as those associated with eating a well-balanced diet made up of conventional foods.
- When foods are reduced to their basic chemical composition and all that is considered is their capacity to deliver important functional components, it undermines the important distinction that has always existed in nutrition between processed and unprocessed foods.
- Inserting chemical compounds into highly processed food products risks conferring drug-like properties on these products and creating a 'magic bullet' approach to disease prevention, to the overall detriment of people's health.
- The higher prices demanded for functional foods could create a category of unaffordable products for everyone.

Summary

The basic premise of functional foods is that by consuming certain food components, the consumer's risk of disease is reduced and health/well-being is enhanced. Future success of the industry will depend on continued research into potentially beneficial components, availability of valid biomarkers of their functional effects, a strong regulatory framework overseeing health claims and effective and truthful communication of benefits to consumers.

Table 74.2 Examples of indicators of physiological function and disease risk.

Target	Biomarker
Gastrointestinal health	Gastrointestinal hormones, viscosity; transit time; composition of intestinal flora
Immune system	Delayed-type hypersensitivity response, phagocytosis, respiratory burst, lymphocyte proliferation, incidence and severity of infections
Athletic/physical performance	Muscle mass, muscle glycogen, substrate (CHO/fat) oxidation, endurance performance, muscle damage markers, hydration status, gastrointestinal tolerance
Cognitive function	Working memory, reaction times, attention, visual information processing, reasoning
Cardiovascular disease	Blood pressure, LDL cholesterol : HDL cholesterol, intima–media thickness, flow-mediated dilatation
Cancer	Oxidative DNA damage, DNA repair integrity, cytotoxicity and genotoxicity, apoptosis, natural killer cells, cytokines, lymphocyte proliferation
Obesity	BMI, body fat, fat distribution, energy intake and expenditure
Diabetes	Glucose tolerance, fasting blood glucose, insulin sensitivity
Bone health	Bone growth, bone mineral density, calcium kinetics

75 Phytochemicals

Aims

1 To identify the major categories of phytochemicals, their key structural features and typical dietary sources
2 To consider their potentially beneficial effects in humans

Plants produce a vast array of compounds called phytochemicals for physiological functions such as growth and repair, pigmentation, pollination, photo-protection and pathogen and predator resistance. Most phytochemicals are not nutrients for humans, but many are being investigated because they might explain the associations between higher intakes of fruits, vegetables and whole grains and the reduced risk of chronic disease.

The major classes of phytochemicals include carotenoids, polyphenols, glucosinolates and phytosterols. Appendix A3 shows the basic chemical structures. Typical examples, dietary sources and possible beneficial effects are shown in Table 75.1.

Carotenoids

Carotenoids are pigments involved in photosynthesis in plants, algae and some microorganisms. Over 750 carotenoids have been identified in nature, but only about 25 have been detected in human tissues. Sources include green vegetables, orange, yellow and red fruits and vegetables and some seafood.

Structurally, carotenoids can be divided into two

Hydrocarbons (e.g. α- and β-carotene, lycopene) contain no hydroxyl (OH) groups and are very hydrophobic.

Xanthophylls (e.g. lutein, zeaxanthin, β-cryptoxanthin) contain one or more OH groups and are less hydrophobic.

The degree of hydrophobicity is important because it affects the way carotenoids are partitioned within lipid environments such as membranes and lipoproteins, and this can affect their biological activity.

Some carotenoids have provitamin A activity due to the presence of one or more β-ionone rings also, carotenoids possess antioxidant properties and may protect cell membranes and plasma lipoproteins against lipid free radicals, and the skin and eyes against the harmful effects of UV light. A key feature of carotenoids is their ability to cooperate with other antioxidants such as vitamins C and E and glutathione.

Most research on carotenoids has been directed towards various forms of cancer and CVD. Research is also ongoing into the possible protective role of lutein and zeaxanthin against eye disorders such as age-related macular degeneration and cataracts.

Polyphenols

Polyphenols protect plants against photosynthetic stress, reactive oxygen species, wounds, herbivores and pathogens. Dietary sources include fruits, vegetables, cereals and beverages. Over 8000 plant phenolics have been identified, and these have been categorised into over 10 classes by chemical structure. The major classes are flavonoids, phenolic acids, stilbenes and lignans.

Flavonoids

Over 5000 flavonoids, making this the largest polyphenol class. Early interest in flavonoids was stimulated by the discovery of the 'French paradox' (i.e. low CVD mortality rate in Mediterranean countries associated with red wine consumption, despite a high saturated fat intake).

Generally, flavonoids consists of two aromatic rings (A and B) joined by an oxygenated C-ring. The nature of the C-ring subdivides into six families: flavanols, flavonols, flavones, isoflavones (known as phyto-oestrogens), flavanones and anthocyanidins. Within each family, differences in the number and nature of the substituents on the rings (e.g. H, OH or OCH_3 groups) give rise to the individual flavonoid monomers.

Flavonoids may be present in foods as glycones (in which a sugar is attached) or as aglycones. They may also be present as dimers, trimers, oligomers and longer-chain polymers.

Flavonoids may be protective against a wide variety of chronic diseases including CVD, cancer, diabetes, osteoporosis, asthma, Alzheimer's disease and Parkinson's disease. A range of biological effects have been reported: antioxidant activity, oestrogenic/anti-oestrogenic activity, neuroprotection, carcinogen detoxification and effects on vascular function, gene expression and apoptosis.

Phenolic acids and derivatives

Phenolic acids are present in all fruits and vegetables and account for about one-third of the total polyphenol content of the diet. They are particularly abundant in acid-tasting fruits. Caffeic acid, gallic acid and ferulic acid are commonly consumed phenolic acids. Chlorogenic acid, a derivative of caffeic acid, is a major polyphenol in coffee and black tea. Curcumin, derived from ferulic acid, is the major yellow pigment in turmeric and mustard. In addition to their role as antioxidants, this class of compounds is under investigation for their possible beneficial effects against cancer, diabetes, inflammation, hypertension and hepatotoxicity. Curcumin, in particular, has demonstrated potent anticancer properties in a variety of human cancer cell lines and animal carcinogenesis models.

Stilbenes

Stilbenes contain two phenyl moieties joined by a 2-carbon methylene bridge. Most stilbenes are synthesised by plants only in response to injury or infection. Resveratrol (the most extensively studied stilbene) is found in grapes, berries, peanuts and wine and may be a major contributor to the 'French paradox'. Its cardio-protective, anti-inflammatory, anti-ageing and antitumour effects are currently under investigation.

Lignans

Lignans are diphenolic compounds found in flaxseed, rye, sesame seeds and brassica vegetables. Although most lignans pass through the gastrointestinal tract without being absorbed, some are converted by intestinal bacteria to enterolignans (enterodiol and enterolactone), which can be absorbed through the enterohepatic circulation. Lignans are under investigation for their possible role in the prevention of cardiovascular and neurodegenerative diseases as well as cancer. In addition, some lignans have anti-inflammatory properties and several are considered to be phyto-oestrogens.

Nutrition at a Glance, Second Edition. Edited by Sangita Sharma, Tony Sheehy and Fariba Kolahdooz.
© 2016 John Wiley & Sons, Ltd. Published 2016 by John Wiley & Sons, Ltd.

Table 75.1 Examples of phytochemicals that may have beneficial biological effects.

Component	Examples	Sources	Possible beneficial effects
Carotenoids	α- and β-carotene	Carrots, pumpkins, sweet potatoes, spinach	Antioxidant role, immunological stimulants, anticancer agents, transcriptional regulators, anti-inflammatory activity
	Lutein, zeaxanthin	Green leafy vegetables, corn	
	Lycopene	Tomatoes, apricots, watermelon	
	β-Cryptoxanthin	Pumpkin, red peppers, oranges	
	Astaxanthin	Salmon, shrimp, lobster, crab	
Flavonoids			
• Flavanols	Catechin, epicatechin	Tea, chocolate, apples, grapes, red wine	Free radical scavenging, metal chelation, vasodilation, reduced platelet aggregation, carcinogen detoxification, effects on gene expression and apoptosis, neuroprotection
• Flavonols	Quercetin, kaempferol	Onions, kale, broccoli, cocoa, tea, red wine	Oestrogenic/anti-oestrogenic effects, cholesterol-lowering and anti-inflammatory effects
• Flavones	Apigenin, luteolin	Citrus fruits, celery, spinach, peppers	
• Isoflavones	Genistein, daidzein	Soybeans, peanuts, chickpeas	
• Flavanones	Hesperetin, naringenin	Oranges, tangerines, grapefruits, lemons, limes	
• Anthocyanidins	Cyanidin, delphinidin	Elderberries, blueberries, blackberries	
Phenolic acids and derivatives	Caffeic acid	Apples, plums, tomatoes, grapes	Anti-inflammatory, antibacterial, antioxidant, antihypertensive, anti-mutagenic activity; protection against hepatotoxicity; induction of apoptosis; inhibition of angiogenesis and tumour metastasis
	Ferulic acid	Wheat bran, rice bran	
	Chlorogenic acid	Apples, pears, carrots, coffee, black tea	
	Curcumin	Turmeric, mustard	
Stilbenes	Resveratrol	Grapes, berries, peanuts, red wine	Cardio-protective, anti-inflammatory, anti-ageing, antitumour effects
Lignans	Secoisolariciresinol, matairesinol, pinoresinol, lariciresinol, sesamin	Flaxseed, rye, cabbage, kale, broccoli, sesame seeds	Cardio-protective, neuroprotective, anticancer, anti-inflammatory effects; phyto-oestrogens
Glucosinolates	Indoles, thiocyanates, isothiocyanates	Brussels sprouts, cabbage, cauliflower, turnips, radishes, kale, rocket	Carcinogen inactivation, protection against DNA damage, apoptosis induction, angiogenesis inhibition, anti-inflammatory effects
Phytosterols	β-Sitosterol, campesterol, stigmasterol	Vegetable oils, nuts, seeds, grains, added to margarines and some dairy products	Cholesterol-lowering; anticancer, anti-atherosclerotic, anti-inflammatory effects; immune modulation; antioxidant activity

Glucosinolates

Glucosinolates are sulphur-containing compounds present in cruciferous vegetables (e.g. cabbage, cauliflower, broccoli, radishes). During food preparation, cooking, chewing and digestion, they are broken down to various biologically active compounds including indoles, thiocyanates and isothiocyanates. The possible role of glucosinolates in cancer, CVD and neurological disease prevention is under intense investigation.

Phytosterols

Phytosterols can be obtained from vegetable oils, nuts, seeds and grains. They are also the functional ingredients in cholesterol-lowering food products. Phytosterols are currently being investigated for their possible beneficial effects against cancer, inflammatory conditions (e.g. osteoarthritis) and immune function (e.g. asthma).

Interpreting the evidence

Evidence continues to grow about the potential health benefits of phytochemicals; however, this evidence must be interpreted with caution.
• Phytochemicals (even within the same category) exist in many forms, and may have different biological effects of all forms are the same;
• Food composition data for most phytochemicals are inadequate.
• For most phytochemicals, little is known about their bioavailability.

This is important because just because something is consumed, that does not necessarily mean that it is absorbed. And if it is not absorbed then it cannot have a protective effect (at least systemically).
• Following consumption, the concentration of a phytochemical in plasma or tissues is high enough to explain any observed effects.
• The health effects of some phytochemicals could be due to metabolites rather than the compounds themselves. Alternatively, generalised induction of detoxifying enzymes following consumption of phytochemicals may help inactivate carcinogens, free radicals, or other harmful compounds.
• For unabsorbed phytochemicals, microbial metabolites might have beneficial effects in the large intestine, or elsewhere.
• If the relationship between phytochemical intake and a particular disease is being studied using biomarkers, the biomarker must be a valid measure of the disease process.

Summary

Despite enormous interest in the role of phytochemicals in chronic disease prevention, the real contribution of such compounds to human health protection and the mechanisms through which they operate remain unclear. The structural complexity of phytochemicals, limitations of food composition databases and uncertainty about the bioavailability and metabolism of most phytochemicals make it difficult to precisely relate dietary intakes to chronic disease outcomes. Much more research is needed across a broad range of disciplines before any specific dietary recommendations for phytochemicals can be made.

76 Genetically modified foods

Aims

1 To explore the definition of genetically modified (GM) foods
2 To examine the advantages and controversies surrounding genetically modified foods

Genetically modified organisms and foods

Genetic modification aims to create desirable traits within the organism. This process alters the genetic makeup of the organism and therefore is termed 'genetic engineering' or 'recombinant DNA technology'. A genetically modified organism (GMO) is developed by altering the organism's genetic material (i.e. DNA) by transferring specific genes from one organism to another, either within the same species or between unrelated species. These altered organisms are utilised for agricultural, medical, research and environmental management purposes. GM plants and animals then become GM foods available for consumption by other animals and people.

Some of the most common GM crop varieties include corn, soybeans, sugar beets and canola. Potatoes, rice, wheat, squash, papaya, cranberries, raspberries and cantaloupe are also available as GM crops. The future of GM food crops includes apples that don't brown, coffee that contains less caffeine, melons with an increased shelf life, bananas that don't have worm parasites or viruses, sunflower oil with less saturated fat and cabbage that can defend itself from caterpillars.

Examples of GM animals include GM pigs that have lower saturated fat, higher unsaturated fat and less harmful phosphorous in their manure. GM animals are also involved in the production of pharmaceuticals, such as proteins expressed in milk from sheep, cows and goats, which provide antimicrobials that target bacteria like *Salmonella*.

Emergence of GMO

Traditionally, farmers utilised selective breeding to produce crops that expressed the desirable traits; however, this technique takes time and does not always produce the desired outcome. Applying modern genetic modification technologies allows food producers to create crops with the desired traits with more efficiency and accuracy (Table 76.1).

GMOs have increased in use since their emergence on the market in 1994. Initially, GMOs were marketed as a way to protect crops and, thus, increase yield. It was the belief that the increase in yield garnered by this new technology was a way to solve world hunger. Food producers have increasingly utilised these GM seeds and crops due to their many agricultural advantages over traditional crops.

Health benefits of GM foods

Beyond the traditional agricultural advantages of GMO, vigorous research on and utilisation of advanced genetic engineering have led to some health benefits of GM foods (Table 76.2).

Controversies concerning GM foods

Once modified genes are released into the environment, it is impossible to remove them. Some negative health (Table 76.3), environmental (Table 76.4) and socio-economic (Table 76.5) consequences of GMOs are the basis for the controversies and general public unease surrounding the consumption of GM foods. With GM crops, there is concern and debate on their potential to cause gene transfer, outcrossing and allergenicity. Gene transfer refers to the gene flow of GM crops genes into the digestive tract that may lead to adverse health effects, outcrossing refers to the gene flow of GM crops into staple crops, and lastly, allergenicity refers to the gene flow of common allergens originating from crops.

Compared to GM plants, GM animals have proven to be an even more contentious issue. In addition to the many similar concerns raised for altering the genetic material in plants, there are also multiple ethical and animal welfare issues that accompany the research and modification of animal DNA.

Table 76.1 Agricultural advantages of genetically modified organisms.

Agricultural benefits	Example
Insect resistance	By introducing a gene from the bacterium *Bacillus thuringiensis* (Bt), plants can produce a toxic protein that targets specific insects
Herbicide tolerance	Some soybeans are genetically modified to be herbicide tolerant. All plants (weeds) other than soybean plants growing within the field are destroyed, which results in a reduction in production cost
Hostility protection	GM crops can be cultivated in hostile growing conditions. In 2001, a tomato variety was developed that disperses salt from the ground into its leaves, preventing the taste of the tomato from being affected by the high level of salinity in the soil. Drought-resistant maize is cultivated in Africa
Cold tolerance	The DNA of cold water fish contains an antifreeze gene that has been introduced into potato and tobacco plants
Disease resistance	In Africa, pathogen-resistant bananas are cultivated on a commercial basis

Nutrition at a Glance, Second Edition. Edited by Sangita Sharma, Tony Sheehy and Fariba Kolahdooz.

Table 76.2 Health benefits of genetically modified organisms.

Health benefits	Example
Production of pharmaceuticals	Tomatoes, potatoes and bananas are targeted for introducing DNA for vaccines and medications. Producing edible versions of vaccines and medications will be especially beneficial for developing countries in which refrigeration and storage of vaccines and medication can be an issue
Development of phytoremediation	A species of poplar tree has been developed that removes heavy metals from the soil
Improved nutrition	The level of β-carotene is artificially increased in 'golden' rice, which reduces vitamin A deficiency

Table 76.3 Health concerns from consuming genetically modified foods.

Concerns	Example
Allergic reaction	An allergen from Brazil nuts was unknowingly incorporated into a developmental strain of soybeans, and when discovered, the produce had to be abandoned
Unwanted gene transfer	To verify a successful gene transfer, antibiotic-resistant genes are inserted into GMOs as a marker. If this gene was then transferred to pathogenic bacteria in the environment, these bacteria could become antibiotic resistant
Mixing of GM and non-GM foods in the food supply	A strain of Bt corn not approved for human consumption and intended for use as animal feed entered the food supply in a fast food chain of restaurants
Unknown health effects	Some animal studies are reporting adverse health effects, such as abnormalities in the digestive tracts of rats. The severity of adverse health effects with increased length and extent of exposure to GM foods is unknown

Table 76.4 Environmental concerns surrounding genetically modified organisms.

Concerns	Example
Cross-pollination between GMO and non-GMO leading to genetic pollution and outcrossing	Genetic pollution may result in a decrease in the genetic diversity and sustainability of a species and potentially harmful strains introduced into the crops meant for human consumption. Outcrossing may cause the offspring to outcompete other species, changing their traditional role in the ecosystem and even replacing conventional species used by farmers. Herbicide-tolerant 'superweeds' are created by the undesirable transfer of herbicide-tolerant genes from GMOs to weeds
Decreased pesticide effectiveness	Insects may become resistant to pesticides if pesticide-resistant genes added to GMOs are unexpectedly transferred to their DNA
Mutation	Inserted genes may cause harmful mutations within the organism itself. There is uncertainty as to how stable inserted genes will be over several generations
Unknown impact on birds, insects and soil microorganisms	GMO may harm pollinators such as bees and animals that traditionally feed on the crops such as birds. Fungi in the soil and rumen bacteria may also be impacted

Table 76.5 Socio-economic concerns with genetically modified foods.

Concerns	Example
Economic cost to farmers	GMO are often patented to ensure a profit after the costly research and development process. Suicide genes (genes that would cause seeds from mature crops to be sterile) are used by the agribusiness as a way to inhibit patent infringement, ensuring that farmers purchase new seeds every year. This can cause large increases in farming cost for small farmers and farmers in developing countries
Unintended consumption of animals	Cross-species insertion is common when developing GMOs. This can have significant implications for individuals of certain cultural and religious groups. The insertion of genes from pigs into plant produce would result in Muslims unknowingly consuming haraam or prohibited food

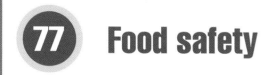

77 Food safety

Aims

1 To define safe food
2 To identify various sources of food hazards and introduce hazard analysis and critical control point (HACCP)
3 To introduce current issues around food safety

Safe food

Food safety encompasses a number of important elements (Figure 77.1). These include:
• The use of safe production, transportation, processing, handling and storage procedures
• Maintenance of adequate nutrient content during processing
• Freedom from chemical, microbial and biological (including genetic) hazards
• Provision of appropriate guidance on use before the end of the food's shelf life

Different people may define food safety differently. For instance, the food industry may describe safe food differently than the general public.

Food hazards

Food hazards are biological, chemical or physical agents associated with food and food production that have the potential to threaten food safety. They may cause adverse effects in the digestive tract (e.g. diarrhoea and/or vomiting) as well as in other physiological systems (e.g. reproductive and nervous systems). They can also lead to cancer, behavioural and cognitive impairments and if left untreated, even death.

Biological hazards

Biological hazards include bacteria (e.g. *Salmonella*, *Campylobacter jejuni* and *Escherichia coli*), parasites (e.g. *cryptosporidium*, *cryptospora* and *trematodes*), viruses (e.g. *hepatitis A*, *Norwalk* and *rotaviruses*), yeasts and moulds.

These microbial pathogens can cause harm by two mechanisms:
1 By colonising inside the gastrointestinal tract of humans and invading organs (infections)
2 By producing toxins (intoxications)

The survival of pathogens in food depends on intrinsic and extrinsic factors (Table 77.1).

Table 77.1 Example of intrinsic and extrinsic factors that influence the survival of pathogens in food.

Intrinsic factors	Extrinsic factors
pH of the food	Heat treatment
Moisture content of the food	Storage temperature
Oxidation–reduction (redox) potential	Relative humidity of the environment
Nutritional content	Presence and concentration of gases
Antimicrobial constituents	Presence and activity of other microorganisms
Biological structure	

Chemical hazards

Chemical hazards may occur naturally, during food processing, storage and preparation and through agricultural and industrial contamination.

Naturally occurring chemical hazards include:
• Mycotoxins (e.g. aflatoxin) and shellfish/mushroom toxins
• Heavy metals (e.g. cadmium, lead and mercury), which may be found naturally in water or plants or accumulate in animals (e.g. mercury in fish)

Food production, processing, storage and preparation may introduce chemical hazards in a number of ways, including:
• Excessive utilisation of veterinary drugs such as antibiotics and hormones
• Contamination of foods by cleaners and sanitisers, either on the farm (e.g. milk) or in the factory
• Excessive use of food additives (e.g. preservatives, colours and allergens)
• Excessive nutrient fortification
• Cross-contamination with food allergens (e.g. nuts) within food production facilities
• Undesirable chemical changes (e.g. formation of *trans*-fatty acids)

Environmental chemical contamination may occur in two mechanisms:
• Low-level contamination in the long term, due to gradual deposition of harmful chemicals
• High-level contamination in the short term, resulting from an accidental release of chemicals

Chemical contaminants may adversely affect the environment, including water, crops and livestock.

Agricultural contaminants include pesticides such as dichlorodiphenyltrichloroethane (DDT) and related compounds. Human industrial activities may also utilise harmful chemicals (e.g. coolants such as polychlorinated biphenyls (PCBs)) and contaminate the environment.

Physical hazards

Physical hazards are foreign objects such as glass, metal, wood and bone in food from accidental or intentional contact or poor food processing practices. Not all foreign objects are hazardous, as in the case of hair or some insects that are undesirable but unlikely to cause injuries.

Ensuring food safety

Food is exposed to hazards from its production to consumption. Therefore, practices to ensure food safety must be carried out throughout the various steps involved in the food supply chain (Figure 77.2).

Hazard analysis and critical control point

In response to increasing concern about food safety, hazard analysis and critical control point (HACCP) is widely accepted by many public health agencies (e.g. World Health Organization), consumers and industries.

HACCP is defined as 'a logical system to identify hazards and/or critical situations and to produce a structured plan to control these situations'.

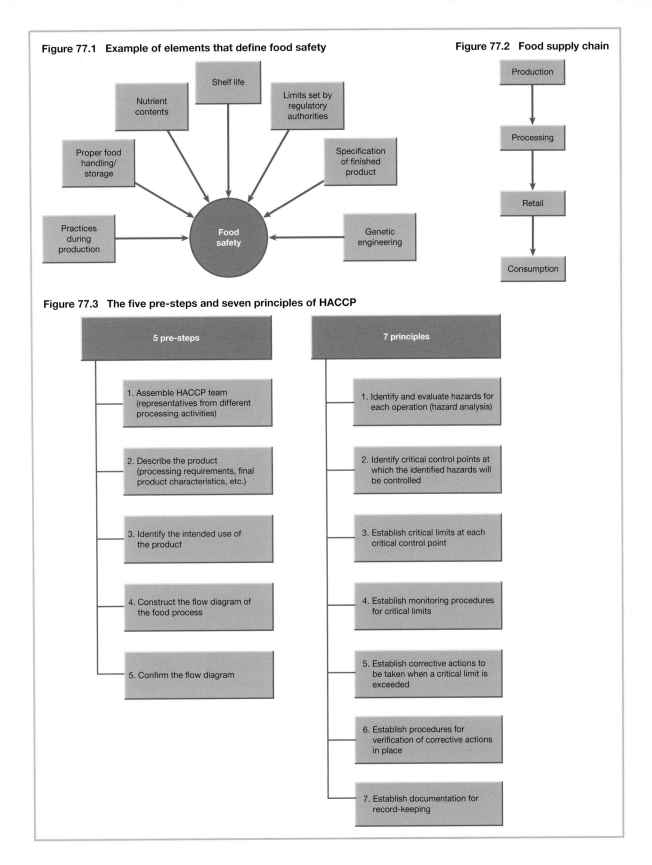

Figure 77.1 Example of elements that define food safety

Nutrient contents

Shelf life

Limits set by regulatory authorities

Proper food handling/ storage

Specification of finished product

Practices during production

Genetic engineering

Food safety

Figure 77.2 Food supply chain

Production

Processing

Retail

Consumption

Figure 77.3 The five pre-steps and seven principles of HACCP

5 pre-steps

1. Assemble HACCP team (representatives from different processing activities)

2. Describe the product (processing requirements, final product characteristics, etc.)

3. Identify the intended use of the product

4. Construct the flow diagram of the food process

5. Confirm the flow diagram

7 principles

1. Identify and evaluate hazards for each operation (hazard analysis)

2. Identify critical control points at which the identified hazards will be controlled

3. Establish critical limits at each critical control point

4. Establish monitoring procedures for critical limits

5. Establish corrective actions to be taken when a critical limit is exceeded

6. Establish procedures for verification of corrective actions in place

7. Establish documentation for record-keeping

The seven principles of HACCP must be documented in a HACCP plan and monitored continuously or regularly according to facility protocol (Figure 77.3).

Current issues in food safety

Agricultural/industrial chemical agents and food additives may be used extensively to increase shelf life and enhance the visual appeal of foods, but may threaten food safety.

In particular, antimicrobial agents used in food production can contribute to antimicrobial resistance of pathogens and increase the risk of food-borne diseases in humans.

The centralisation of food production, mass production of foods and internationalisation of food distribution may allow rapid and worldwide distribution of contaminated food.

Some food hazards can bioaccumulate, and the final consumers in the food chain (i.e. humans) may be affected severely.

Appendix A1: Structures of the fat-soluble vitamins A, D, E and K

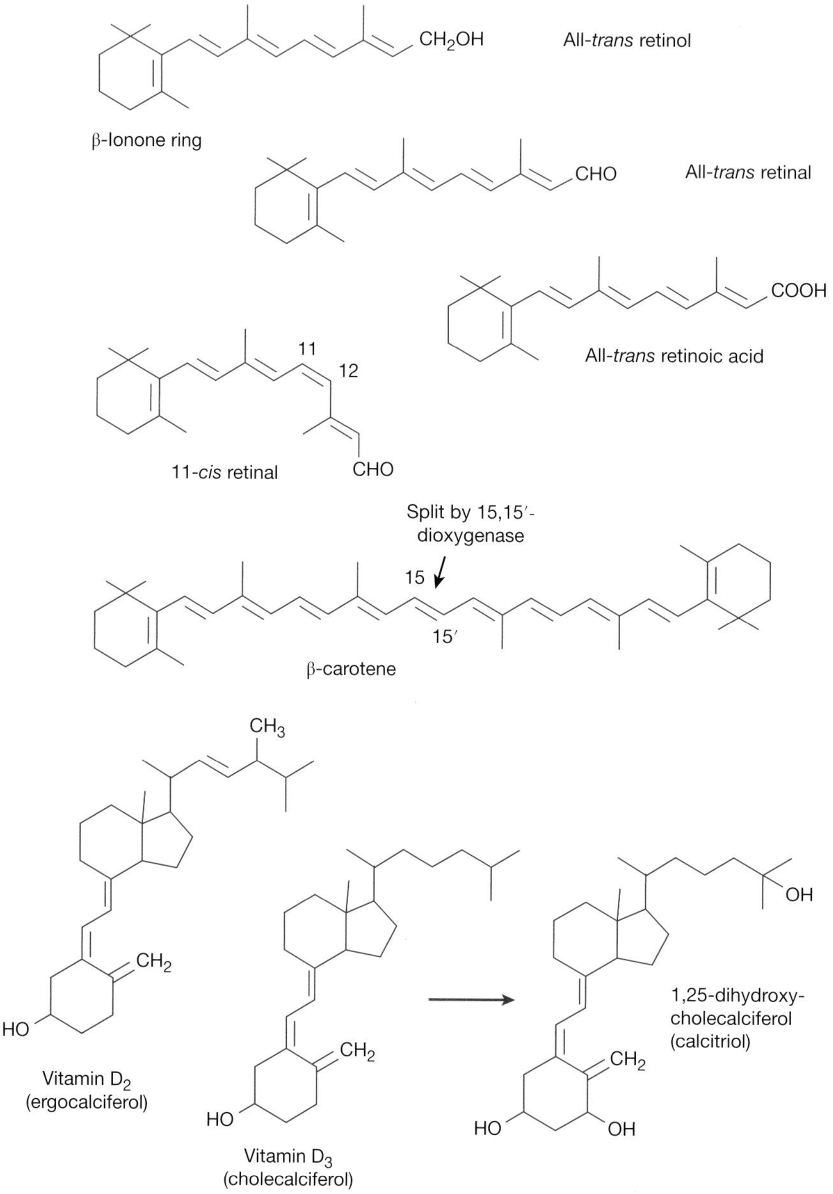

CH₂OH — All-*trans* retinol

β-Ionone ring

CHO — All-*trans* retinal

COOH — All-*trans* retinoic acid

11-*cis* retinal — CHO

Split by 15,15′-dioxygenase

β-carotene

Vitamin D₂ (ergocalciferol)

Vitamin D₃ (cholecalciferol)

1,25-dihydroxy-cholecalciferol (calcitriol)

Nutrition at a Glance, Second Edition. Edited by Sangita Sharma, Tony Sheehy and Fariba Kolahdooz.
© 2016 John Wiley & Sons, Ltd. Published 2016 by John Wiley & Sons, Ltd.

Basic tocopherol structure

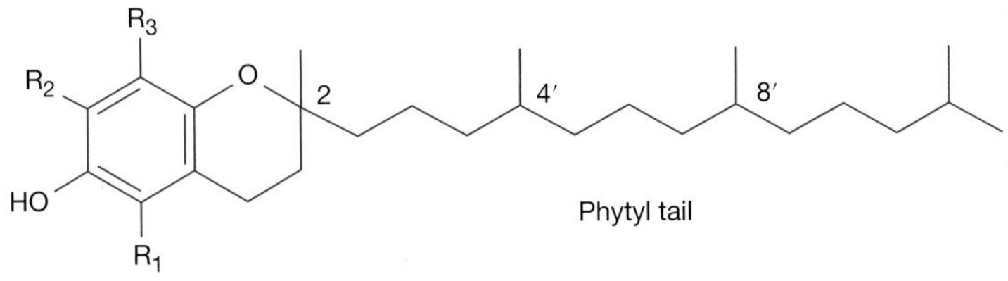

Phytyl tail

Chromanol ring

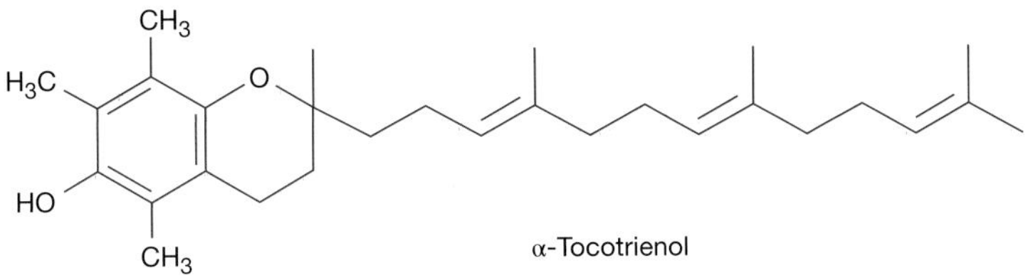

α-Tocotrienol

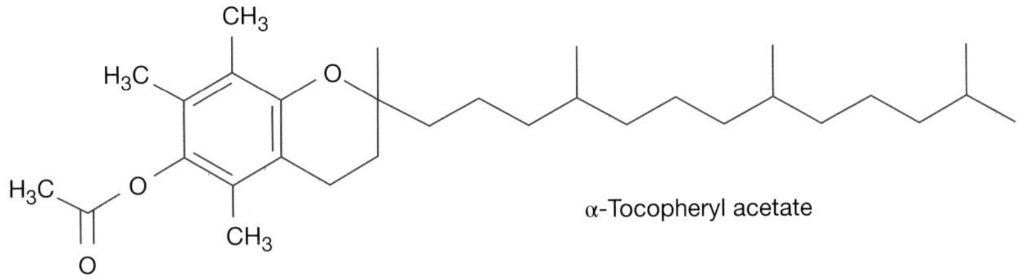

α-Tocopheryl acetate

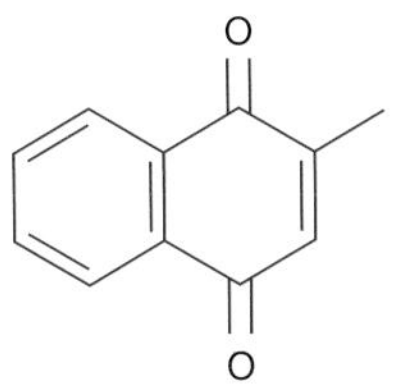

Menadione (vitamin K$_3$)

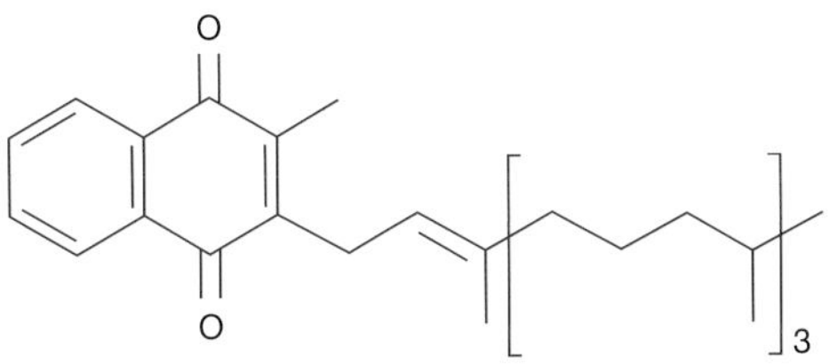

Isoprene

Phylloquinone (vitamin K$_1$)

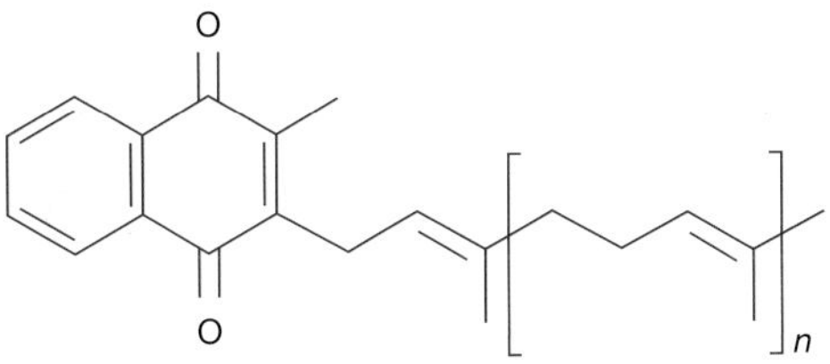

Menaquinone (vitamin K$_2$)

Appendix A2: Structures of the water-soluble vitamins: Thiamin, riboflavin, niacin, vitamin B$_6$, biotin, pantothenic acid, folic acid, vitamin B$_{12}$ and vitamin C

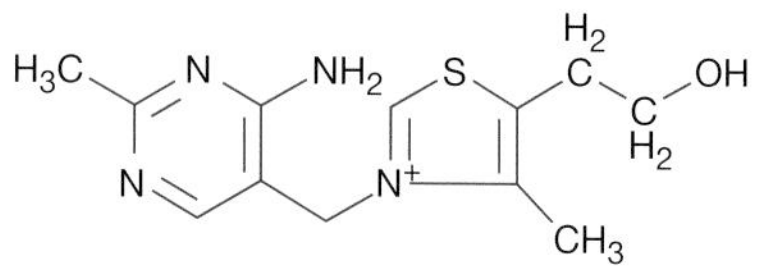

Thiamin

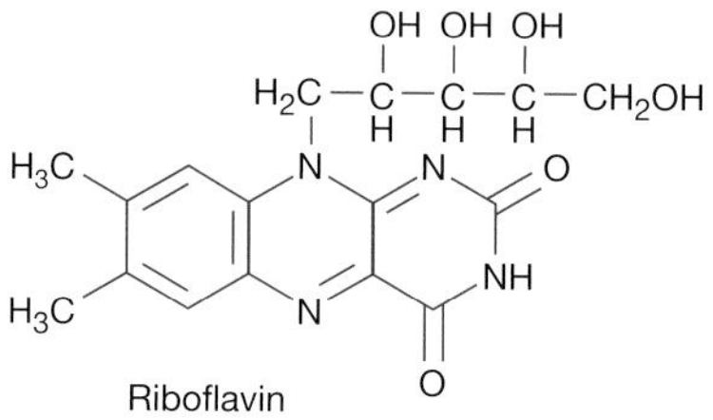

Riboflavin

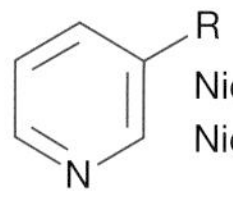

Nicotinic acid: R = COOH
Nicotinamide: R = CONH$_2$

Niacin

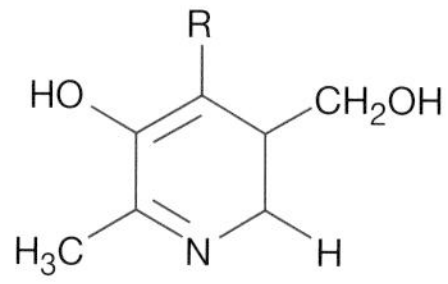

Pyridoxine: R = CH$_2$OH
Pyridoxal: R = CHO
Pyridoxamine: R = CH$_2$NH$_2$

Vitamin B$_6$

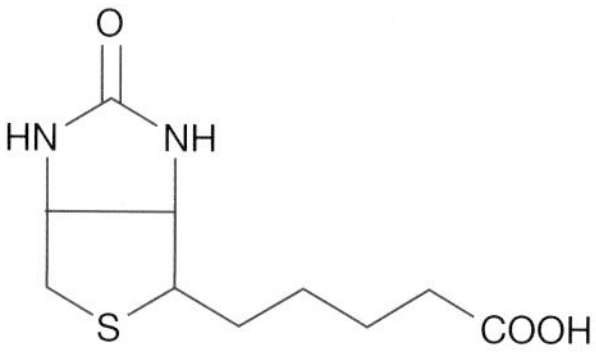

Biotin

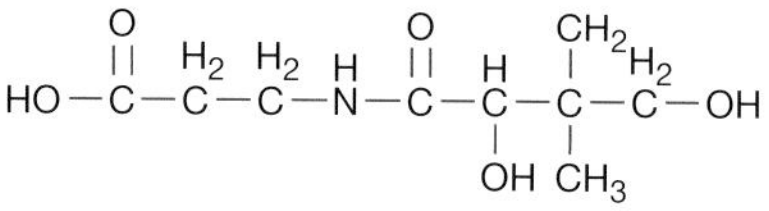

Pantothenic acid

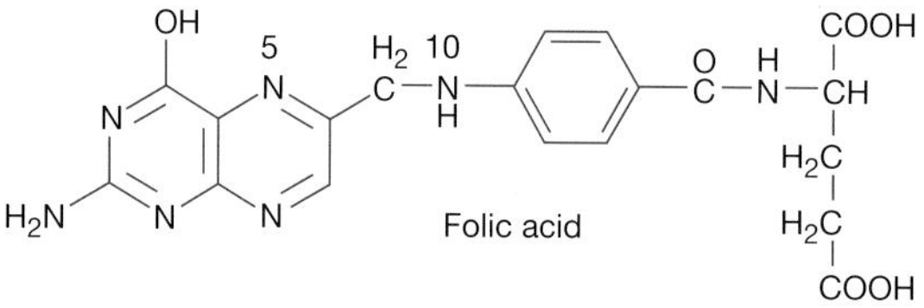

Folic acid

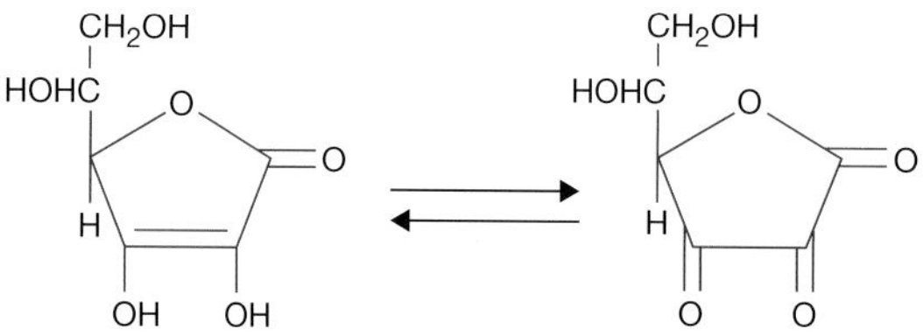

Ascorbic acid

Dehydroascorbate

Nutrition at a Glance, Second Edition. Edited by Sangita Sharma, Tony Sheehy and Fariba Kolahdooz.
© 2016 John Wiley & Sons, Ltd. Published 2016 by John Wiley & Sons, Ltd.

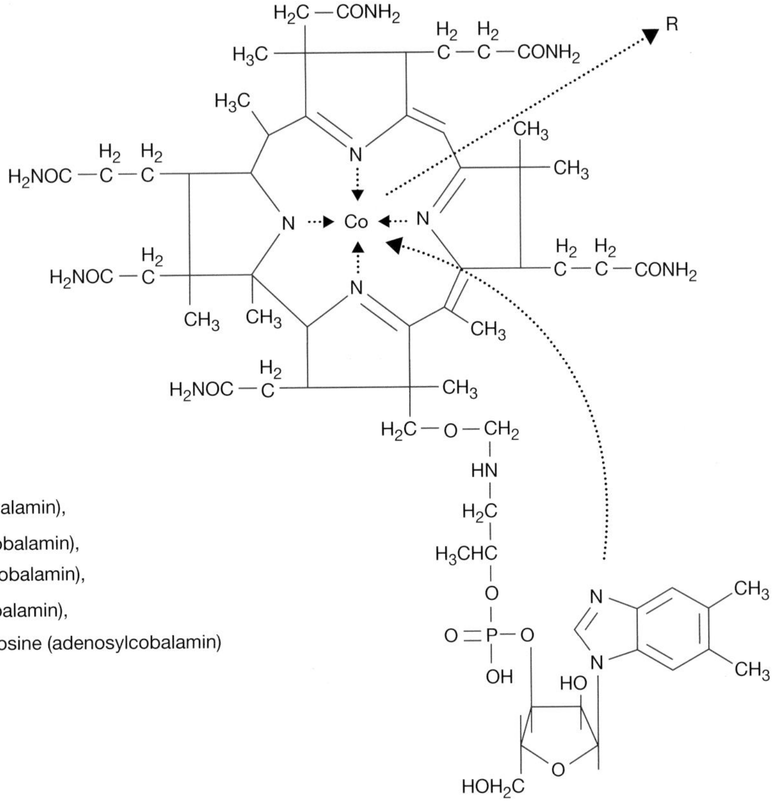

Vitamin B$_{12}$

R = CN (cyanocobalamin),

CH$_3$ (methylcobalamin),

OH (hydroxocobalamin),

H$_2$O (aquocobalamin),

5'-deoxyadenosine (adenosylcobalamin)

Appendix A3: Structures of the major classes of phytochemicals

Basic flavonoid structure

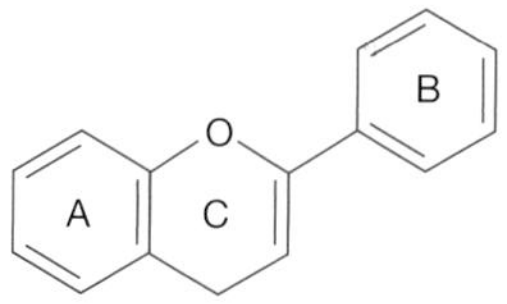

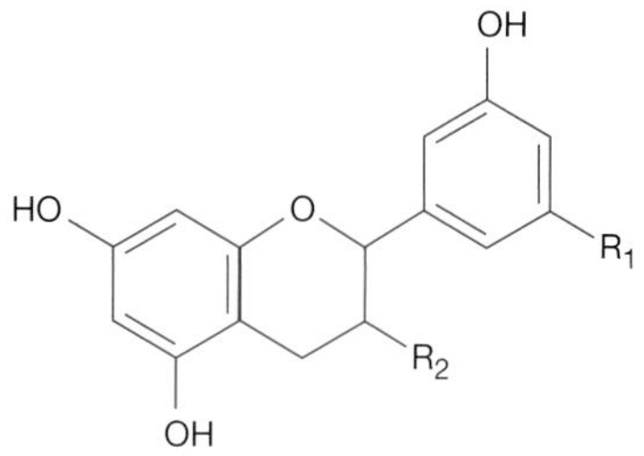

Flavanols
Catechin: $R_1 = H$, $R_2 = OH$

Epigallocatechin: $R_1 = OH$, $R_2 = OH$

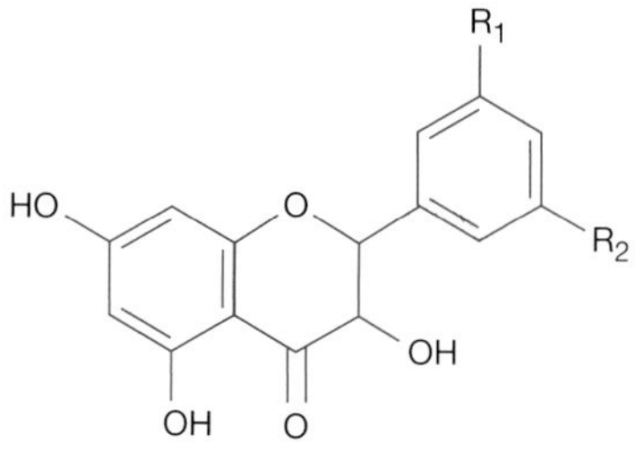

Flavonols
Quercetin: $R_1 = OH$, $R_2 = H$

Kaempferol: $R_1 = H$, $R_2 = H$

Myricetin: $R_1 = OH$, $R_2 = OH$

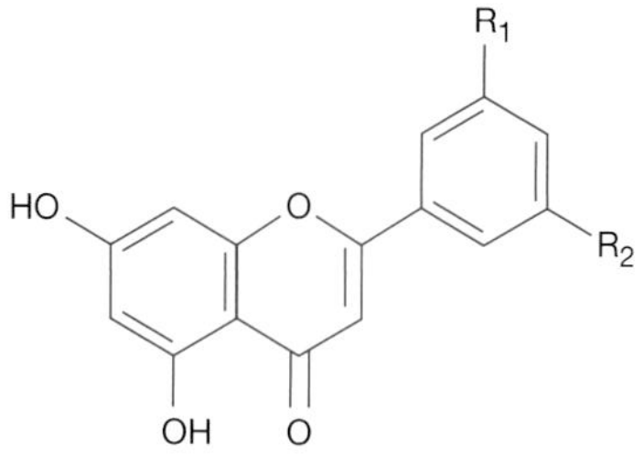

Flavones
Apigenin: $R_1 = H$, $R_2 = H$

Luteolin: $R_1 = OH$, $R_2 = H$

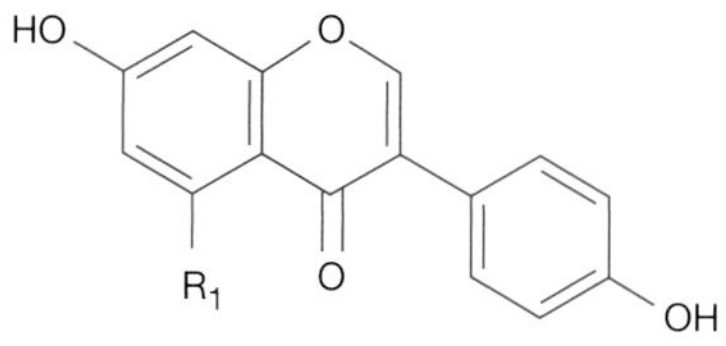

Isoflavones (phyto-oestrogens)
Genistein: $R_1 = OH$

Diadzein: $R_1 = H$

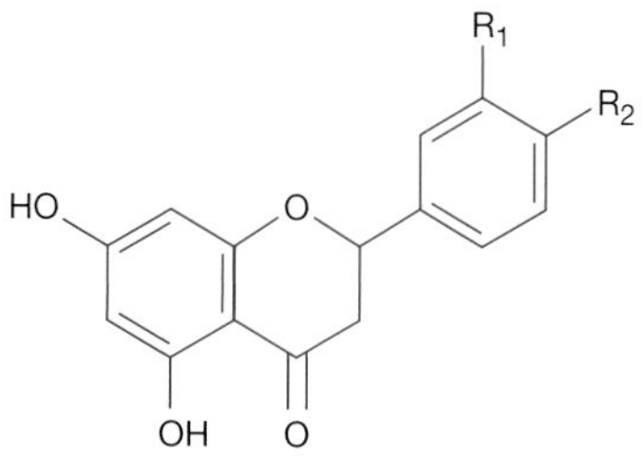

Flavonones
Hesperetin: $R_1 = OH$, $R_2 = OCH_3$

Naringenin: $R_1 = H$, $R_2 = OH$

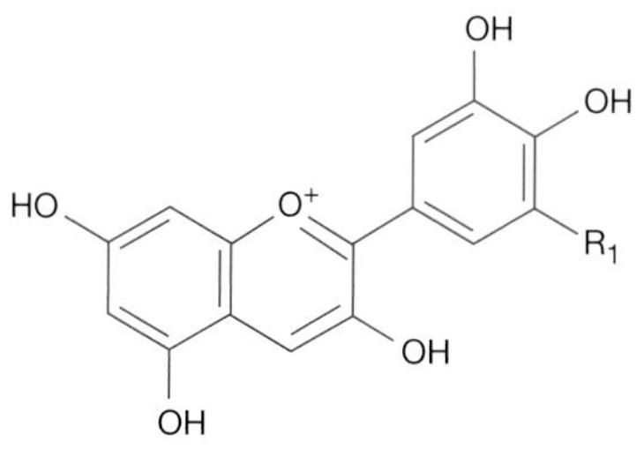

Anthocyanidins
Cyanidin: $R_1 = H$

Delphinidin: $R_1 = OH$

Nutrition at a Glance, Second Edition. Edited by Sangita Sharma, Tony Sheehy and Fariba Kolahdooz.
© 2016 John Wiley & Sons, Ltd. Published 2016 by John Wiley & Sons, Ltd.

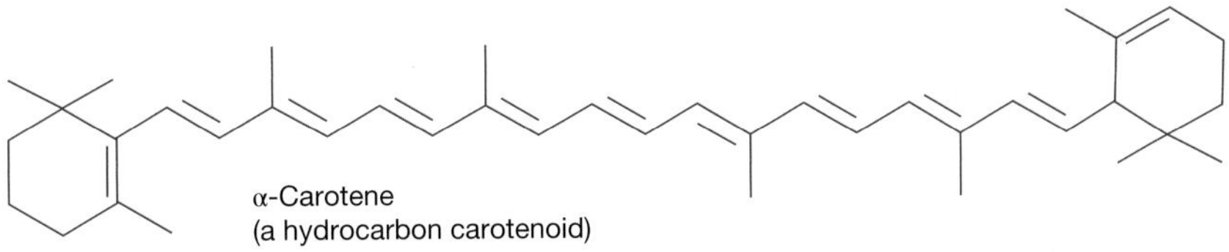

α-Carotene
(a hydrocarbon carotenoid)

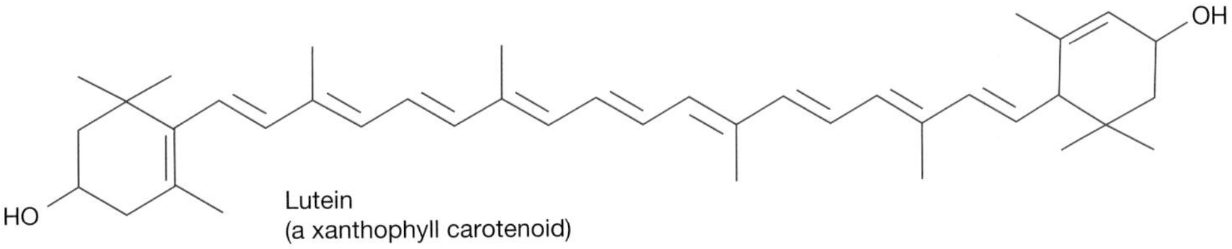

Lutein
(a xanthophyll carotenoid)

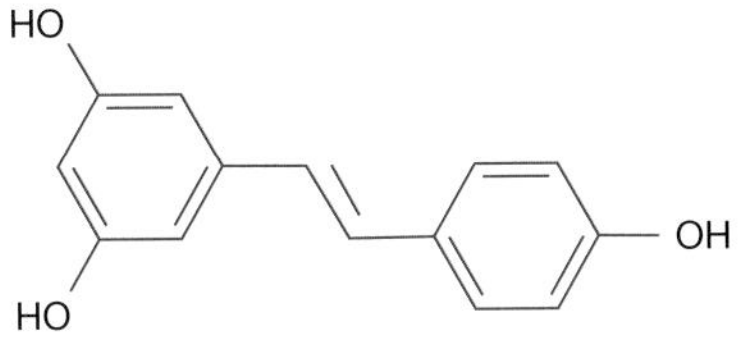

trans-resveratrol
(a stilbene)

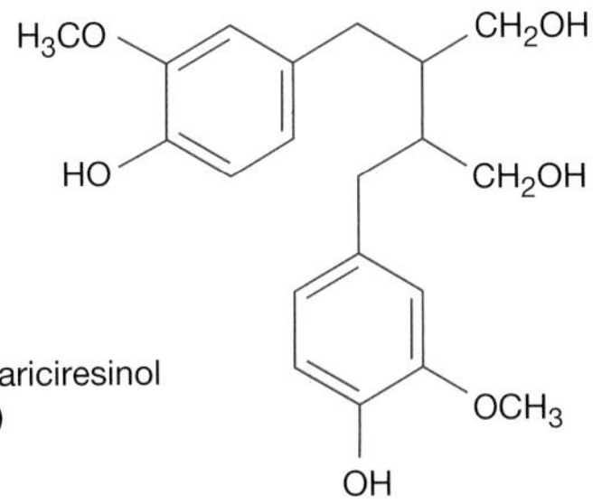

Secoisolariciresinol
(a lignan)

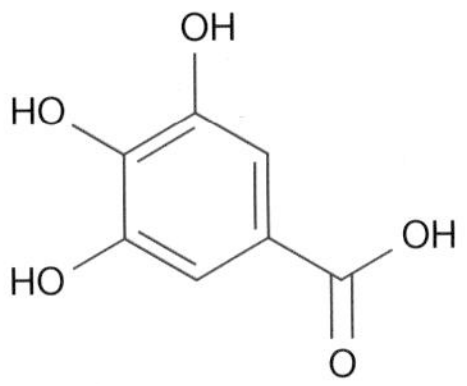

Gallic acid

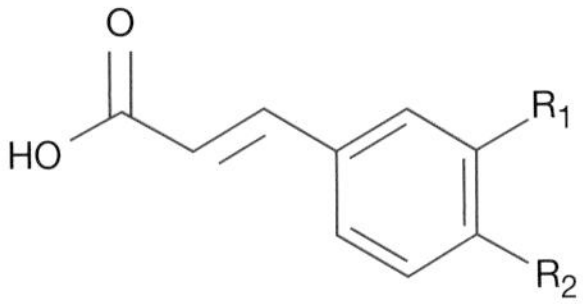

Caffeic acid: R_1 and R_2 = OH
Ferulic acid: R_1 = OCH$_3$, R_2 = OH

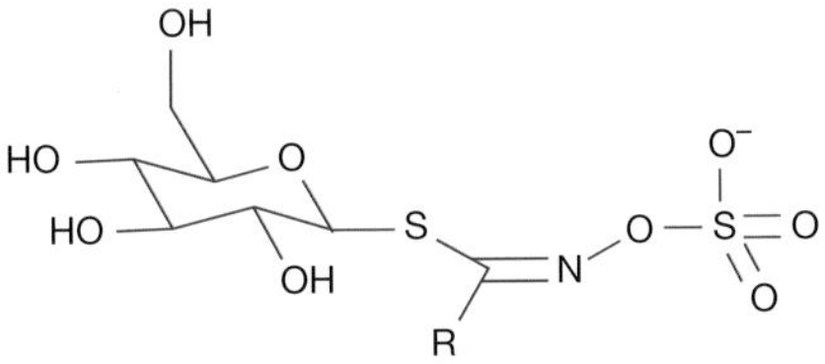

Basic glucosinolate structure

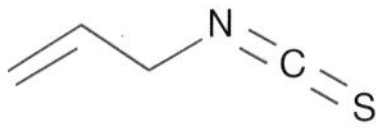

Allyl isothiocyanate

Bibliography

Alkerwi, A., Sauvageot, N., Pagny, S., Beissel, J., Delagardelle, C. & Lair, M.L. (2012) Acculturation, immigration status and cardiovascular risk factors among Portuguese immigrants to Luxembourg: findings from ORISCAV-LUX study. *BMC Public Health*, 12, 864.

Bacon, R.T. & Sofos, J.N. (2003) Characteristics of biological hazards in foods. In: R. H. Schmidt & &Rodrick, G.E. (eds), *Food Safety Handbook*, pp. 157–195. John Wiley & Sons, Inc., Hoboken.

Bahreini, N., Noor, M.I., Koon, P.B., *et al.* (2013 Aug) Weight status among Iranian adolescents: comparison of four different criteria. *Journal of Research in Medical Sciences*, 18 (8), 641–646.

Barasi, M. (2003) *Human Nutrition: A Health Perspective*. Hodder Arnold, London.

Bhandari, S.D. (2003) Hazards resulting from environmental, industrial, and agricultural contaminants. In: R. H. Schmidt & G. E. Rodrick (eds), *Food Safety Handbook*, pp. 291–321. John Wiley & Sons, Inc., Hoboken.

Blundell, J.E., Burley, V.J., Cotton, J.R. & Lawton, C.L. (1993 May) Dietary fat and the control of energy intake: evaluating the effects of fat on meal size and postmeal satiety. *American Journal of Clinical Nutrition*, 57 (5 Suppl), 772S–777S.

Booth, B.T. & Vogel, K.P. (2006) Revegetation priorities. *Rangelands*, 28 (5), 24–30.

Cade, J., Thompson, R., Burley, V. & Warm, D. (2002 Aug) Development, validation and utilisation of food-frequency questionnaires – a review. *Public Health Nutrition*, 5 (4), 567–587.

Cade, J.E., Burley, V.J., Warm, D.L., Thompson, R.L. & Margetts, B.M. (2004 Jun) Food-frequency questionnaires: a review of their design, validation and utilisation. *Nutrition Research Reviews*, 17 (1), 5–22.

Camire, M.E. & Kantor, M.A. (1999 Jul) Dietary supplements: nutritional and legal considerations. *Food Technology*, 53 (7), 87–96.

Canadian Celiac Association (2007) *Celiac Disease – What Is It?* Retrieved 2015 Aug 18 from http://celiac.ca/pdfs/celiac%20disease%20what%20is%20it.pdfpdf [accessed on 26 August 2015].

Canadian Celiac Association (2014) *About Celiac Disease.* Retrieved 2015 Aug 18 from http://celiac.ca/pdfs/celiac%20disease%20what%20is%20it.pdf [accessed on 26 August 2015].

Canadian Circumpolar Institute (2014) *Northern Research Licensing and Permits.* Canadian Circumpolar Institute. Retrieved 2014 Jan 30 from http://www.cci.ualberta.ca/en/GrantsandScholarships/NorthernResearchLicensingandPe.aspx [accessed on 26 August 2015].

Casey, L. (2013 Aug) Caring for children with phenylketonuria. *Canadian Family Physician*, 59 (8), 837–840.

Charkow, R. (2011, Mar 8) Genetically modified foods: the facts and debates. *CBC News.* Retrieved 2015 Aug 18 from http://www.cbc.ca/news/technology/genetically-modified-foods-the-facts-and-debates-1.1031789 [accessed on 26 August 2015].

Chiu, M., Austin, P.C., Manuel, D.G. & Tu, J.V. (2012 Jan) Cardiovascular risk factor profiles of recent immigrants vs long-term residents of Ontario: a multi-ethnic study. *Canadian Journal of Cardiology*, 28 (1), 20–26.

Combellack, A. (2009 Dec 7) *Food safety hazards.* Retrieved 2015 Aug 18 from http://www.foodsafetyindia.com/2009/12/food-safety-hazards.html [accessed on 26 August 2015].

Council for International Organization of Medical Sciences (2002) *International ethical guidelines for biomedical research involving human subjects.* Council for International Organizations of Medical Sciences. Geneva. Retrieved 2015 Aug 19 from http://www.cioms.ch/publications/layout_guide2002.pdf [accessed on 26 August 2015].

David Suzuki Foundation (2014) *Understanding GMO.* Retrieved 2015 Aug 18 from http://davidsuzuki.org/what-you-can-do/queen-of-green/faqs/food/understanding-gmo// [accessed on 26 August 2015].

Deeks, J.J., Dinnes, J., D'Amico, R., *et al.* (2003) Evaluating non-randomised intervention studies. *Health Technology Assessment*, 7 (27), iii–173.

Deena, S. (2007) Randomisation (or random allocation). Bandolier: evidence based thinking about health care. Retrieved 2013 Jul 2 from http://www.medicine.ox.ac.uk/bandolier/booth/glossary/RCT.html [accessed on 26 August 2015].

Dekker, L.H., Snijder, M.B., Beukers, M.H., *et al.* (2011) A prospective cohort study of dietary patterns of non-western migrants in the Netherlands in relation to risk factors for cardiovascular diseases: HELIUS-Dietary Patterns. *BMC Public Health*, 11, 441.

DerMarderosian, A. (2013 Aug) Overview of dietary supplements. *The Merck Manual for Health Care Professionals.* Retrieved 2015 Aug 19 from http://www.merckmanuals.com/professional/special-subjects/dietary-supplements/overview-of-dietary-supplements [accessed on 26 August 2015].

Department of Health (1991) Report on health and social subjects 41: dietary reference values for food energy and nutrients for the United Kingdom. Report of the panel on dietary reference values of the committee on medical aspects of food policy. The Stationary Office, London.

Dewey, K. (2005) Guiding principles for feeding non-breastfed children 6-24 months of age. World Health Organization, Geneva. Retrieved 2015 Aug 18 from http://whqlibdoc.who.int/publications/2005/9241593431.pdf [accessed on 26 August 2015].

Diaz, J.M. & Fridovich-Keil, J.L. (2014, Jul 14) *Genetically modified organism (GMO).* Retrieved 2015 Aug 18 from http://www.britannica.com/science/genetically-modified-organism [accessed on 26 August 2015].

Dickson, B.C., Streutker, C.J. & Chetty, R. (2006 Oct) Coeliac disease: an update for pathologists. *Journal of Clinical Pathology*, 59 (10), 1008–1016.

Dinsdale, H., Ridler, C. & Ells, L. (2011) *A simple guide to classifying body mass index in children.* National Obesity Observatory, Oxford. Retrieved 2015 Aug 18 from http://www.noo.org.uk/uploads/doc/vid_11601_A_simple_guide_to_classifying_BMI_in_children.pdf [accessed on 26 August 2015].

Duijts, L. (2012 Jan) Fetal and infant origins of asthma. *European Journal of Epidemiology*, 27 (1), 5–14.

European Food Safety Authority (2012) Population reference intakes for protein. *European Food Safety Journal*, 10 (2), 2557.

Eurostat (2013) *Migration and migrant population statistics.* Retrieved 2013 Aug 13 from http://ec.europa.eu/eurostat/statistics-explained/index.php/Main_Page [accessed on 26 August 2015].

Federal Ministry of Education and Research. (2010 Nov 4) *Disease-resistant bananas, drought-tolerant maize.* Retrieved 2015 Aug 18 from http://www.gmo-safety.eu/news/1242.disease-resistant-bananas-drought-tolerant-maize.html [accessed on 26 August 2015].

Nutrition at a Glance, Second Edition. Edited by Sangita Sharma, Tony Sheehy and Fariba Kolahdooz.
© 2016 John Wiley & Sons, Ltd. Published 2016 by John Wiley & Sons, Ltd.

Food Allergy Research & Education (2014) *About food allergies*. Retrieved 2015 Aug 18 from http://www.foodallergy.org/about-food-allergies [accessed on 26 August 2015].

Food and Agriculture Organization of the United Nations (2003 Mar) *Weighing the GMO arguments: against*. Retrieved 2015 Aug 18 from http://www.fao.org/english/newsroom/focus/2003/gmo8.htm [accessed on 26 August 2015].

Food Safety Programme (2002) *WHO global strategy for food safety: safer food for better health*. World Health Organization, Geneva. Retrieved 2015 Aug 21 from http://apps.who.int/iris/bitstream/10665/42559/1/9241545747.pdf [accessed on 26 August 2015].

Forsdahl, A. (1977) Are poor living conditions in childhood and adolescence an important risk factor for arteriosclerotic heart disease? *British Journal of Preventive and Social Medicine*, 31 (2), 91–95.

Gibney, M.J., Margetts, B.M., Kearney, J.M. & Arab, L. (2004) *Public Health Nutrition*. Blackwell Publishing, Oxford.

Gibson, R.S. (2005) *Principles of Nutritional Assessment* (2nd edn.). Oxford University Press, New York.

Gonzalez-Casanova, I., Sarmiento, O.L., Gazmararian, J.A., *et al*. (2013 May) Comparing three body mass index classification systems to assess overweight and obesity in children and adolescents. *Revista Panamericana de Salud Publica*, 33 (5), 349–355.

Griffiths, A.J., Wessler, S.R., Lewontin, R.C. & Carroll, S.B. (2008) *Introduction to Genetic Analysis* (9th edn.). W. H Freeman & Company, New York.

Gurley, B. (2014 August 28) Dietary Supplement. *Encyclopaedia Britannica*. Retrieved 2015 Aug 18 from http://www.britannica.com/topic/dietary-supplement [accessed on 26 August 2015].

Halfdanarson, T.R., Litzow, M.R. & Murray, J.A. (2007 Jan 15) Hematologic manifestations of celiac disease. *Blood*, 109 (2), 412–421.

Health Canada (2012 Jul 24) *Frequently asked questions – biotechnology and genetically modified foods*. Retrieved 2015 Aug 18 from http://www.hc-sc.gc.ca/fn-an/gmf-agm/fs-if/faq_1-eng.php#p2p2 [accessed on 26 August 2015].

Health Canada (2014 May 27) *Nutrition for healthy term infants: recommendations from birth to six months*. Retrieved 2015 Aug 19 from http://www.hc-sc.gc.ca/fn-an/nutrition/infant-nourisson/recom/recom-6-24-months-6-24-mois-eng.phpphp [accessed on 26 August 2015].

Hinkle, L.E. (1973) Coronary heart disease and sudden death in actively employed American men. *Bulletin of the New York Academy of Medicine*, 49 (6), 467–474.

Holmboe-Ottesen, G. & Wandel, M. (2012) Changes in dietary habits after migration and consequences for health: a focus on South Asians in Europe. *Food & Nutrition Research*, 56.

Institute of Medicine and National Research Council of the National Academies (2013) *Implementing guidelines on weight gain & pregnancy*. Retrieved 2013 Aug 19 from http://www.nap.edu/catalog/18292/implementing-guidelines-on-weight-gain-and-pregnancy [accessed on 26 August 2015].

International Confederation of Dietetic Associations (2008) *International code of ethics and code of good practice*. International Confederation of Dietetic Associations. Retrieved 2015 Aug 19 from http://www.internationaldietetics.org/Downloads/ICDA-Code-of-Ethics-and-Code-of-Good-Practice.aspx [accessed on 26 August 2015].

Jackson, K.M. & Nazar, A.M. (2006 Apr) Breastfeeding, the immune response, and long-term health. *Journal of the American Osteopathic Association*, 106 (4), 203–207.

Koike, H., Hama, T., Kawagashira, Y., *et al*. (2012 Jul) The significance of folate deficiency in alcoholic and nutritional neuropathies: analysis of a case. *Nutrition*, 28 (7–8), 821–824.

Krishnaswamy, K., Naidu, A.N., Prasad, M.P. & Reddy, G.A. (2002 May) Fetal malnutrition and adult chronic disease. *Nutrition Reviews*, 60 (5 Pt 2), S35–S39.

Kumanyika, S. (2006 Feb) Nutrition and chronic disease prevention: priorities for US minority groups. *Nutritions & Reviews*, 64 (2 Pt 2), S9–S14.

Lalkhen, A. & McCluskey, A. (2008) Clinical tests: sensitivity and specificity. *Continuing Education in Anaesthesia, Critical Care & Pain*, 8 (6), 221–223.

Leung, G. & Stanner, S. (2011) Diets of minority ethnic groups in the UK: influence on chronic disease risk and implications for prevention. *Nutrition Bulletin*, 36 (2), 161–198.

Levitt, N.S., Lambert, E.V., Woods, D., Hales, C.N., Andrew, R. & Seckl, J.R. (2000 Dec) Impaired glucose tolerance and elevated blood pressure in low birth weight, nonobese, young South African adults: early programming of cortisol axis. *Journal of Clinical Endocrinology & Metabolism*, 85 (12), 4611–4618.

Mahan, L.K., Escott-Stump, S., & Raymond, J.L. (2012) *Krause's Food & The Nutrition Care Process* (13th edn.). Elsevier/Saunders, St. Louis.

Martin, D.C. & Yankay, J.E. (2013 Apr) *Refugees and Asylees: 2012*. US Department of Homeland Security. Retrieved 2013 Aug 19 from http://www.dhs.gov/sites/default/files/publications/ois_rfa_fr_2012.pdf [accessed on 26 August 2015].

Mayo Clinic (2014a Apr 5) *Healthy lifestyle: nutrition and healthy eating – nutritional supplements*. Retrieved 2015 Aug 19 from http://www.mayoclinic.org/healthy-lifestyle/nutrition-and-healthy-eating/basics/nutrition-basics/hlv-20049477?reDate=19082015 [accessed on 26 August 2015].

Mayo Clinic (2014b Feb 12) *Diseases and conditions: food allergy – symptoms*. Retrieved 2015 Aug 18 from http://www.mayoclinic.org/diseases-conditions/food-allergy/basics/symptoms/con-20019293 [accessed on 26 August 2015].

Mitchell, C. (2010, December 1) Company asks USDA to approve GM apples. *Food Safety News*. Retrieved 2015 Aug 18 from http://www.foodsafetynews.com/2010/12/company-asks-usda-to-approve-gm-apples/#.VdOAVvmjNcY [accessed on 26 August 2015].

National Center for Complementary and Alternative Medicine (NCCAM) (2013 Mar) *Using dietary supplements wisely*. National Institutes of Health. Retrieved 2015 Aug 19 from https://nccih.nih.gov/health/supplements/wiseuse.htm [accessed on 26 August 2015].

National Research Council (2005) *Dietary Reference Intakes for Energy, Carbohydrate, Faiber, Fat, Fatty Acids, Cholesterol, Protein, and Amino Acids*. The National Academies Press, Washington, DC.

Newbold, K.B. & Danforth, J. (2003 Nov) Health status and Canada's immigrant population. *Social Science & Medicine*, 57 (10), 1981–1995.

Newslow, D. (2003) Hazard Analysis Critical Control Point (HACCP). In: R. H. Schmidt & G. E. Rodrick (eds), *Food Safety Handbook*, pp. 363–379. John Wiley & Sons, Inc., Hoboken.

Nuffield Council on Bioethics (2014) *Possible benefits of GM crops in developing countries*. Retrieved 2015 Aug 19 from http://nuffieldbioethics.org/wp-content/uploads/2014/07/GM-Crops-2-Chapter-3-Current-and-potential-uses-of-GM-Crops-in-developing-countries.pdf [accessed on 26 August 2015].

Nutritional Supplements (2008) *Gale Encyclopedia of Medicine*. Retrieved 2015 Aug 19 from http://medical-dictionary.thefreedictionary.com/Nutritional+Supplements [accessed on 26 August 2015].

Ormandy, E.H., Dale, J. & Griffin, G. (2011) Genetic engineering of animals: ethical issues, including welfare concerns. *Canadian Veterinary Journal*, 52 (5), 544–550.

Otten, J.J., Hellwig, J.P. & Meyers, L.D. (2006) *Dietary Reference Intakes: The Essential Guide to Nutrient Requirements*. National Academies Press, Washington, DC.

Oxford Dictionaries (2013) *Definition of ethics in English*. Oxford University Press. Retrieved 2015 Aug 19 from http://www.oxforddictionaries.com/definition/english/ethics [accessed on 26 August 2015].

Pelegrini, A., Silva, D.A., Gaya, A.C. & Petroski, E.L. (2013) Comparison of three criteria for overweight and obesity classification in Brazilian adolescents. *Nutrition Journal*, 12, 5.

Perez-Escamilla, R. (2011 May) Acculturation, nutrition, and health disparities in Latinos. *American Journal of Clinical Nutrition*, 93 (5), 1163S–1167S.

Regev-Tobias, H., Reifen, R., Endevelt, R., *et al*. (2012 Jan) Dietary acculturation and increasing rates of obesity in Ethiopian women living in Israel. *Nutrition*, 28 (1), 30–34.

Reid, A.P. (2003) Hazards associated with nutrient fortification. In: R. H. Schmidt & G. E. Rodrick (eds), *Food Safety Handbook*, pp. 265–275. John Wiley & Sons, Inc., Hoboken.

Rodrick, G.E. & Schmidt, R.H. (2003) Physiology and survival of foodborne pathogens in various food systems. In: R. H. Schmidt & Rodrick, G.E. (eds), *Food Safety Handbook*, pp. 138–156. John Wiley & Sons, Inc., Hoboken.

Romon, R. (2001) Evaluation de l'apport alimentaire. In: A. Basdevant, M. Laville & E. Lerebours (eds), *Traité de nutrition clinique de l'adulte*, 109–120 pp. Flammarion Médecine Sciences, Paris.

Rosen, L., Manor, O., Engelhard, D. & Zucker, D. (2006 Jul) In defense of the randomized controlled trial for health promotion research. *American Journal of Public Health*, 96 (7), 1181–1186.

Rosenmoller, D.L., Gasevic, D., Seidell, J. & Lear, S.A. (2011) Determinants of changes in dietary patterns among Chinese immigrants: a cross-sectional analysis. *International Journal of Behavioral Nutrition and Physical Activity*, 8, 42.

Rupp, H. (2003) Chemical and physical hazards produced during food processing, storage, and preparation. In: R. H. Schmidt & Rodrick, G.E. (eds), *Food Safety Handbook*, pp. 233–263. John Wiley & Sons, Inc., Hoboken.

Rutishauser, I.H. (2005 Oct) Dietary intake measurements. *Public Health Nutrition*, 8 (7A), 1100–1107.

Rytina, N. (20133) *Estimates of the Legal Permanent Resident Population in 2012*. US Department of Homeland Security. Retrieved 2013 Aug 19 from http://www.dhs.gov/sites/default/files/publications/ois_lpr_pe_2012.pdf [accessed on 26 August 2015].

Sakko, K. (2002 May) *The debate over genetically modified foods*. Retrieved 2015 Aug 18 from http://www.actionbioscience.org/biotechnology/sakko.html [accessed on 26 August 2015].

Sanou, D., O'Reilly, E., Ngnie-Teta, I. *et al.* (2014 Feb) Acculturation and nutritional health of immigrants in Canada: a scoping review. *Journal of Immigrant and Minority Health*, 16 (1), 24–34.

Satia, J.A. (2010) Dietary acculturation and the nutrition transition: an overview. *Applied Physiology, Nutrition and Metabolism*, 35, 219–223.

Schweihofer, J. (2013 Jul 18) Biological, chemical and physical hazards assessed with HACCP. Michigan State University Extension and Sarah Wells, MSU departments of Animal Science & Food Science and Human Nutrition. Retrieved 2015 Aug 19 from http://msue.anr.msu.edu/news/biological_chemical_and_physical_hazards_assessed_with_haccp [accessed on 26 August 2015].

Seward II, R.A. (2003a) Characterization of food hazards. In: R. H. Schmidt & G. E. Rodrick (eds), *Food Safety Handbook*, pp. 11–18. John Wiley & Sons, Inc., Hoboken.

Seward II, R.A.(2003b) Definition of food safety. In: R. H. Schmidt & G. E. Rodrick (eds), *Food Safety Handbook*, pp. 3–9. John Wiley & Sons, Inc., Hoboken.

Sibbald, B. & Roland, M. (1998 Jan 17) Understanding controlled trials. Why are randomised controlled trials important? *British Medical Journal, Journal*, 316 (7126), 201.

Specchio, J.J. (2003) Hazards from natural origins. In: R. H. Schmidt &G. E. Rodrick (eds), *Food Safety Handbook*, pp. 213–231. John Wiley & Sons, Inc., Hoboken.

Statistics Canada (2011) National Household Survey: Immigration, Place of Birth, Citizenship, Ethnic Origin, Visible Minorities, Language and Religion. Statistics Canada. Retrieved 2013 Aug 19 from http://www.statcan.gc.ca/daily-quotidien/130508/dq130508b-eng.htm [accessed on 26 August 2015].

Steckler, A. & McLeroy, K.R. (2008 Jan) The importance of external validity. *American Journal of Public Health*, 98 (1), 9–10.

Stein, K.F. & Corte, C. (2003 Apr) Reconceptualizing causative factors and intervention strategies in the eating disorders: a shift from body image to self-concept impairments. *Archives of Psychiatric Nursing*, 17 (2), 57–66.

Tashiro, M., Yasuoka, J., Poudel, K.C., Noto, H., Masuo, M. & Jimba, M. (2014 Feb) Acculturation factors and metabolic syndrome among Japanese-Brazilian men in Japan: a cross-sectional descriptive study. *Journal of Immigrant and Minority Health*, 16 (1), 68–76.

Thompson, F.E. & Subar, A.F. (2013) Dietary assessment methodology. In: A. M. Coulston, C. J. Boushey & M. G. Ferruzzi (eds), *Nutrition in the Prevention and Treatment of Disease* (3rd edn., pp. 5–46). Elsevier Academic Press, Oxford.

Tsai, S.F., Chen, S.J., Yen, S.J., *et al.* (2014 Jun 19) Iron deficiency anemia in young children with predominant breastfeeding. *Pediatrics and Neonatology*, 55 (6), 466–469.

United States Department of Agriculture (2013) *Recent trends in GE adoption*. United States Department of Agriculture. Retrieved 2014 Jun 3 from http://www.ers.usda.gov/data-products/adoption-of-genetically-engineered-crops-in-the-us/recent-trends-in-ge-adoption.aspx#.U7WITZRdXTo [accessed on 26 August 2015].

United States Department of Agriculture (2014) *Genetically engineered animals*. United States Department of Agriculture. Retrieved 2015 Aug 19 from http://www.fda.gov/AnimalVeterinary/DevelopmentApprovalProcess/GeneticEngineering/GeneticallyEngineeredAnimals/ucm113597.htm [accessed on 26 August 2015].

United States Food and Drug Administration (2014a) *Questions & answers on food from genetically engineered plants*. United States Food and Drug Administration. Retrieved 2015 Aug 19 from http://www.

fda.gov/Food/FoodScienceResearch/Biotechnology/ucm346030.htm [accessed on 26 August 2015].

United States Food and Drug Administration (2014b Apr 10) *What is a dietary supplement?* US Food and Drug Administration. Retrieved 2015 Aug 19 from http://www.fda.gov/aboutfda/transparency/basics/ucm195635.htm [accessed on 26 August 2015].

United States Food and Drug Administration (2014c) *FDA takes final step on infant formula protections*. U.S. Food and Drug Administration. Retrieved 2015 Aug 19 from http://www.fda.gov/downloads/ForConsumers/ConsumerUpdates/UCM400238.pdf [accessed on 26 August 2015].

Webb, P. & Bain, C. (2011) *Essential Epidemiology: An Introduction for Students and Health Professionals* (2nd edn., pp. 222–234). Cambridge University Press, Cambridge.

WebMD (2012 Aug 2) *Vitamins and supplements lifestyle guide*. Retrieved 2015 Aug 19 from http://www.webmd.com/vitamins-and-supplements/lifestyle-guide-11/supplement-faq [accessed on 26 August 2015].

WebMD (2014 Jun 29) *Dietary supplements (herbal medicines and natural products) – topic overview*. Retrieved 2015 Aug 18 from http://www.webmd.com/food-recipes/dietary-supplements-topic-overview [accessed on 26 August 2015].

Webster-Gandy, J., Madden, A. & Holdsworth, M. (2011) *Oxford Handbook of Nutrition and Dietetics* (2nd edn., p. 840). Oxford University Press, Oxford.

Whitman, D.B. (2000, Apr 20) Genetically Modified Foods: Harmful or Helpful?. *CSA Discovery Guide*. Retrieved 2015 Aug 18 from http://www.fhs.d211.org/departments/science/mduncan/bioweb/Biotechnology/Genetically%20Modified%20Foods.pdf [accessed on 26 August 2015].

Willet, W. (1998) *Nutritional Epidemiology* (2nd edn.). Oxford University Press, New York.

Wit, J.M. & Boersma, B. (2002 Dec) Catch-up growth: definition, mechanisms, and models. *Journal of Pediatric Endocrinology and Metabolism*, 15 (Suppl 5), 1229–1241.

World Cancer Research Fund/American Institute for Cancer Research (2007). *Food, Nutrition, Physical Activity, and the Prevention Of Cancer: A Global Perspective*. AICR, Washington, DC.

World Health Organization (2010) *Health of Migrants – The Way Forward: Report of a global consultation*, Madrid, Spain, 3–5 March 2010. World Health Organization, Geneva. Retrieved 2013 Aug 19 from http://www.who.int/hac/events/consultation_report_health_migrants_colour_web.pdf [accessed on 26 August 2015].

World Health Organization (2011) *Standards and Operational Guidance for Ethics Review of Health-Related Research with Human Participants*. WHO Press, Geneva.

World Health Organization (2014a) *Food Safety*. World Health Organization. Retrieved 2015 Aug 21 from http://www.who.int/mediacentre/factsheets/fs399/en/ [accessed on 26 August 2015].

World Health Organization (2014b) *Foodborne disease surveillance: general information*. World Health Organization. Retrieved 2014 Mar 18 from http://www.who.int/foodborne_disease/resistance/general/en/ [accessed on 26 August 2015].

World Health Organization (2014c) *Frequently asked questions on genetically modified foods*. World Health Organization. Retrieved 2015 Aug 21 from . http://www.who.int/foodsafety/areas_work/food-technology/Frequently_asked_questions_on_gm_foods.pdf?ua=1 [accessed on 26 August 2015].

World Health Organization (2014d) *Infant and young child feeding*. World Health Organization. Retrieved 2015 Aug19 from http://www.who.int/mediacentre/factsheets/fs342/en/ [accessed on 26 August 2015].

World health Organization Expert Consultation (2004 Jan 10) Appropriate body-mass index for Asian populations and its implications for policy and intervention strategies. *Lancet*, 363 (9403), 157–163.

World Medical Association (2013) *Declaration of Helsinki – Ethical Principles for Medical Research Involving Human Subjects*. World Medical Association. Retrieved 2015 Aug 19 from http://www.wma.net/en/30publications/10policies/b3/index.html [accessed on 26 August 2015].

Ziegler, A.G., Schmid, S., Huber, D., Hummel, M. & Bonifacio, E. (2003 Oct 1) Early infant feeding and risk of developing type 1 diabetes-associated autoantibodies. *Journal of American Medical Association*, 290 (13), 1721–1728.

Index

Nutrition at a Glance, Second Edition. Edited by Sangita Sharma, Tony Sheehy and Fariba Kolahdooz.
© 2016 John Wiley & Sons, Ltd. Published 2016 by John Wiley & Sons, Ltd.